Health-related votive tablets from Japan

To Kiichiro Tsutani

Health-related votive tablets from Japan

Ema for healing and well-being

Peter A.G.M. De Smet
Ian Reader

LEIDEN PUBLICATIONS

Contents

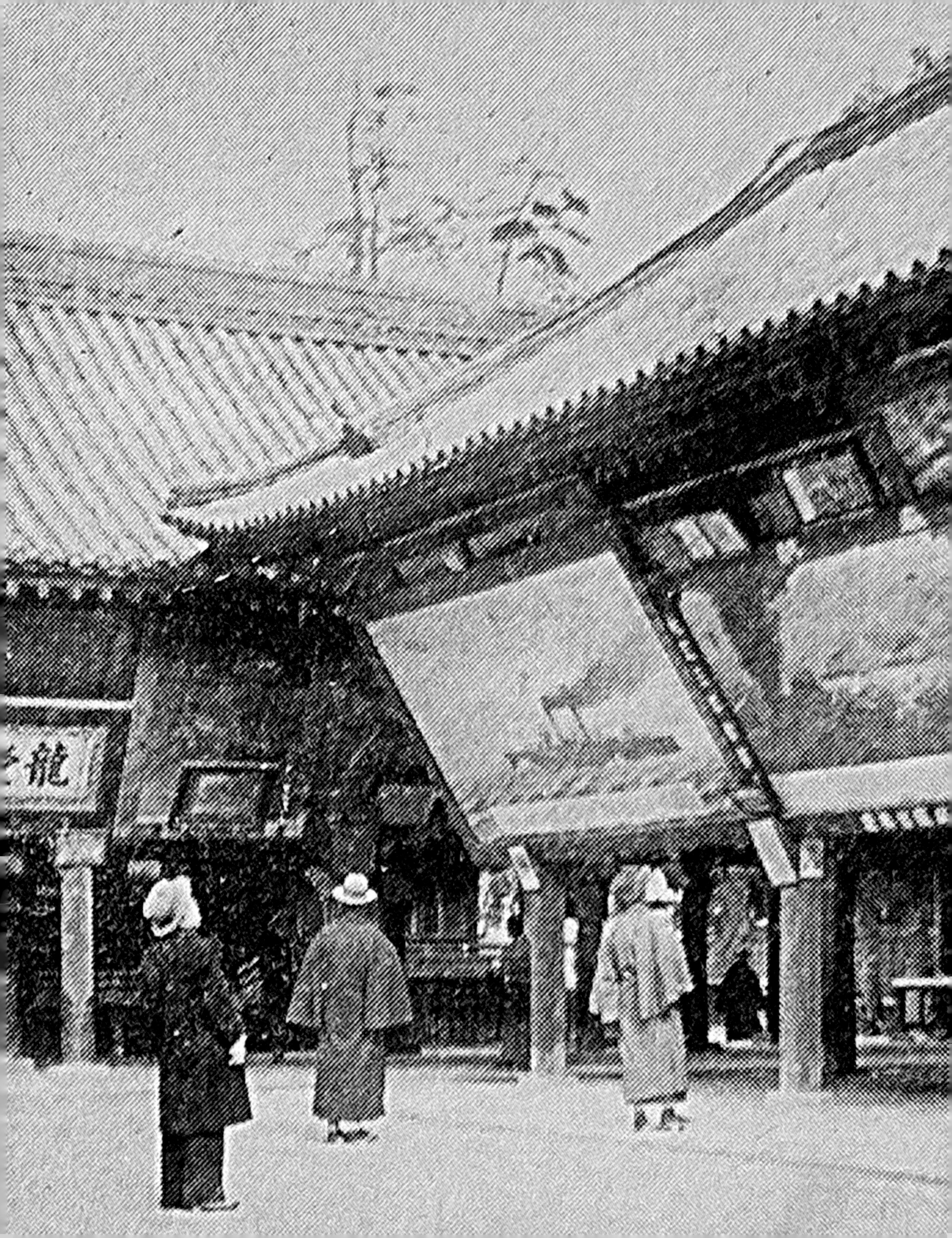
龍

Foreword
Messages to the Gods

Ema, or wooden wishing plaques as they are known in Japan, are generally found at temples and shrines dedicated to *kami* (gods) or Buddhist figures of worship.

They are eloquent expressions of folk art, which contain prayers, requests and words of gratitude. On one side the *ema* are hand-painted or a print is applied; on the other side of the tablet a message or request to the gods is written. This does not mean that the Japanese believe that the gods will answer their prayers or solve their problems. Rather, writing *ema* offers a sense of comfort and support in difficult times. Addressing *kami or* Buddhist figures of worship also gives the feeling that every effort was made to reach the individual's ultimate goal. It is believed that writing to the gods strengthens one's self-confidence and writing on *ema* is regarded as a positive act in the eyes of the Japanese. The number one request on *ema* is from students asking for help with an exam. It is followed by requests for success in business and for the good health and safety of family. These requests are seen as acts of gratitude and good intentions towards parents and teachers. The general meaning of the *ema* resembles lighting a candle or intercession in church. Both are acts to show compassion and love for others. Often a request is made for ailing family or friends and writing *ema*, much like lighting a candle in church, evokes a sense of comfort and peace. Both *ema* and the rituals preformed in church lend themselves to self-expression, making it easier to overcome difficulties. To make room for new *ema* the old ones are often burned. This burning can be compared to lighting a candle in church and symbolises the release of the request written on *ema*.

The present population of Japan is ageing rapidly and now has the highest number of elderly citizens. Requests for *boke fūji* – defeating of dementia – on *ema* have increased significantly. Another well-known medical problem in Japan is dental decay. There are numerous temples and shrines where one can pray for the relief or prevention of dental ailments.

As director of a museum devoted to Japan, and in particular to the relationship between the Dutch and Japanese, it gives me great pleasure to dedicate an exhibition in Japan Museum SieboldHuis to a special group of *ema*: Japanese votive tablets with lifecycle-related and health-related designs and purposes. It is particularly significant when one considers that our museum is named after the physician Philipp Franz von Siebold (*17 February 1796 Wurzburg, Germany – 18 October 1866 Munich*). Siebold's love for Japan played an important role in the development of Western sciences in Japan, as well as in Western knowledge of Japan. He introduced many new surgical procedures and techniques at his clinic near Deshima and gained lasting fame for his contributions in the field of medicine. In Japan he was known as the miracle doctor for his new and innovative cataract operations. He also successfully promoted the use of surgical forceps in difficult deliveries. In addition, Siebold introduced a number of Japanese medical procedures to the West, including *moxa* techniques and acupuncture.

This is the first time that an English book dedicated solely to small *ema* (15 x 9 cm) with an emphasis on the rich diversity of health-related *ema* with concise but informative texts on their medical as well as cultural background is published. There have been Japanese books on *ema* in general, but so far there has been neither an English book about contemporary *ema* in general nor a comprehensive Japanese book about health-related *ema*.

First and foremost I would like to thank author and *ema* collector Peter De Smet. He is a Dutch university professor of pharmacy and collected with great passion almost all the prayers for health and healing depicted in this book. He also gathered most of the information about their medical and cultural context. I would also like to thank co-author professor Ian Reader who is a specialist in Japanese religions, and Kiichiro Tsutani for his valuable contribution. Sincere thanks also go to The Association for Health Economics Research and Social Insurance and Welfare, Tokyo, Japan for its financial contribution to this catalogue.

This exhibition (17 March 2017 – 11 June 2017), catalogue and the accompanying events would not have been possible without the dedication of the staff and volunteers, Eva Trimp and Teatske Kramer, of Japan Museum SieboldHuis.

The design was in the competent hands of Haico Beukers and Marga Scholma. I am most grateful to Anniek Meinders and Romy Uijen of Leiden University Press for this splendid publication. I would also like to thank the exhibition sponsors, The Association for Health Economics Research and Social Insurance and Welfare, Tokyo, Japan, Panasonic Healthcare, Astellas B.V. and the Friends of the Japan Museum SieboldHuis.

It is extremely satisfying to have had such a committed team working towards the realisation and completion of the book and exhibition – both such powerful expressions of the purpose and goals of Japan Museum SieboldHuis.

This catalogue is dedicated to all those died of cancer, in particular Gido Netters.

Kris Schiermeier
Director Japan Museum SieboldHuis
Leiden, The Netherlands

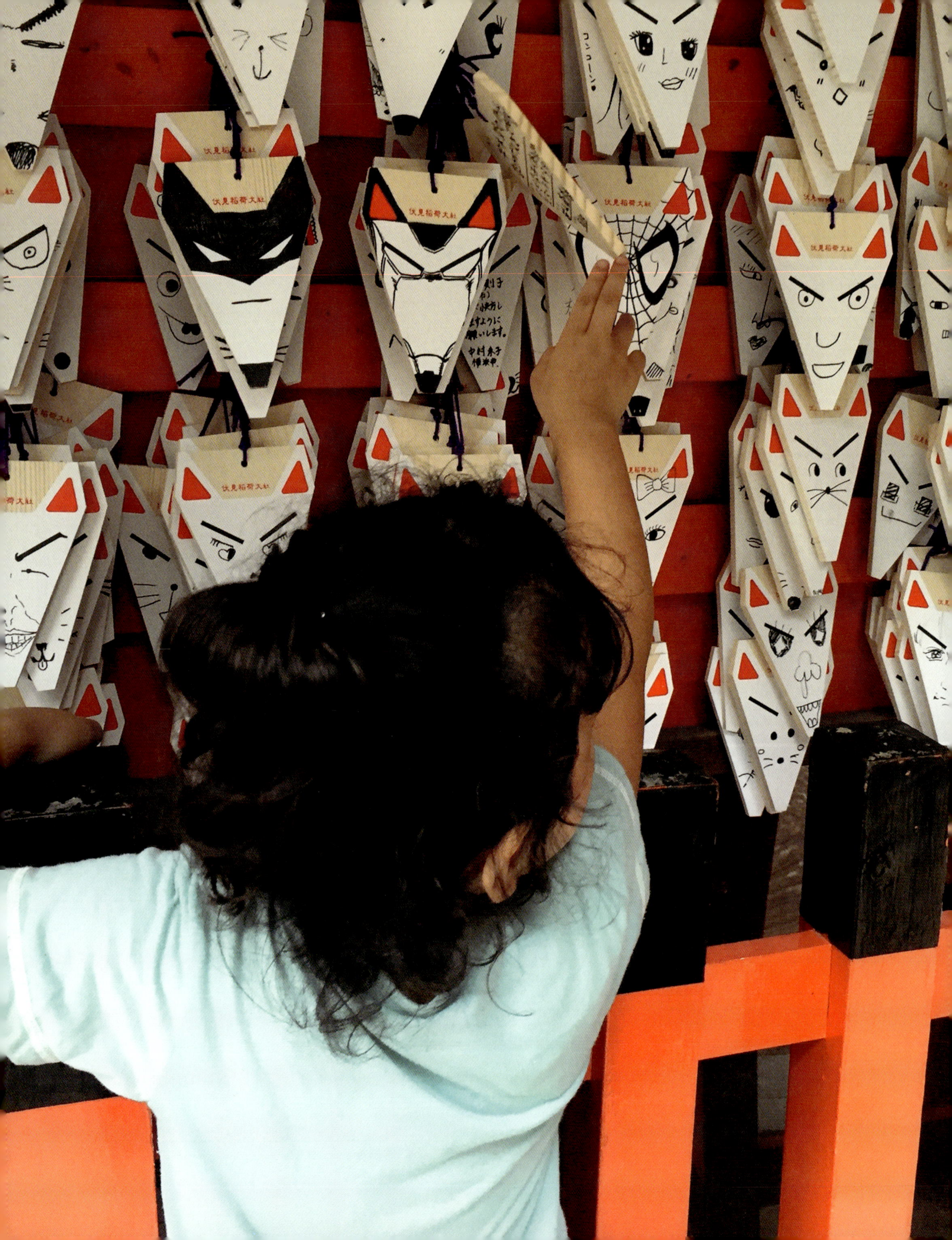
伏見稲荷大社

はじめに
神への祈り

日本で願い事を記した木製の絵馬は神社仏閣で広く見ることができますが、それは信仰の対象となる神や仏に捧げられたものです。

それに書かれているのは祈りや願い、そして感謝の言葉であり、民俗芸術を雄弁に表現するものです。絵馬の片面には手描きまたは印刷の絵柄があり、裏面には神への言葉や願いが書かれています。これは、神が祈りに答え問題を解決すると日本人が信じていることを意味するものではありません。むしろ絵馬に書くことにより困難なときの慰めと支えを得るのです。崇敬する神仏に祈るときには、人は最終目標を達成するためあらゆる努力をしたという気持ちにもなります。神に願いを書くことは自信を深めることと考えられ、絵馬に書くことは日本人の目には積極的な行為と映るのです。絵馬に書かれた願い事で最も多いのは学生が試験に合格することを願うもので、その次に多いのが商売繁盛、健康と家内安全を祈願したものです。これらの願いは両親や先生に対する感謝・善意のしるしであると見なされています。絵馬が一般的に意味するものは、教会で蝋燭を灯したり神へのとりなしを求めるのに似ています。いずれも他者への思いやりと愛情を示す行為なのです。家族や友人の病気平癒を願い絵馬を書くことは、教会で蝋燭を灯すのに似ており安らかな気持ちを呼び起こします。絵馬も教会で行われる儀式も自己を表現する手段を提供し、困難を乗り越えるのを楽にしてくれます。新しい絵馬を掲げる場所を作るため古い絵馬はしばしば燃やされます。この絵馬焚きは教会での蝋燭点灯と比較することができ、絵馬に書かれた願い事の解放を象徴しています。

今日の日本では急速に高齢化が進み、現在は高齢者の数が最高となっています。そこで「ぼけ封じ」を願う絵馬が非常に多くなってきています。その他に日本では歯に関する医療問題が有名で、歯痛を鎮めたり防ぐために祈りを捧げる寺社が数多くあります。

日本、特に日蘭関係を専門とするこの日本博物館シーボルトハウスにおいて、絵馬を集めた「日本の奉納額：人の一生と健康に関する絵柄とご利益」の特別展を開催することは館長として欣快の至りです。特に当博物館が医師フィリップ・フランツ・フォン・シーボルト（1796年2月17日ドイツ、ヴュルツブルク - 1866年10月18日ミュンヘン）に因んで名付けられたことを考えれば意義深いものがあります。シーボルトの日本への愛情は、日本における西洋科学の発展ならびに西洋の日本に対する知識の深まりにとって重要な役割を果たしました。シーボルトはさまざまな新しい外科手術やその技術を出島に近い彼の診療所で紹介し、その名声は医学分野での貢献により長く伝えられました。日本でシーボルトは革新的な白内障手術を施し、"奇跡の医師"として知られるようになります。彼は難産のときに使用する外科鉗子も普及させ、鍼灸など日本のさまざまな治療法を西洋に伝えました。

小型絵馬 (15 x 9 cm) に特化した英語の本が出版されたのは初めてのことで、この本では健康に関する絵馬の多様性を紹介するとともに、医学的および文化的背景について簡潔ながら有益な情報の詰まったテキストを添えています。絵馬全般に関する本は日本にはありますが英語の本はありません。また健康に関する絵馬についての包括的な日本語の本もないのが現状です。

著者であり絵馬の収集家であるペーター・デ・スメット氏にまず深く感謝したいと思います。彼はオランダの大学の薬学教授で、この本で採り上げているほぼすべての健康と癒しに関する絵馬を大変な熱意をもって収集されました。また絵馬の医学的・文化的背景に関する情報もそのほとんどを収集しています。また日本の宗教の専門家である共著者のイアン・リーダー教授にも感謝いたします。津谷喜一郎氏からは貴重なご意見を賜りました。東京の医療経済研究・社会保険福祉協会からこのカタログに対する資金援助を戴いたことに深甚の感謝をいたします。

本展覧会（2017年3月17日から2017年6月11日）ならびにカタログ、関連行事は、日本博物館シーボルトハウスのスタッフやボランティアのエヴァ・トリンプ氏、テーツケ・クラーマー氏の尽力がなければ実現しませんでした。

デザインは経験豊かなハイコ・ボイカース氏とマルハ・スホルマ氏の手によるものです。この素晴らしい出版についてはライデン大学出版局のアニーク・マインダース氏とローミー・アウエン氏に感謝いたします。本展覧会のスポンサーとなっていただいた東京の医療経済研究・社会保険福祉協会、Panasonic Healthcare、Astellas B.V.、日本博物館シーボルトハウス友の会にも謝意を表します。

本の出版と展覧会実現のためにこれほど献身的な働きをするチームが得られたことは大きな喜びであり、できあがった本と展覧会の両者は日本博物館シーボルトハウスの目指すものをみごとに体現しています。

この目録をヒド・ネッテル氏をはじめ、ガンで亡くなったすべての方々に捧げます。

クリス・スヒールメイヤー
日本博物館シーボルトハウス館長
オランダ、ライデン

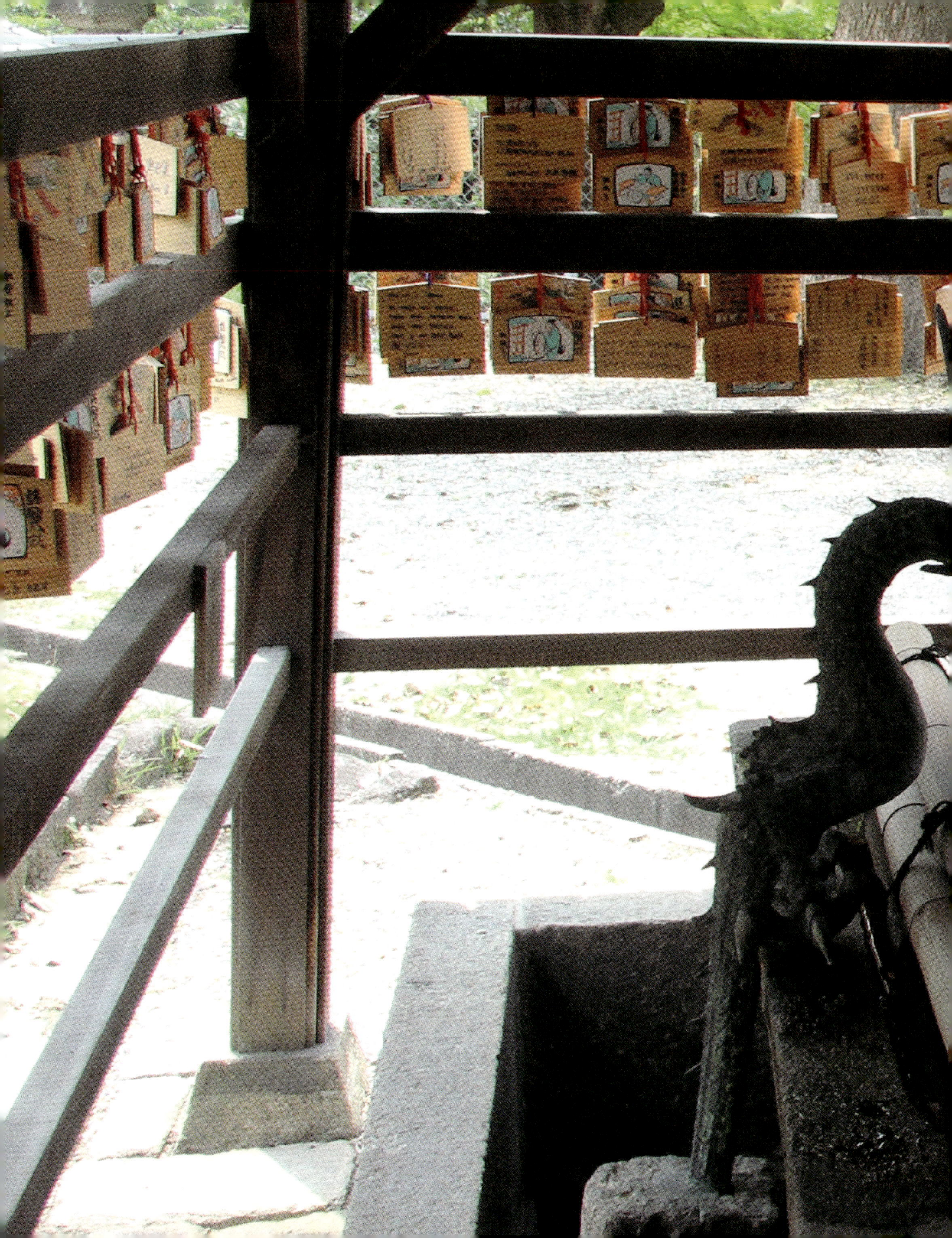

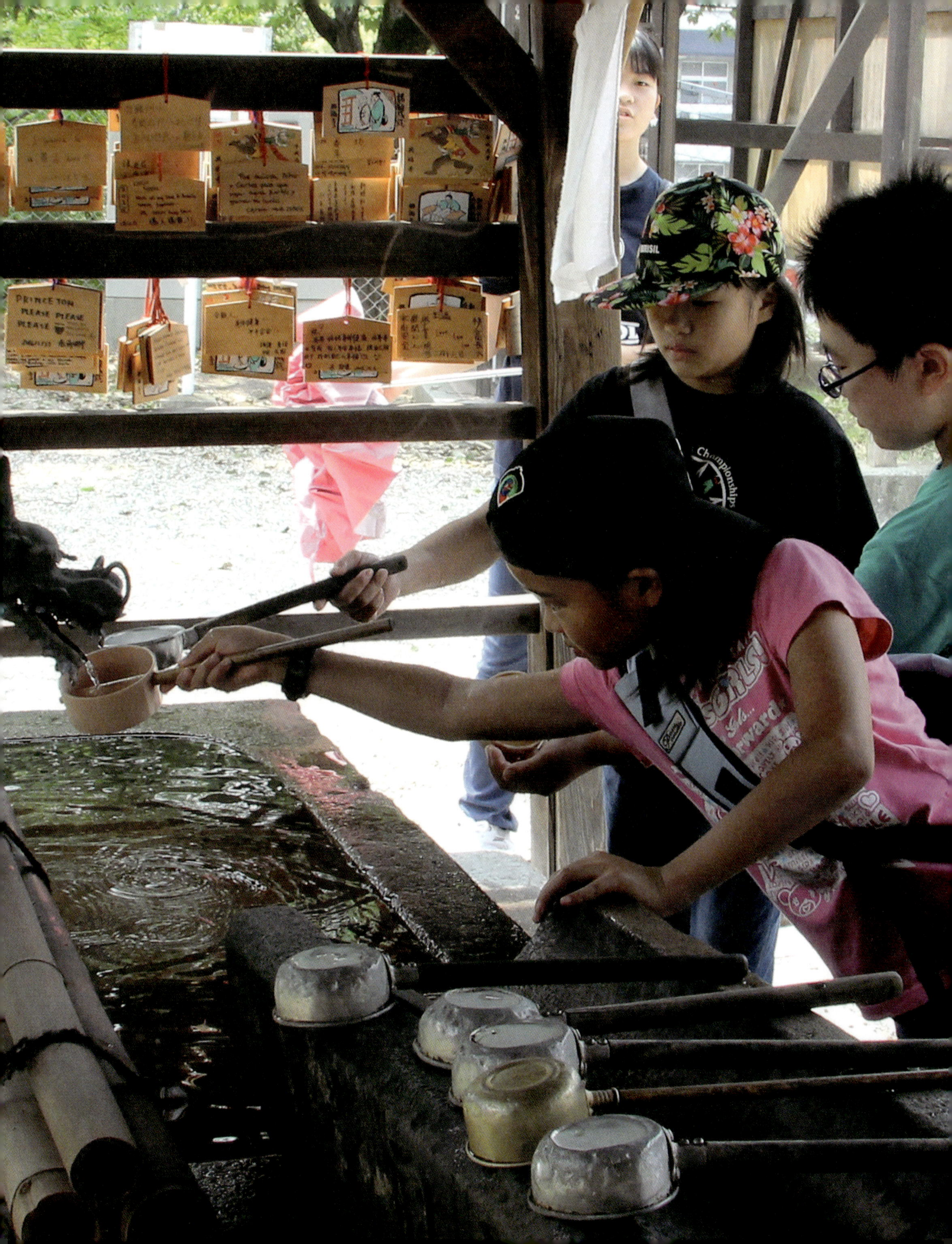
PRINCETON
PLEASE PLEASE
PLEASE
Championships

Abbreviations of key references

Below is a list of abbreviations that refer to the key references throughout the book. In the text the abbreviations are hyphenated with the relevant page number(s).

AE Ashikaga E. Votive pictures: a Japanese superstition. Western Folklore 1954;13:29-33

AJ Jannetta AB. Diseases of the early modern period in Japan. In Kiple KF, (ed): The Cambridge world history of human disease. Cambridge: Cambridge University Press, 1993:385-389

BB Bocking B. A popular dictionary of Shinto. London: Routledge, 2005

EO Ohnuki-Tierney E. Illness and culture in contemporary Japan: an anthropo-logicalview. Cambridge: Cambridge University Press, 1984

FS Starr F. Ema. Transactions of The Asiatic Society of Japan 1920;48:1-22

GG1 Grebe G. Omamori – Japanese amulets. Available at: http://omamorifromjapan.blogspot.nl/ [accessed 27 May 2016]

GG2 Grebe G. Japan – shrines and temples. Available at: http://japanshrinestemples.blogspot.nl/ [accessed 27 May 2016]

GG3 Greve G. Special galleries ... Daruma museum (03) Introducing Japanese culture. Available at: http://daruma-museumgallery.blogspot.nl/ [accessed 27 May 2016]

GK Goriyaku kotomeguri. Available at: http://www.goriyaku.kotomeguri.com/ [accessed 27 May 2016]

GS De Garis F, Sakai A. We Japanese, being descriptions of many of the customs, manners, ceremonies, festivals, arts and crafts of the Japanese, besides numerous other subjects. Yokohama: Yamagata press, 1950

HD Holtom DC. Japanese votive pictures (the ikoma ema). Monumenta Nipponica 1938;1:154-164

HS Snow HK. Ema: display practices of Edo period votive paintings. Thesis. Stanford: Stanford University, 2010. Available at: https://searchworks.stanford.edu/view/8714846 [accessed 27 May 2016]

HSJ Historical Statistics of Japan. Tokyo: Statistics Bureau, Ministry of Internal Affairs and Communications. Chapter 2 Table 23-b: Summary of vital statistics – ratio (1872-2004). Available at: http://www.stat.go.jp/data/chouki/zuhyou/02-23-b.xls [Accessed 27 May 2016]

IH1 Iwai H. Ema (12 history and human culture). Tokyo: Hosei University Printing Office, 1974

IH2 Iwai H. Ema ni negai o. Tokyo: Nigensha, 2007

IJ Ishiko J. Koema zufu fujikomerareta minshu no inori. Tokyo: Haga Shoten, 1972

IO Okkes IM, Polderman GO, Fryer GE, Yamada T, Bujak M, Oskam SK, Green LA, Lamberts H. The role of family practice in different health care systems: a comparison of reasons for encounter, diagnoses, and interventions in primary care populations in the Netherlands, Japan, Poland, and the United States. J Fam Pract 2002;51:72-73

IR Reader I. Letters to the gods – the form and meaning of ema. Japanese Journal of Religious Studies 1991;18:23-50

IY Iiazawa T, Yasuda N. Gendai no ema. Tokyo: Tokuma Shoten Publishing Co., 1978

JE Embree JF. Sanitation and health in a Japanese village. Journal of the Washington Academy of Sciences 1944;34:97-108

JM Joya M. Mock Joya's Things Japanese. 6th revised edn. Tokyo News Service, 1971

KJ Kawada J. 59. Ema votive boards. In Le Fur Y, (ed): Musée du quai Branly: the collection: art from Africa, Asia, Oceania, and the Americas. Paris: Flammarion, 2009, pp 158-159+462

KM Kondō M. Negai uranai omajinai. Mito: Ibaraki Kenritsu Rekishikan [Ibaraki History Museum], 2000

KU Encyclopedia of Shinto. Kokugakuin University, Tokyo. Available at: http://k-amc.kokugakuin.ac.jp/DM/dbTop.do;-jsessionid=1B9695B313567D2A9152D-C59C8019E01?class_name=col_eos [accessed 27 May 2016]

LF Frédéric L. Japan encyclopedia. Cambridge: Harvard University Press, 2002

MA Ashkenazi M. Handbook of Japanese mythology. Santa Barbara: ABC-CLIO, 2003

MH Marukawa H. On a kind of established form of invocation peculiar to Japanese religions – The votive offering of the ema to gods: its origin and development. Tenri journal of religion 1961;No.3:39-57

ML Lock MM. East Asian medicine in urban Japan: varieties of medical experience. Berkeley: University of California Press, 1984

MS Schumacher M. A to Z photo dictionary. Japanese Buddhist statuary. Gods, goddesses, Shinto kami, creatures and demons. Available at: http://www.onmarkproductions.com/html/buddhism.shtml [accessed 27 May 2016]

NM Naito Museum of Pharmaceutical Science and Industry. Ema. Available at: http://www.eisai.co.jp/museum/history/b0800/0100.html [accessed 27 May 2016]

OM Anonymous. Rino Ino people – Omi ema. Issue 84. Otsu Misasagi: Otsu City Museum of History, 1991

OT Ohtow T. Yéma, or votive tablets. Contemporary Japan 1942;11: 585-598

PH05 Anonymous. Japan's experiences in public health and medical systems: towards improving public health and medical systems in developing countries. Tokyo: Japan International Cooperation Agency, 2005: Chapter 1 and Appendix. Available at: http://jica-ri.jica.go.jp/IFIC_and_JBICI-Studies/english/publi-cations/reports/study/topical/health/ [accessed 27 May 2016]

RT Reader I, Tanabe Jr. GJ. Practically religious: worldly benefits and the common religion of Japan. Honolulu: University of Hawai'i Press, 1998

SH Sato Y, Hanawa T, Arai M, Cyong J-C, Fukuzawa M, Mitani K, Ogihara Y, Sakiyama T, Shimada Y, Toriizuka K, Yamada T. Introduction to Kampo Japanese traditional medicine. Tokyo: Elsevier Japan, 2005

SY15 Japan Statistical Yearbook 2015. Tokyo: Statistics Bureau, Ministry of Internal Affairs and Communications. Chapter 2 Table 25: Standardized vital rates and reproduction rates (1925-2012). Available at: http://www.stat.go.jp/data/nenkan/back64/zuhyou/y0225000.xls [accessed 27 May 2016] Chapter 21 Table 15: Deaths and death rates by leading causes of death (1975-2012) Available at: http://www.stat.go.jp/data/nenkan/back64/zuhyou/y2115000.xls [accessed 27 May 2016]

SY16 Japan Statistical Yearbook 2016. Tokyo: Statistics Bureau, Ministry of Internal Affairs and Communications. Chapter 26 Table 22A: Religious organisations, clergymen and adherents (1990-2013). Available at: http://www.stat.go.jp/data/nenkan/zuhyou/y652622a00.xls [accessed 27 May 2016]

TS Ema (II) small votive tablets. Handbook of the Tenri Sankōkan Museum collec-tions no.18. Tenri: Tenri Sankokan Museum, 1978

TT Takeshima T, Kumada M, Mise J, Ishikawa Y, Yoshizawa H, Nakamura T, Okayama M, Kajii E. Reasons for encounter and diagnoses of new out-patients at a small community hospital in Japan: an observational study. Int J Gen Med 2014;7:259-269

US United States War Department. Medical and sanitary data on Japan. The Department, 1945

VO Von Ortenberg A. Ema: Motiv und Hintergrund japanischer Votivtafeln. München: Iudicium Verlag, 2013

WF Farris WW. Diseases of the premodern period in Japan. In Kiple KF, (ed): The Cambridge world history of human disease. Cambridge: Cambridge University Press, 1993:376-385

Additional references are listed in the notes at the end of each section. In most cases, websites have been excluded because of their volatile nature. The reader can retrieve such sources by searching Google Images for 絵馬 (*ema*) in combination with the Japanese term for the sanctuary, the *ema* design, or its intended benefit (e.g., disease or illness).

001

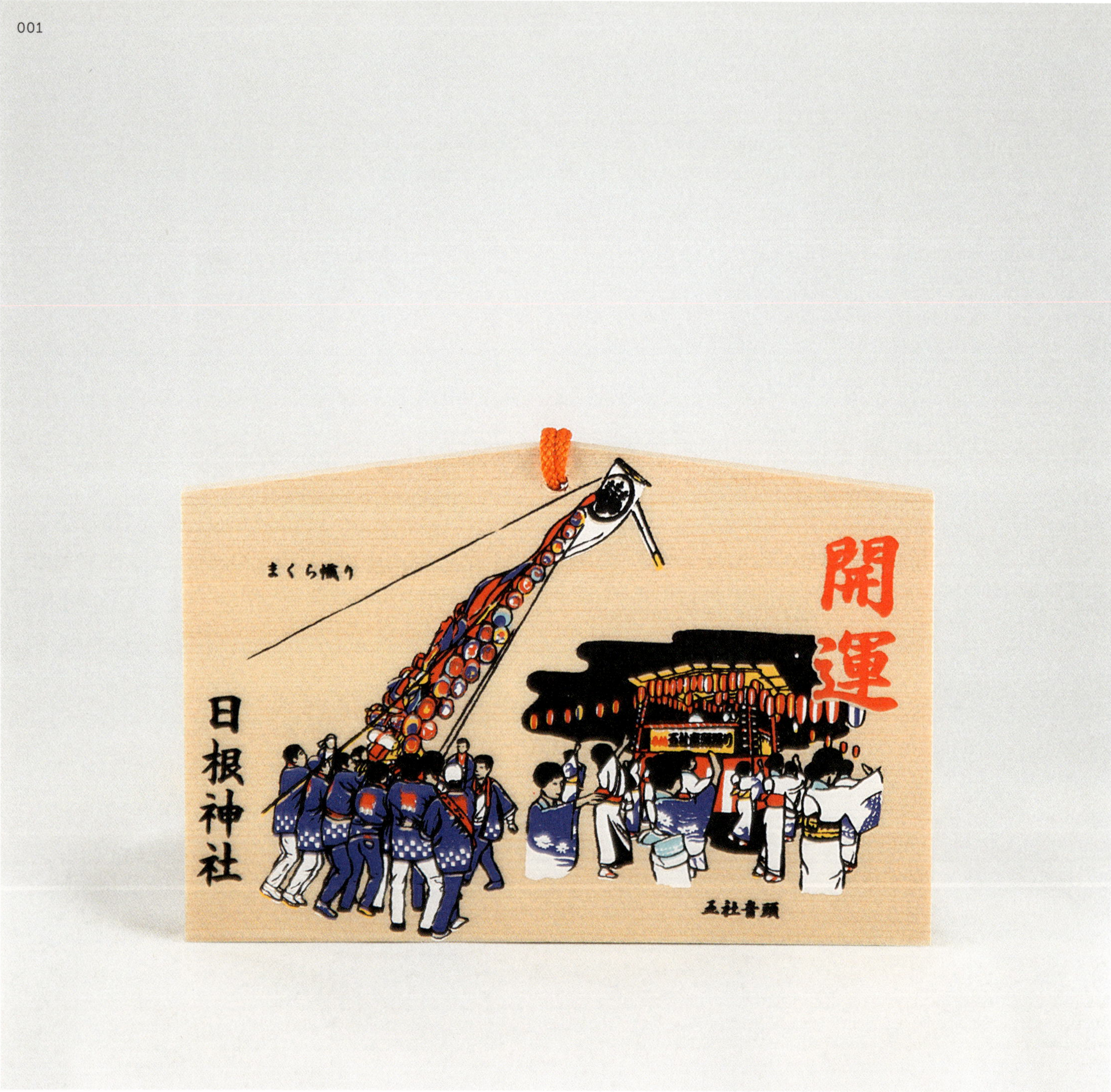

002

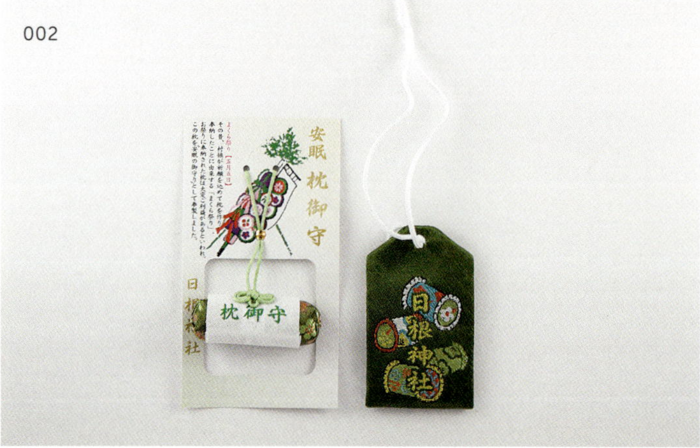

003

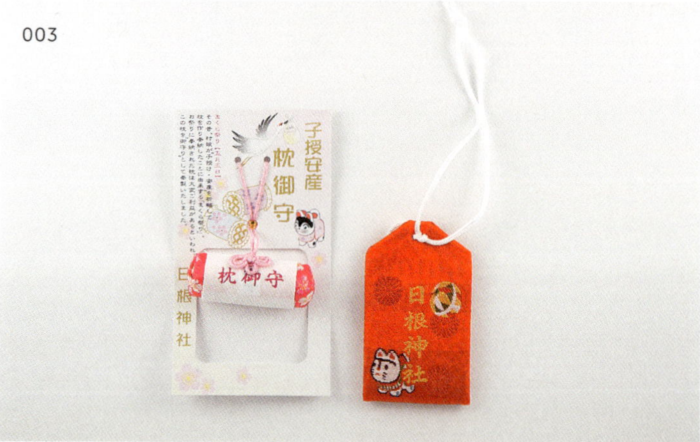

1 Introduction 紹介 (*Shōkai*)

001–003
Religious objects from *Hine Jinja* 日根神社
a Shinto shrine in Izumisano, Osaka Prefecture.
Early 21st century.
001
Votive tablet (*ema*). W. 15.9 cm
The inscriptions read:
開運 = *kaiun* (opening up good luck)
五社音頭 = *Goshaondo* (type of chorus song)
まくら幟り= *makura nobori* (pillow banner)
日根神社 = *Hine Jinja*
002
Charms (*mamori*) for *anmin* (quiet sleep)
003
Charms (*mamori*) for *anzan* (easy delivery)

Hine Jinja is visited for *kosazuke* (child wish), *anzan* (easy delivery), and *anmin* (quiet sleep). The shrine sells special charms and pillow covers for quiet sleep (plate 002). Sleep disorders such as *fumin* (insomnia) are a common complaint in Japanese outpatients [IO; TT]. The *ema* shown here (plate 001) may be used for any of the above-mentioned wishes. Its left side shows a parade during the annual *Makura Matsuri* (Pillow Festival) at the shrine. Men in *happi* coats carry a five metre bamboo pole to which colourful pillows are attached. According to some, this may have come from the legendary offering of rice bags tied to green bamboo sticks to soldiers going to battle, while others interpret the bags as symbols of *kodakara* (the treasure that is children). The right side of the *ema* shows a special dance during another festival at the shrine, *Yu Matsuri* (Hot Water Festival).

Many Shinto shrines and Buddhist temples in Japan sell charms (*mamori* and *fuda*) that can be taken home as a symbol and container of the sacred power of the Shinto deity (*kami*) or Buddhist figure of worship who is enshrined there (see the section on health-related charms on p.61). In many cases, the same sanctuaries also sell small wooden votive tablets known as *ema*, which are meant to be left on a rack at the shrine or temple. The front of these tablets is usually decorated with a picture, but one can write a personal wish or need on the reverse and then hang the tablet on the rack in the hope that the enshrined *kami* or buddha will fulfil this particular desire or request [IR; RT-178].

004

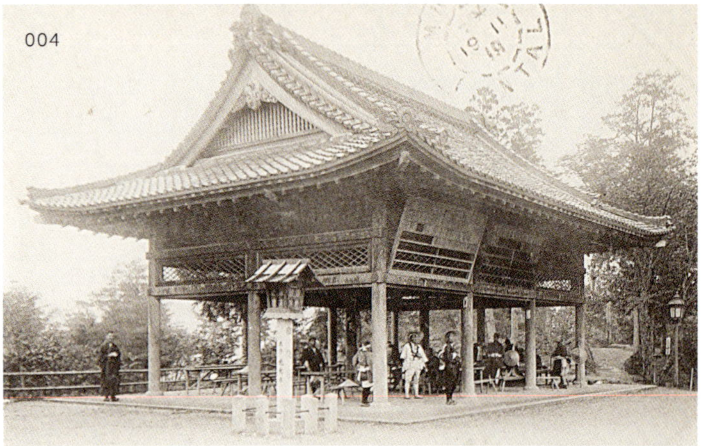

005

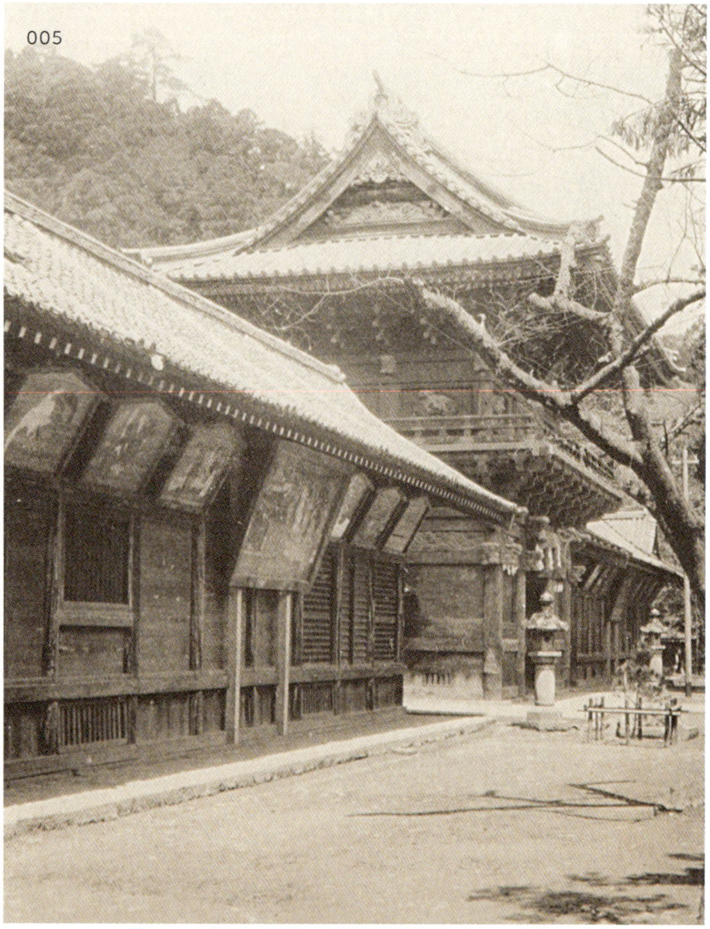

006

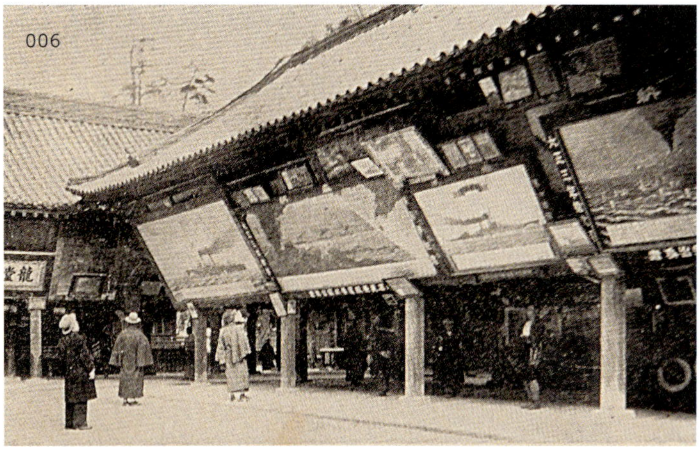

007

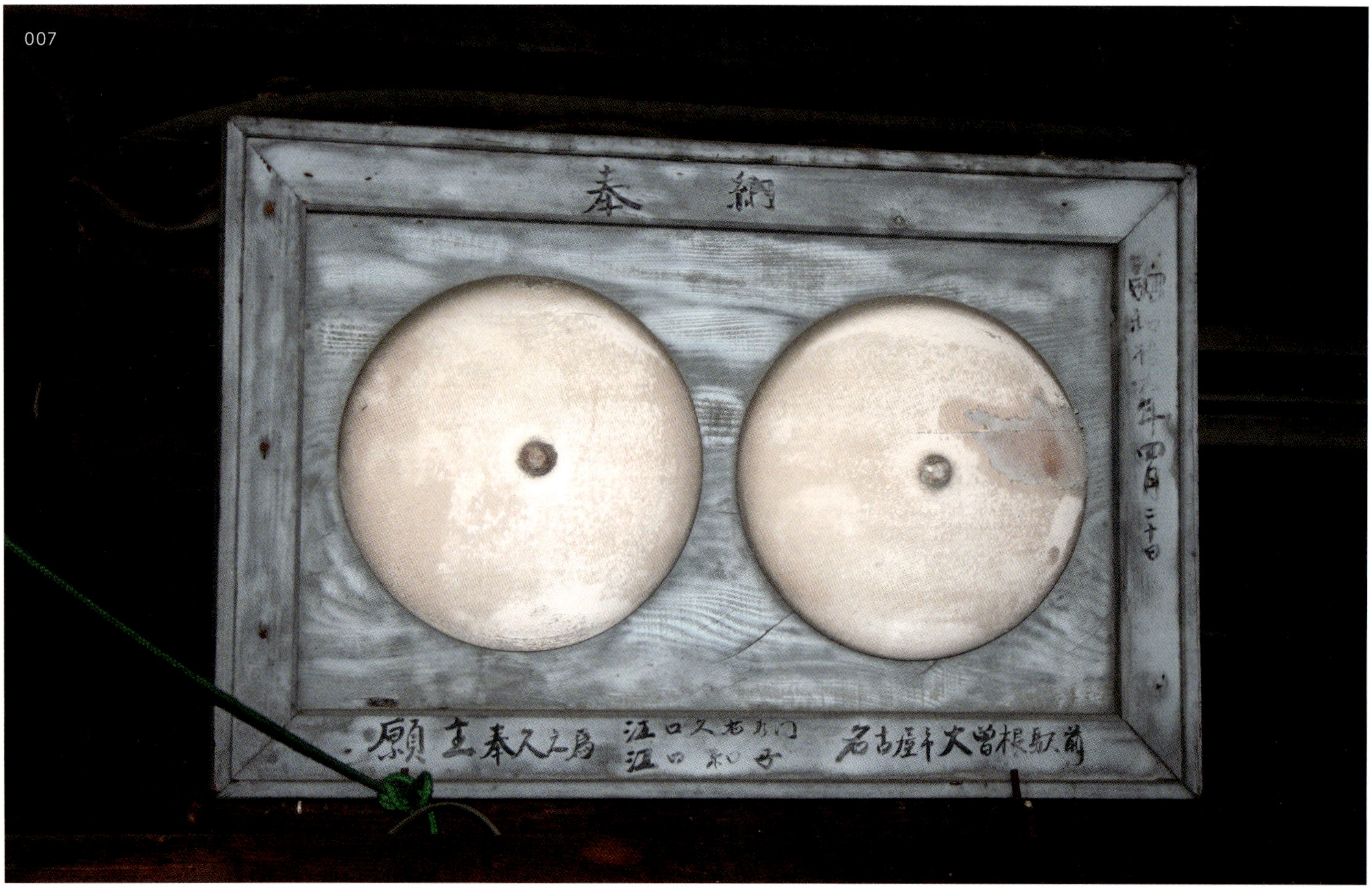

Historic view

The word *ema* literally means "horse picture" (*e* for picture and *ma* for horse). Until recently, it was commonly assumed that the earliest *ema* always had an isolated horse as their design and that one had started to offer these tablets to the gods instead of offering real horses. This view is no longer easy to defend. The oldest *ema*-like tablets come from the 8th century (Nara period) and are thus older than any literary suggestion that they were substitutes for real horses (see Table 1 for a historic timeline of Japan). In addition, two of these earliest *ema* have a different design: one represents a *sarukomahiki* (monkey leading a horse) whereas the other one depicts an *ushi* (cow/ox). It is unresolved whether these early *ema*-like tablets were already used specifically as votive offerings or served more generally as *fuda* (charms) [IR; HS; 2].

The use of *ema* is well-documented in medieval texts and illustrations. Their development may have reached a turning point in the 15th century, when they became larger and started to depict subjects other than horses more often. In the Edo period, the offering of *ema* became more and more popular. *Emashi* (painters of *ema*) and *emauri* (sellers of *ema*) emerged as new professions. Two main categories of *ema* paintings coexisted side by side [HD; OM-10; KJ; HS-1,11,18; IR; GG1-2011/09]:

- *ōema* (large *ema*) which were generally commissioned as single pieces by well-to-do donors from professional painters (including even such famous artists as Hokusai); they were more than 30 cm and sometimes over a metre in width and were displayed in a Shinto *haiden* (front shrine), a Buddhist main hall, or in a special building called *emadō* (*ema* hall); there is some evidence that the use of these *emadō* goes back at least to the mid-15th century;
- *koema* (small *ema*) which were usually simple without the artistic merits of the *ōema*; they were less than one foot long and had either been painted by the donor himself or mass-produced by craftsmen selling their wares to worshipers.

More likely than not, the latter category opened the door for illiterate believers from lower social classes to make votive donations as well.

004
Postcard from the early 20th century showing an *emadō* (*ema* hall) at *Yūki Jinja* 結城神社, Tsu, Mie Prefecture

Prehistoric and ancient Japan		Up to 538 AD
Classical Japan	Asuka period	538-710 AD
	Nara period	710-794 AD
	Heian period	794-1185 AD
Medieval Japan (Feudal Japan)	Kamakura period	1185-1333 AD
	Ashikaga (Muromachi) period	1336-1573 AD
	Azuchi-Momoyama period	1573-1600 AD
Early Modern Japan	Edo period (Tokugawa period)	1600-1868 AD
Imperial Japan (Modern Japan)	Meiji period	1868-1912 AD
	Taishō period	1912-1926 AD
	Shōwa period	1926-1989 AD
	Heisei period	1989-present

Table 1 Historic time periods of Japan [1]

005
Postcard from the early 20th century showing large *ema* at *Shizuoka Sengen Jinja* 静岡浅間神社, Shizuoka, Shizuoka Prefecture

006
Postcard from the early 20th century showing an *emadō* (*ema* hall) at *Kotohiragū* 金刀比羅宮 Kotohira, Kagawa Prefecture.
The principal *kami* (deity) enshrined is associated with seafaring. Today, the shrine offers small *ema* with the design of a sailing ship for *kōkai anzen kigan* (prayer for a safe voyage).

007
Large votive tablet (*ōema*). *Ryūonji* 龍音寺. Komaki, Aichi Prefecture.
Ryūonji has a collection of *ōema* (large votive tablets) depicting female breasts, which dates back to the early 19th century. Such *ema* were intended for the sufficient production and easy flow of breast milk [RT-243]. Today, the temple sells *koema* (small votive tablets) to pray for this purpose or for beautiful breasts (see p.93).

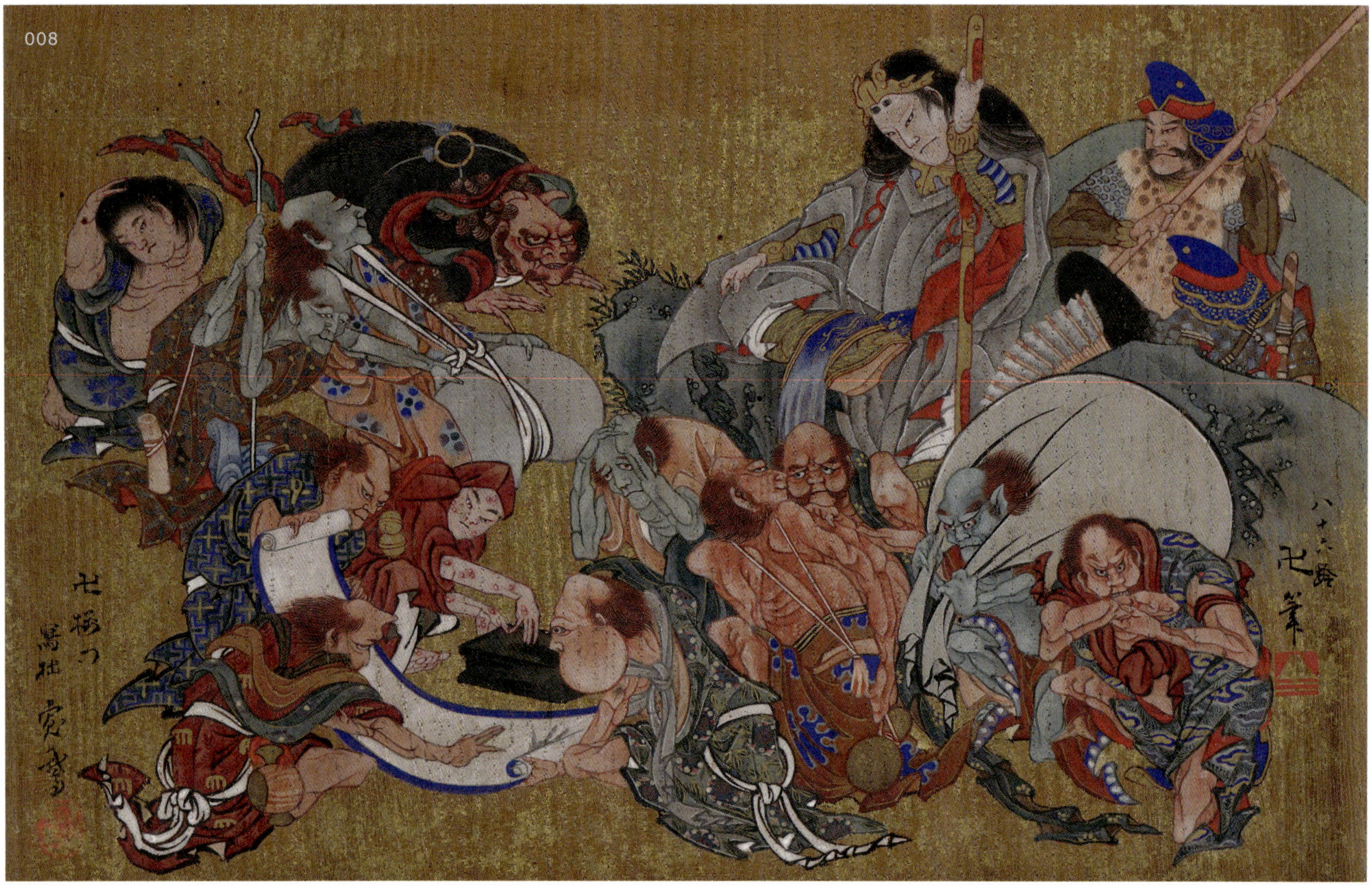

008

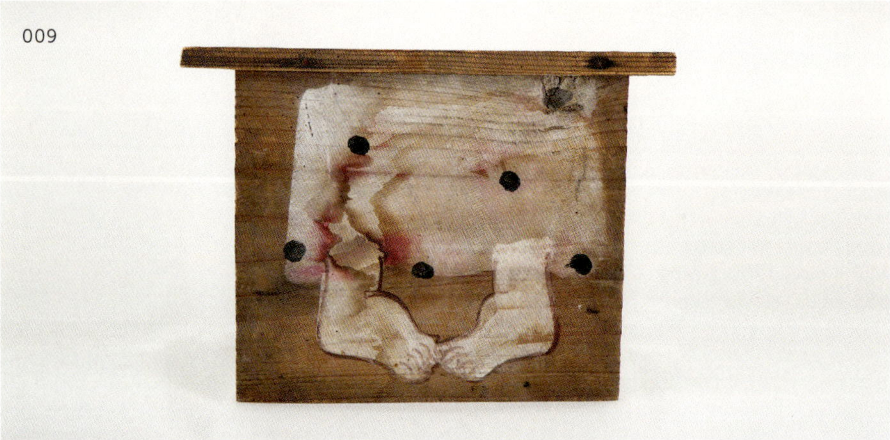

009

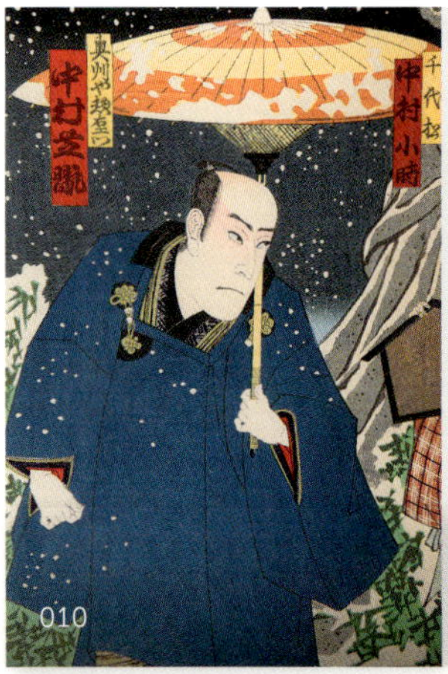

010

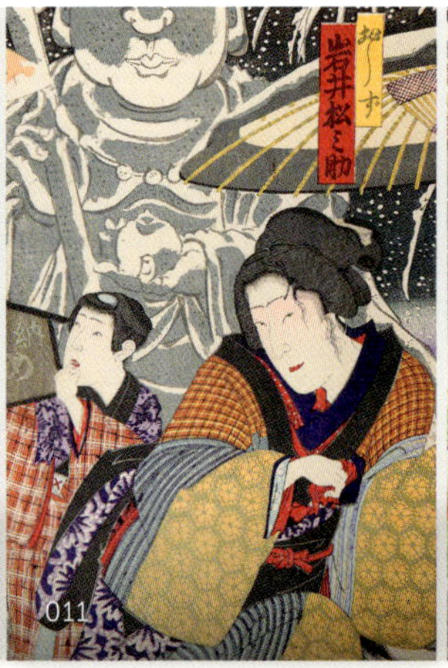

011

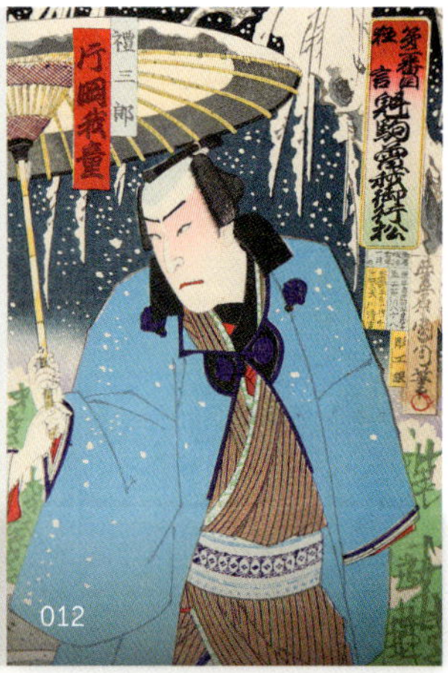

012

008
Susanoo no Mikoto making a pact with spirits of illnesses. Reduced-scale copy of a famous large votive painting by Hokusai in 1845. Copy made by Soga, a pupil of Manjiro, in 1860. 21.5 x 27.5 cms. British Museum (London) inv.no.1881,1210,0.2036

The original *ema* was in *Ushijima Jinja* in the *Mukōjima* part of Edo (the former name of Tokyo) where it was destroyed in the great earthquake of 1923. The spirits that can be identified most easily on this copy are those of measles, smallpox, mumps, elephantiasis and itching. Some of the other spirits possibly represent fevers, leprosy, erysipelas and corpulence [3].

009
Koema (small *ema*). Late 19th or early 20th century (Meiji Period). W. 23.3 cm.

The design on this *ema* is known as *kahanshin* (lower half of the body) and was used for *fujinbyō* (women's illnesses). See p.187 in the section on women's illnesses.

010–012
Woodblock print (*hanga*). Late 19th century. W. 72 cm

This tryptich by *Kunichika* shows a small group of people visiting a sanctuary in winter-time. In the middle, a young girl is carrying a small *ema* to be left at the sanctuary. The *ema* design consists of two facing *hiragana* characters (め = *me* = eye) and was generally used for wishes concerning eye symptoms/complaints (see p.137). This may explain why the girl seems to be looking rather worried. Behind the girl is the large statue of a buddha holding a *hōju* (wish granting jewel).

013

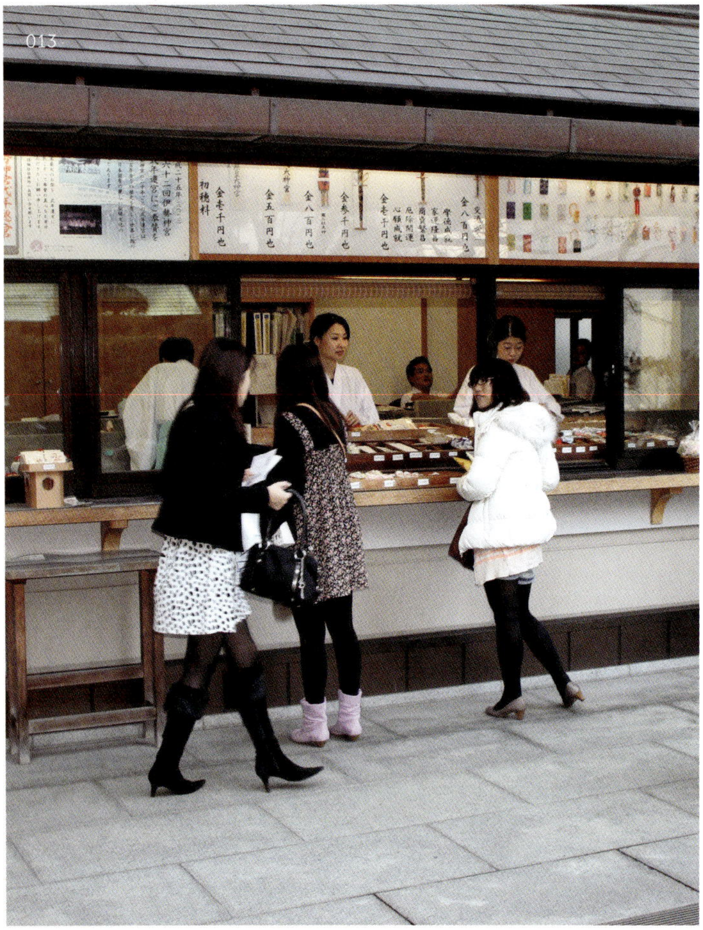

014

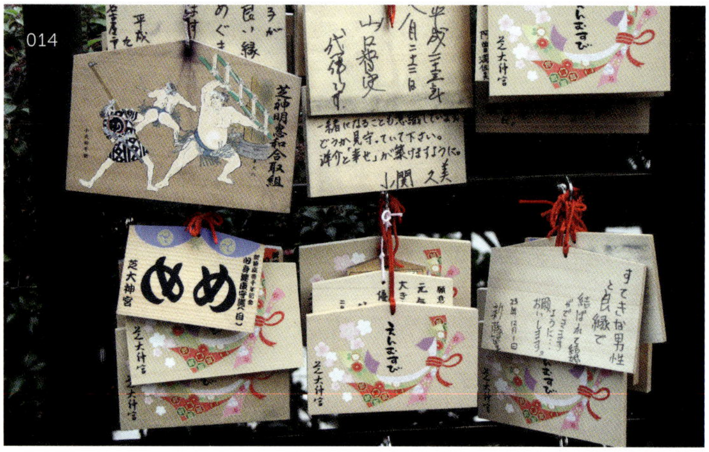

015

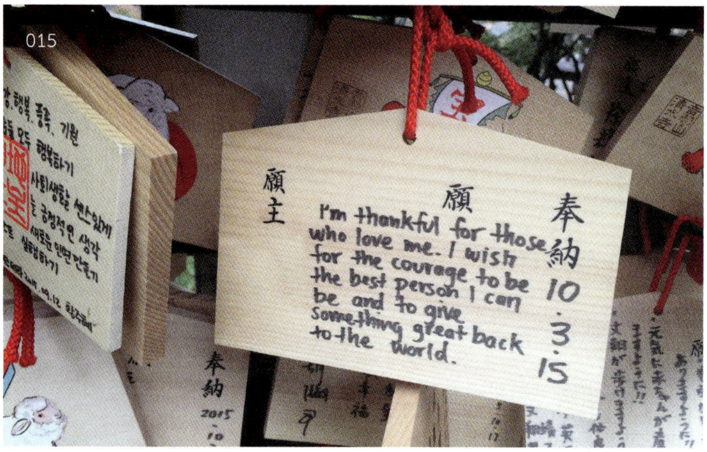

016

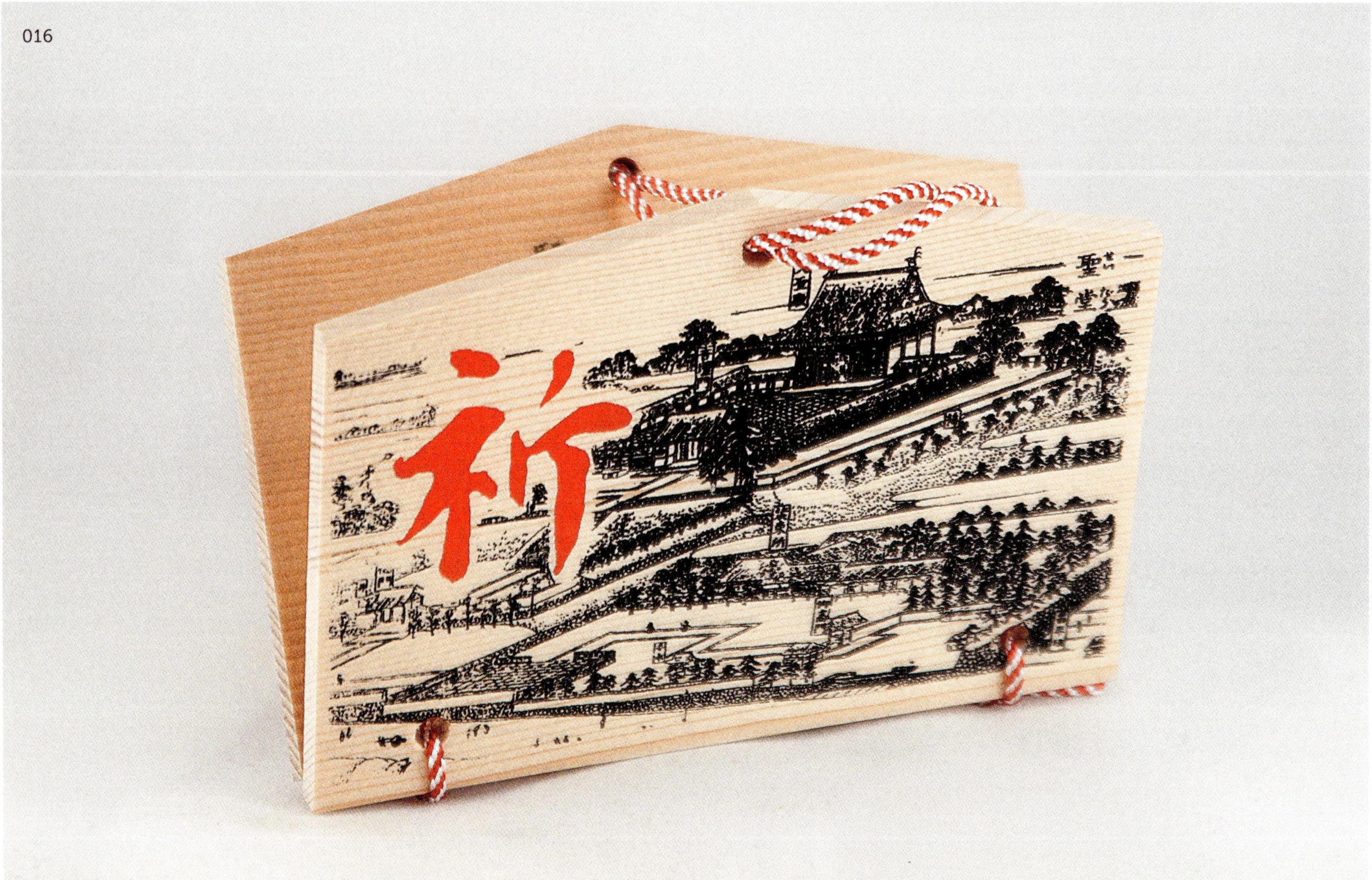

Contemporary practices

The tradition of addressing a Shinto *kami* (deity) or Buddhist figure of worship by writing a personal wish on the reverse of a small *ema* has continued until our time. Usually, applicants buy an *ema* of their choice at a shrine or temple office where a variety of charms (*mamori*) and other religious objects can be acquired. Technically one does not buy these objects, but one makes a donation and gets an *ema* or *mamori* in return. The wish on the reverse does not have to concern one's own problem but may also relate to that of a family member or friend. *Ema* writing can also be applied to acknowledge the fulfilment of a wish, but this seems to happen less often than the submission of a request [IR; KJ; HS].

If a shrine or temple offers more than one particular *ema*, the correct *ema* can easily be selected by looking at the design on the front. In the past, these designs must have been an essential part of the personal message of those who were not literate enough to write their message down on the *ema*. According to surveys conducted between 1877 and 1893, 61% of males and 27% of females in Meiji Japan could sign their own name [4]. As the literacy rate went up to its present level of 99%, emphasis most likely shifted from the meaning of an impersonal picture on the front of the *ema* to the individual messages written on the reverse by petitioners [IR].

These personal messages are quite relevant, of course, to scholars studying religious perceptions and behaviour. In surveys of *ema* writings in the late 20th century, the types of prayers varied with the specialisation(s) of the sanctuaries investigated. Yet it was not uncommon to find requests that were unrelated to the specific *ema* design or intended use. A leading reason for offering *ema* was the wish to pass a difficult entrance exam for a prestigious high school or university. These requests were particularly observed at *Tenjin Jinja* dedicated to the deified *Sugawara no Michizane* (the *kami* of scholarship), but could also be prominent at other shrines [EO-79,137; IR; 5]. The offering of exam-related *ema* by young people (or on their behalf) remains popular today.

After an *ema* has been written upon, it is hung on a special rack at the shrine or temple. This is done in an open unprotected way so that other visitors can read the wish or dedication if they want to. Some shrines and temples consider it impolite for other people to read what is written on these requests, and some even ask that they not be photographed. It has been mostly temples (such as *Nakayamadera* near Osaka) that offer *mizuko kuyō* (religious memorial services for aborted foetuses) that ask one not to read the message or take photos.

However, many shrines and temples take a more relaxed attitude and it is not uncommon to see visitors reading or taking photographs of the *ema* hanging up. Generally speaking, the Japanese attitude towards privacy has been different from that in Western society. Since the Japanese often live and interact at close quarters, they are bound to acquire detailed knowledge of each other. The resulting lack of actual privacy has been counterbalanced and regulated by normative constraints [6]. This may start to change, however, under the influence of the internet, social media and other globalising factors. *Shimogamo Jinja* in Kyoto (which enshrines a deity for matchmaking) has started to hand out red stickers, after the shrine personnel observed that high school students on a school trip were teasing a classmate, who had written a wish for love on an *ema*. According to the shrine, many visitors are now using a sticker to hide their *ema* wishes [7].

After the *ema* have been offered, they are often burnt before New Year to make room for new *ema* and symbolically to send the written wishes up to the *kami* (deities) and buddhas [IR]. Needless to say, this annual destruction is not very helpful if one wants to collect and study *ema*.

013–014
Shiba Daijingū 芝大神宮 Minato Ward, Tokyo
013
Office where the *ema* (votive tablets) of the shrine can be purchased.
014
Rack for hanging the *ema* after a prayer request or other personal message has been written on their reverse.

The *ema* design in the top right corner is intended to pray for *renai jōju* (love fulfilment). The design in the top left corner represents a famous fight that took place at the shrine in 1804 between fire fighters and sumo wrestlers. Directly below this *ema*, there is a votive tablet decorated with two facing *hiragana* characters (め = *me* = eye) to indicate its usefulness to prevent or heal eye symptoms/complaints. The right character is depicted as such, while the left one is shown in reverse (see p.137). *Ema* are often connected with wordplays, so it does not seem coincidental that the old Japanese term for firefighters is め組 = *megumi* (which means *me* group).

015
Kiyomizudera 清水寺 Higashiyama Ward, Kyoto.
Today, the writing of a personal ema message is no longer reserved for Japanese visitors with a religious background. Messages in foreign languages can also be encountered, particularly at famous sanctuaries that attract many international tourists [HS-9].

016
Yushima Seidō 湯島聖堂 Bunkyo Ward, Tokyo.
Early 21st century. W. 15.1 cm
The red character on the front *ema* reads 祈 which means prayer.

Yushima Seidō offers this *awase ema* (joined together *ema*) that can be closed and tightly bound after the message has been written down (the reverses of the two *ema* are blank). Bloggers associate this *ema* with the protection of privacy and the *kojinjōhōhogohō* (personal information protection law of 2003).

Elsewhere, such double *ema* may be recommended for love and marriage (one half of a couple writing on one *ema* and the other half on the other *ema*, after which the two are tied together). This is not the purpose of the double *ema* at *Yushima Seidō*, however, since their main text reads either *gōkaku kigan* (prayer for passing, e.g. an exam) or *daiganjōju* (realisation of a great ambition).

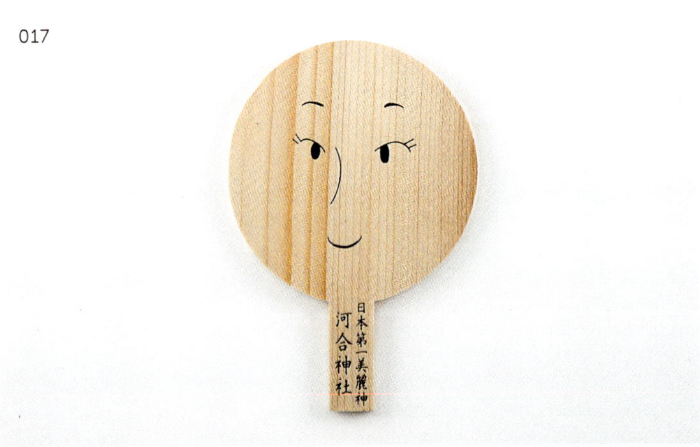

017

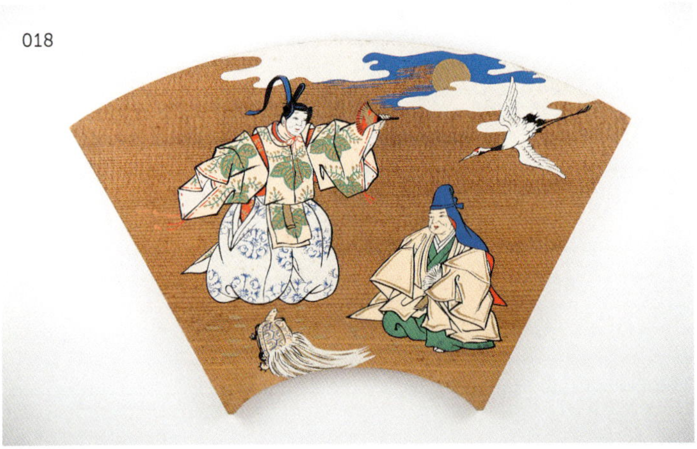
018

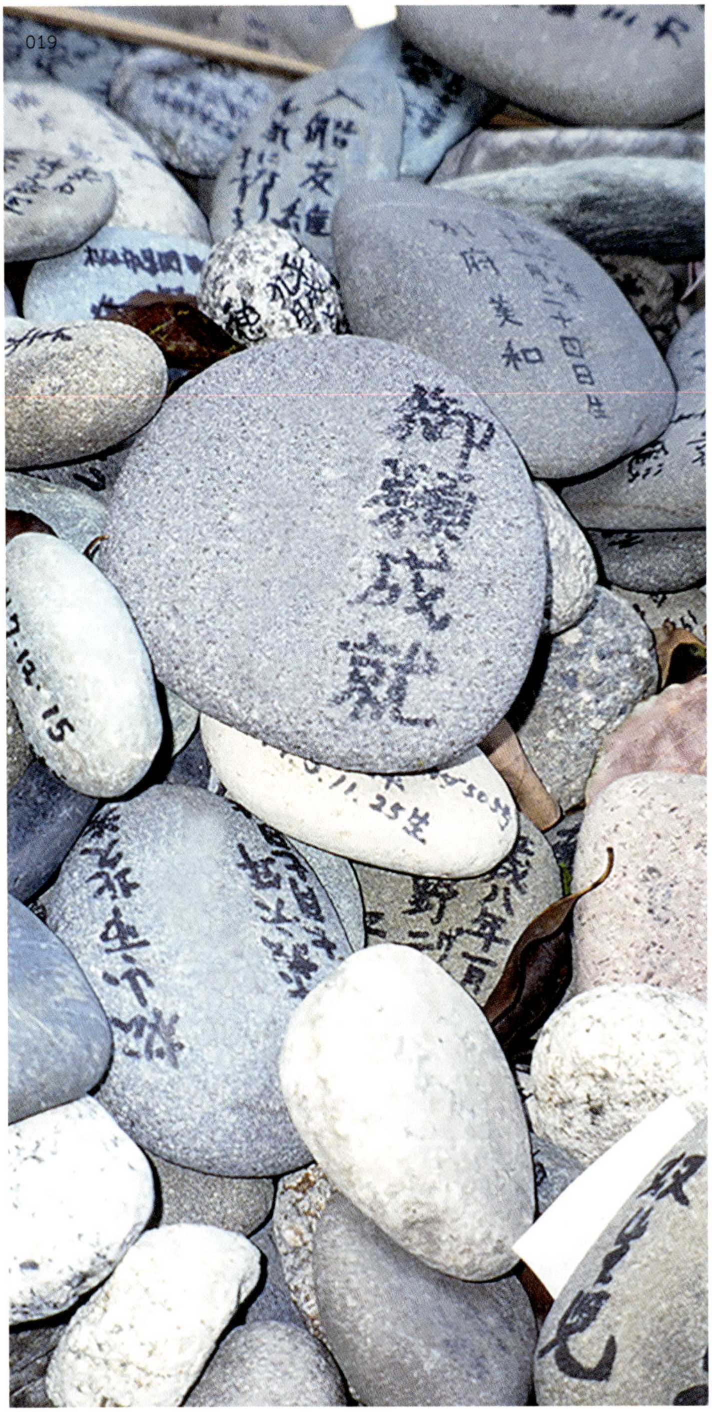
019

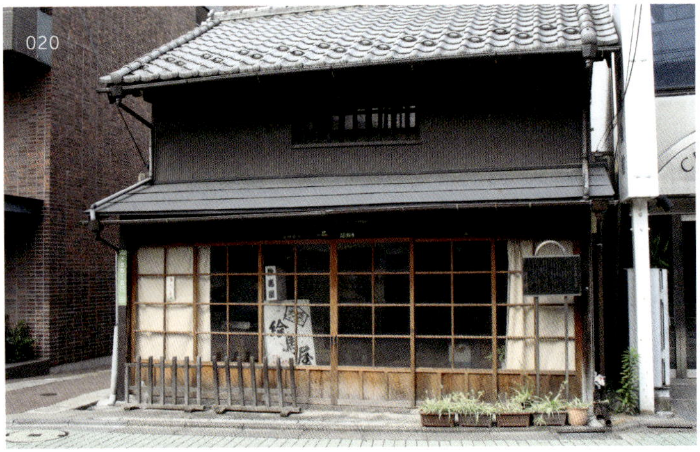

020

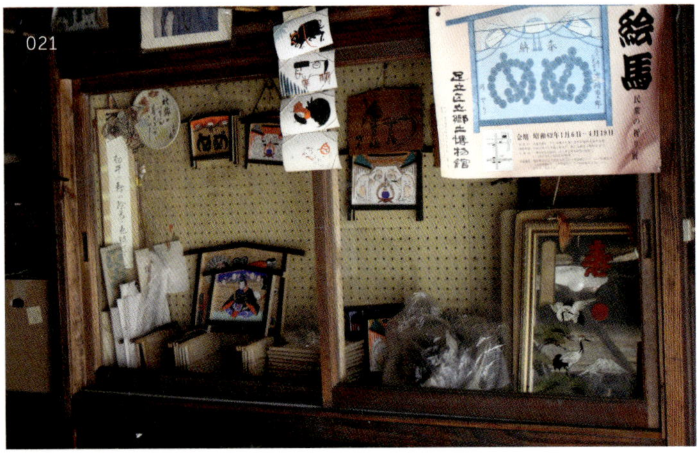

021

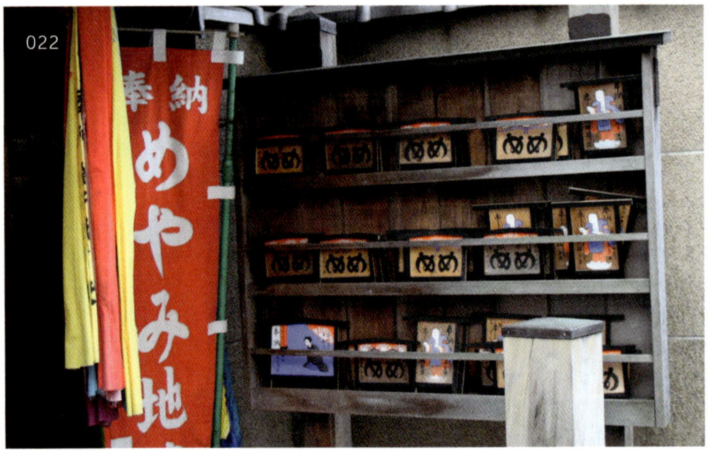

022

Appearances

Contemporary *ema* usually consist of wood and come in different shapes and sizes. The most common type is 10-15 cm wide and has a pentagonal shape that is reminiscent of a stable entrance [OT; HS-1]. Another common shape that is especially seen in *ema* from the early to mid-20th century is the rectangle. Occasionally, *ema* have other shapes, such as a circle, an octagon, a *shamoji* (wooden rice scoop), or the contours of the object that they portray. There are also three-dimensional *ema* and *ema* consisting of naturally occurring materials (such as stone pebbles or abalone shells) [IH1-93; TS; KM].

Mass production of wooden *ema* by means of screen printing emerged in the mid-20th century and largely superseded the earlier hand-painted *ema*. The latter have not completely disappeared, however. For instance, there is one *ema* shop left in Tokyo that still makes and sells hand-painted *ema*.

017
Hand mirror 手鏡 (*tekagami*). *Kawai Jinja* 河合神社 at *Shimogamo Jinja*. 下鴨神社. Sakyo Ward, Kyoto. Early 21st century. W 8.7 cm
The inscriptions on the handle read:
河合神社 = *Kawai Jinja*
日本第一美麗神 = *Nihon Daiichi birei jin*
(the number one deity in Japan for beauty)

Ema design for enhancement of facial beauty. One can paint on the *ema* which part of the face one would like to improve. The shrine also sells *karin sui* (beauty water made from the fruit of the quince tree) for the same purpose [GG1-2013-11-01]. Quinces are also an ingredient of drinks for good health (cf. the sections on health in part three and on respiratory symptoms/complaints in part four).

018
Large fan-shaped *ema* representing *tsurukame* Late 20th century. W. 33.4 cm

Tsurukame is composed of *tsuru* (crane) and *kame* (tortoise/turtle). Both animals are depicted on the *ema* as symbols of longevity (cf. p.103). *Tsurukame* is also the name of a Noh play in which they dance as long-living animals to celebrate the longevity of an ancient Chinese emperor. The latter also participates in the dancing and retreats thereafter to the Hall of Everlasting Life.

019
Prayer pebbles. *Ichijōji* 一乗寺 Kasai, Hyogo prefecture. Late 20th century

Generally speaking, prayer pebbles with written votive messages are offered for various reasons, including good business, fishery and illnesses of the ear [EO-129; KM-31].

020–022
Emaya Yoshidaya 絵馬屋 吉田屋 (Senju, Adachi Ward) is the only shop left in Tokyo where hand-painted *ema* are still made and sold.

020
Exterior of the shop

021
Interior of the shop

022
Booth at the near-by *Chōenji* temple where *ema* from the shop are also offered for sale.

023

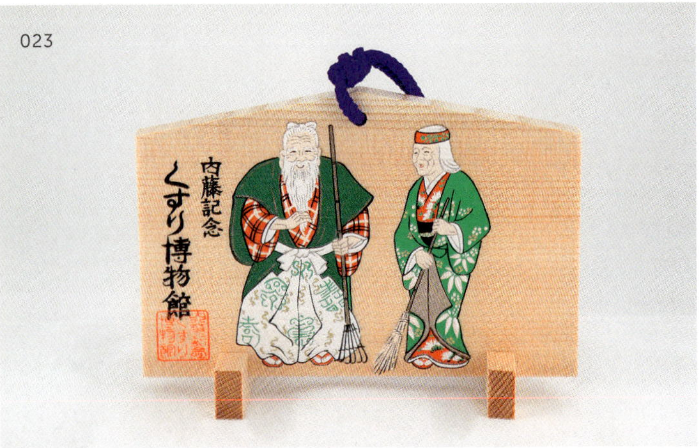

024

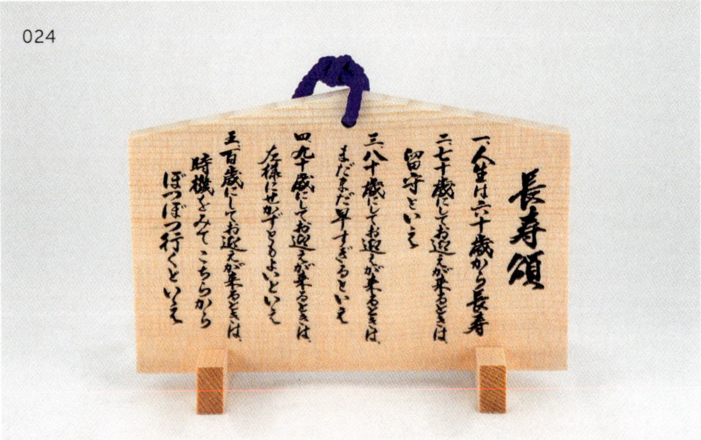

025

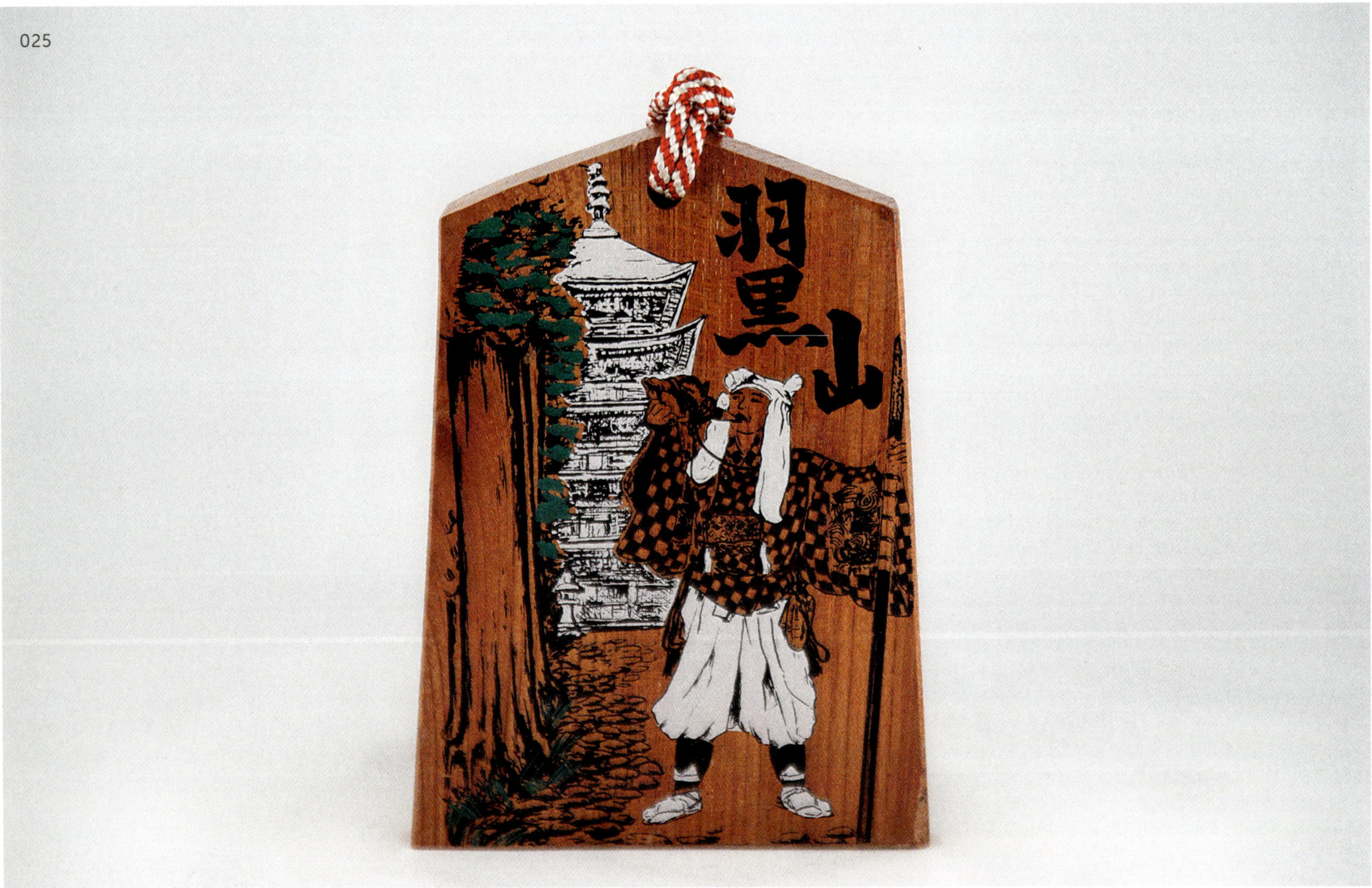

026

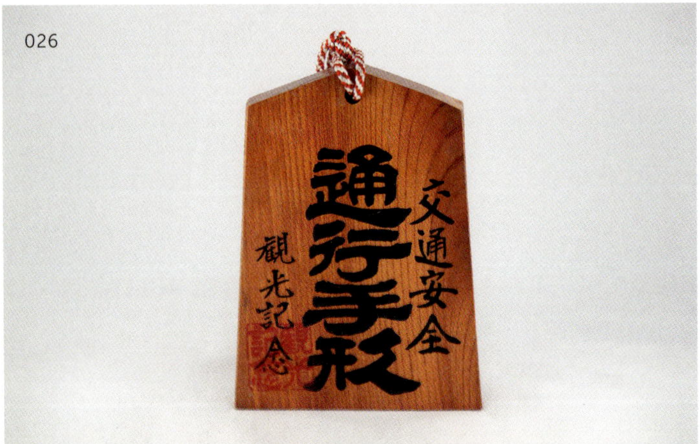

027

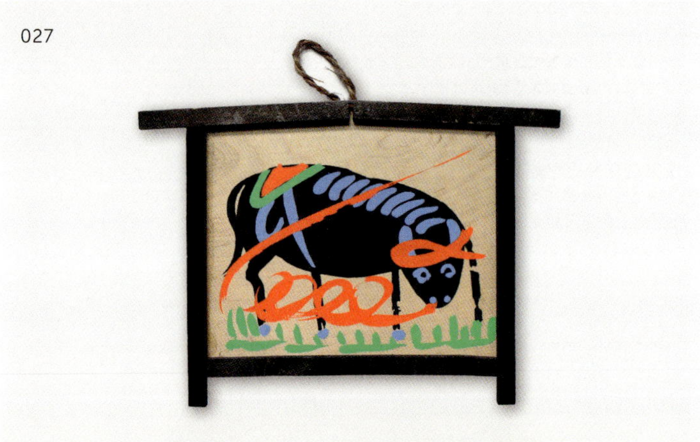

Souvenirs and collectibles

According to Japanese sources, the significance of *ema* as religious votive objects was in substantial decline in the 1960s. In earlier days, there had been a fairly large number of *ema* painters in Tokyo, but this was no longer a profitable trade. At the same time, however, *ema* were gaining ground as objects that were not written upon and left on a rack at the shrine or temple but were taken away to be kept at home [MH; IY-77]. The souvenir function of some *ema* can easily be recognised by their densely printed reverse, which obviously precludes the original function of a message board. When such souvenirs retain the pentagonal shape of an *ema* but are taller than they are wide, they are referred to as *tsūkōtegata*. In the past, when travelling within and between provinces was strictly controlled, such *tsūkōtegata* were used as travel passes.

In the late 20th century, *ema* also became more and more valued as collectibles. A club of *ema* collectors was created that called itself *Nihon ema yūkai* (Japanese *ema* association). Its members were entitled to receive one hand-painted reproduction of an interesting *ema* design every month. Judging from the numbering of these copies, hundreds of different *ema* designs must have been reproduced for this club. The Naito Museum of Pharmaceutical Sciences and Industry (Kakamigahara, Gifu Prefecture) was also interested in hand-painted reproductions and commissioned the *ema* painter *Norihito Yasuda* from Nagoya to produce a large series for the museum. Many *ema* designs in this museum series and various *ema* reproductions for the Japanese collectors' club are health-related and will be discussed in this book. Some *ema* reproductions in the Naito Museum bear such a striking resemblance to the *ema* reproductions for the collectors' club that the question arises whether both may have come from the same source (compare the *ema* design in 027 with the *ema* design of cow/ox and grass (*ushi ya kusa*) in the section on skin illnesses on p.176).

023–024
Ema-shaped souvenir from the Naito Museum of Pharmaceutical Sciences and Industry (Kakamigahara, Gifu Prefecture). 21st century. W. 17.5 cm

The front depicts *jō to uba* (an old man and old woman) as a symbol of *chōju* (longevity) [IH2-14]. The reverse talks about human life from 60, 70, 80, 90, and 100 onwards.

025–026
Tsūkōtegata 通行手形 (travel pass) from Mount Haguro, Dewa Mountains, Yamagata Prefecture. W. 12.7 cm

In the old days, *tsūkōtegata* were sealed statements certifying that the bearer was properly registered and had been granted permission to travel from region to region.

On the front, a *yamabushi* (mountain priest of the *Shugendō* sect) can be recognised from his checkered jacket and his *horagai* (conch shell trumpet). The inscription and the five-storey pagoda in the background (*Gojū-no-tō*) put this scene at Mount Haguro. This is one of the three sacred Dewa peaks believed to represent birth, death and rebirth which have been worshiped for centuries by the *yamabushi*.

The reverse offers so little room for writing that this must be a souvenir and not an *ema* for presenting a personal wish. This is confirmed by the inscriptions:
交通安全 = *kōtsū anzen* (traffic safety)
通行手形 = *tsūkōtegata* (travel pass)
観光記念 = *kankō kinen* (tourist souvenir)

027
Ema hand-painted by *Norihito Yasuda* (Nagoya) on commission from the Naito Museum of Pharmaceutical Sciences and Industry (Kakamigahara, Gifu Prefecture). Museum inv.no. Z22676. Late 20th century.

028

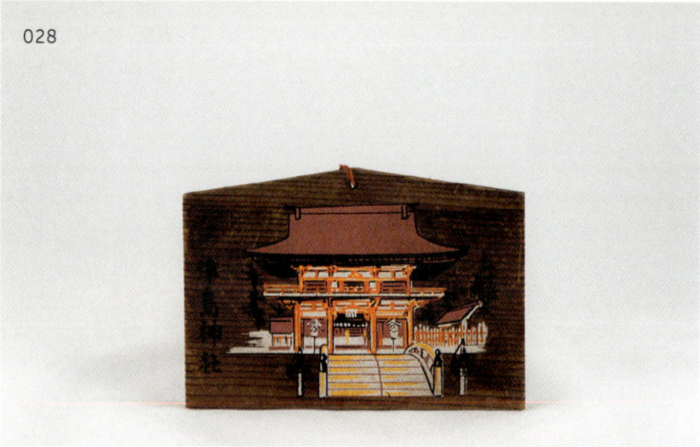

029

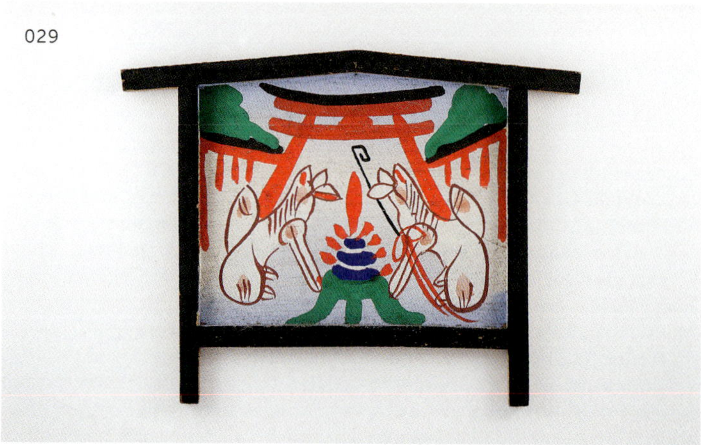

030

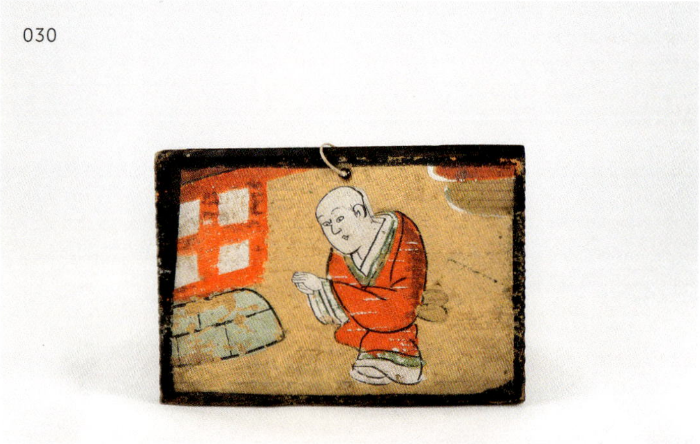

031

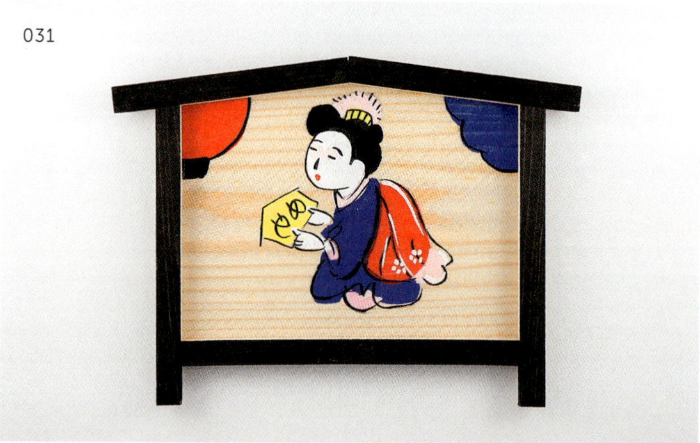

032

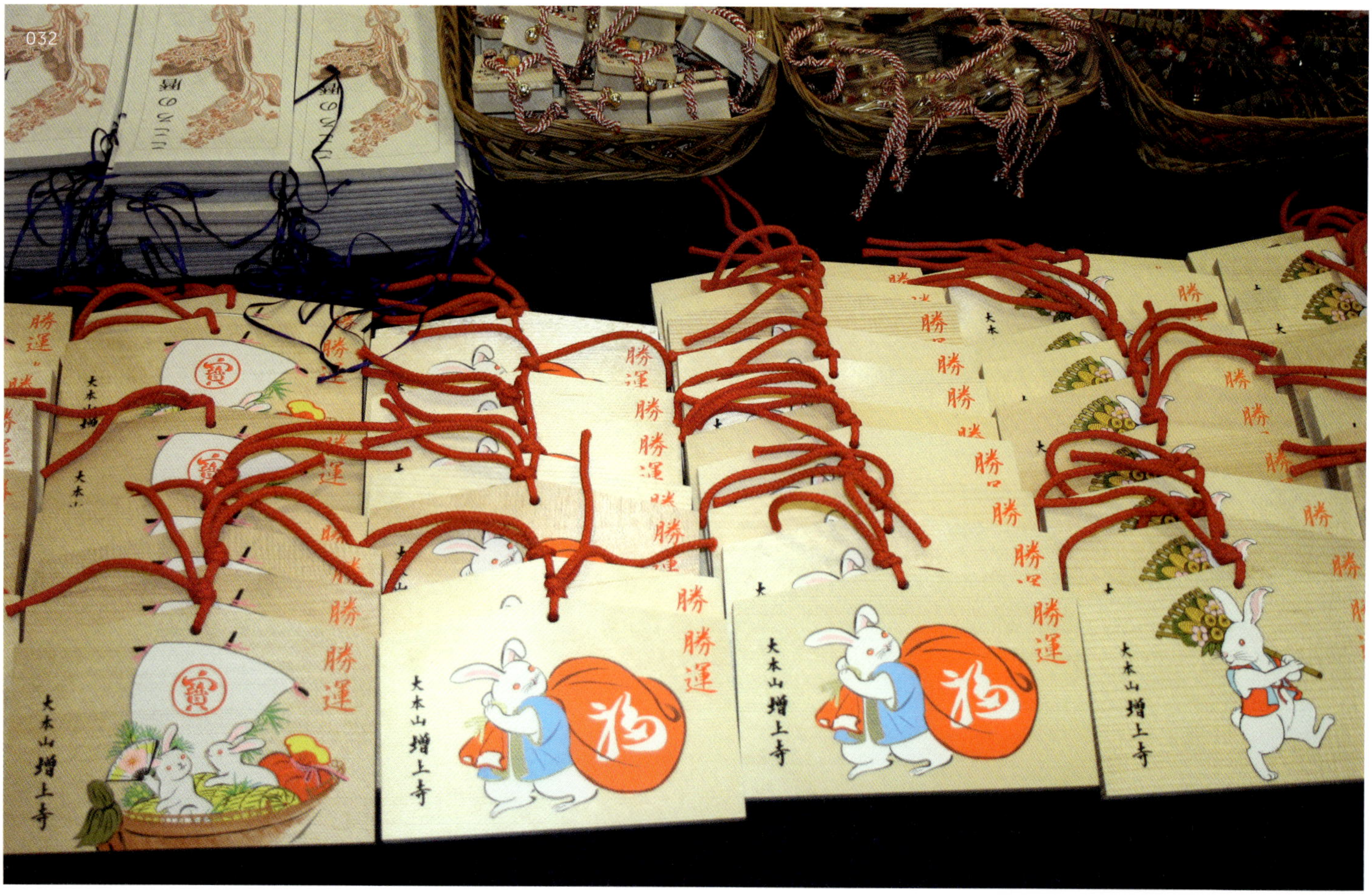

Designs

Common motifs in the designs of small *ema* include [FS; HD; GS; IH1; IH2; IR]:

- a picture of the shrine or temple itself or a scene from its *engi* (legendary foundation story);
- the *kami* (deity) or buddha enshrined at the shrine or temple, a statue or characteristic attribute of that god, or the animal(s) acting as his divine messenger (e.g., a pair of foxes for the Shinto god of rice, *Inari*); cf. the section on figures of worship on p.41)
- a worshiper praying in front of a shrine or making an offering there (such as an *ema* or *mochi* rice cakes);
- the twelve animals of the zodiac cycle; originally, worshipers would select the animal that represented their birth year but now it is much more common that the zodiac animal reflects the current calendar year;
- the representation of one's promise (e.g., the favourite food from which one will abstain) or one's desire (e.g., the sport victory one is interested in, safety of flying, or a padlocked bad habit);
- a festival, dance or ceremony that is taking place at the sanctuary;
- a charm that can be purchased at the shrine or temple (cf. the section on charms on p.61).

The variety in *ema* designs is much larger than these exemplary categories suggest. Motifs range from religious dance paraphernalia and a Japanese *haiku* poem to famous sportspeople and fictional cartoon figures. As the sale of *ema* (and other types of religious objects) is economically important for shrines and temples, these centres strive to offer many attractive and eye-catching designs [IR].

Sometimes, the selection of an *ema* design is underpinned by a play on words that sound similar but have different meanings, for instance, an *ema* in the shape of a pentagon (*gokaku*) for educational success (*gōkaku*). *Ema* designs usually have some relevance to the religious institution at which they are sold. They are commonly inscribed with the name of the sanctuary and the specific benefit (*goriyaku*) that can be acquired from or bestowed by the figure of worship enshrined may also be specified [IR].

The intended use of an *ema* design is not always straight forward, since the same motif may relate to different benefits over time or in different locations. For instance, the meaning of a horse design on an *ema* is not always immediately obvious. The horse can be a zodiac animal representing the calendar year or the birth year of the worshipper, but it can also be a local wooden toy expressing a legendary story. In some parts of Japan, *ema* with horses served to appease the gods in times of drought or abundant rain. Furthermore, *ema* with horses were offered for the well-being of horses in the horse-breeding areas of Japan. There are also shrines (such as *Fujinomori Jinja*, Fushimi Ward, Kyoto) which offer *ema* in relation to horse racing. The explicit purpose of these latter *ema* is not the health of the race horse but *kachiuma* (winning horse).

028
Tsushima Jinja 津島神社 Tsushima, Aichi Prefecture. Late 20th century. W. 12.3 cm
The inscription reads: 津島神社 = *Tsushima Jinja*

Tsushima Jinja heads the network of the *Tsushima* cult, which has *Gozu Tennō* and *Susanoo* as its main deities. *Gozu Tennō* (literally Ox-Headed Heavenly King) is a combinatory Shinto/Buddhist deity. He has been identified with the Shinto deity *Susanoo* who features in the legend of *Somin Shōrai* (see p.65) [KU]. *Gozu Tennō* is also worshipped at *Yasaka Jinja* (Kyoto) where his epidemic-causing power stood at the birth of the annual *Gion* festival (see the entry on *Goryō* festival and *Gion* festival on p.53).

In popular belief, *Gozu Tennō* transformed in the course of time from an epidemic-causing spirit into a tutelary protector against epidemics. On the island of Kyushu, *kitoshi* (healing priests) would make magical paper images of a horned figure called *goddon* (a variation on *Gozu Tennō*) with the power to ward off evil spirits and diseases (such as smallpox). These paper images could be pasted on a wall in the farmhouse or were folded up and worn around the neck as a charm [8].

029
Foxes 狐 (*kitsune*). Hand-painted reproduction for a Japanese club of ema collectors called *Nihon Ema Tomo no Kai* (Friends of Japanese Ema Society). No.311. Late 20th century. W. 18.2 cm. Original design from Naruto Town (now Sanmu City), Chiba prefecture

Foxes are the servants and messengers of *Inari*, the Shinto deity of rice who is associated with agriculture and fertility. *Ema* fox designs may portray a single fox or two foxes beside each other, but more commonly depict two facing foxes (*mukai kitsune*). There is often a *torii* (Shinto shrine gate) in the scene as well. There may be a *nyoi hōju* (wish-fulfilling jewel) between the two foxes that is a symbol of *Inari* and represents financial as well as spiritual wealth. One of the foxes may hold a *kagi* (key) in its mouth that gives access to the rice granary. Together, these two objects symbolize that the feminine (jewel) and the masculine (key) are equally needed for fertility [FS; TS-17,21; IH2-30; GG1-2011/09; MS; 9].

Ema with foxes are generally used to pray for *gokokuhōjō* (abundant harvest) and *shōbai hanjō* (prosperous business). Occasionally, they have also been used for *kosazuke* (being blessed with a child) or *fujinbyō* (women's illnesses) [TS-17,21; IH2-30; NM-Z22665]. Cf. the entries on facing foxes on p.89 and p.195.

030
Man worshipping 男の拝み (*otoko no ogami*)
Origin unclear. Early 20th century. W. 13.1 cm

The man is kneeling in front of a local sanctuary. There are also *ema* designs where the worshipper is a woman, a child, or a mother with child [TS-24; IH2-20].

031
Woman worshipping 女の拝み (*onna no ogami*)
Hand-painted reproduction for a Japanese club of *ema* collectors called *Nihon Ema Tomo no Kai* (Friends of Japanese Ema Society). No.372. Late 20th century. W. 18.3 cm. Original design from *Takedera* (Iino, Saitama Prefecture).

The woman is holding the *ema* design of *mukai me* (facing *me* characters) in her hands that is widely used for *ganbyō heiyu* (recovery from eye illnesses). See the entry on facing *me* characters on p.137.

032
Ema for the year of the rabbit (2011) for sale at *Zōjōji* (Minato Ward, Tokyo).

033

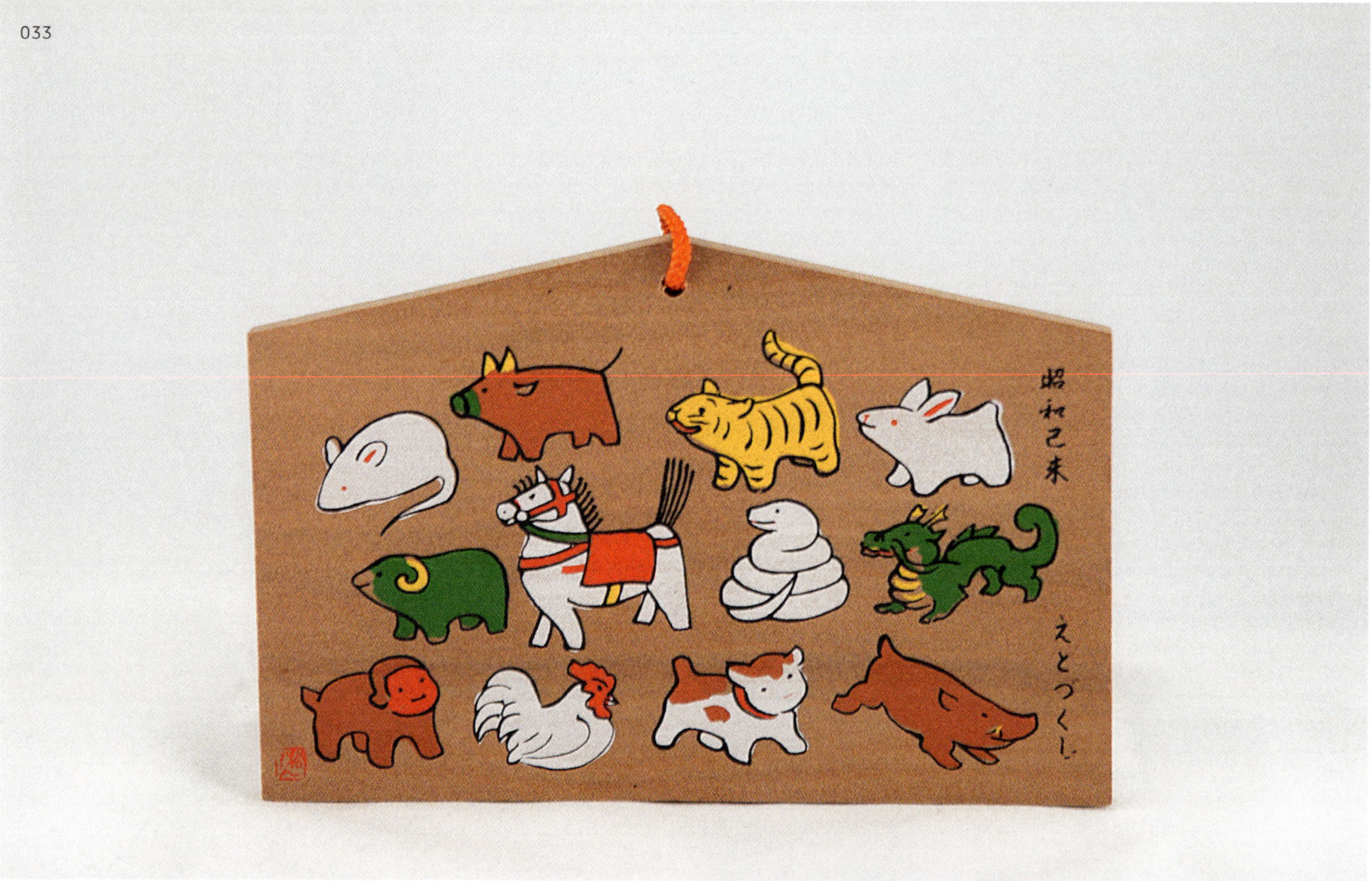

034

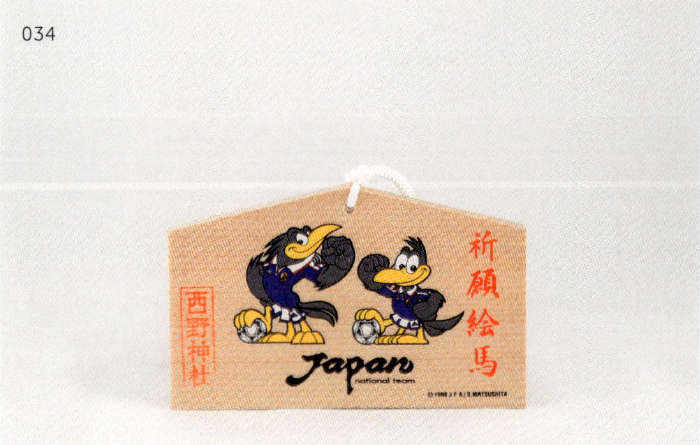

035

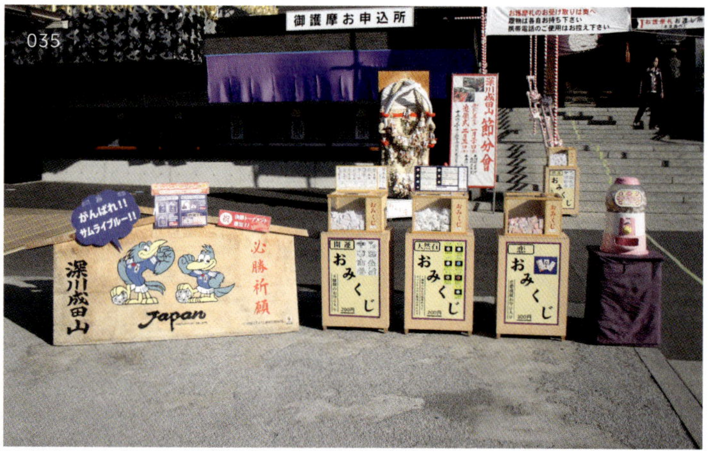

036

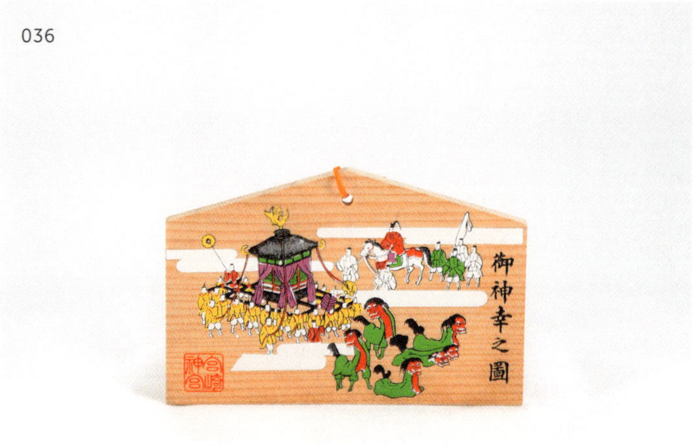

037

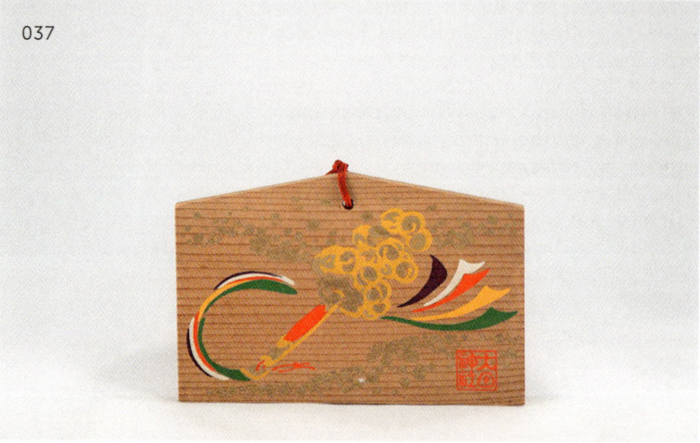

033
All twelve animals of the Chinese zodiac system 十二支の動物 (*jūnishi no dōbutsu*). Late 20th century. W. 17.3 cm.

The individual zodiac animals are: *ne* (rat); *ushi* (ox); *tora* (tiger); *usagi* (hare); *tatsu* (dragon); *mi* (snake); *uma* (horse); *hitsuji* (sheep); *saru* (monkey); *tori* (rooster); *inu* (dog); and *i* (boar) [GS-95; MS].

034
Three-legged crows 八咫烏 (*yatagarasu*) *Nishino Jinja* 西野神社. Sapporo, Hokkaido Prefecture. Early 21st century. W. 13.9 cm
The inscriptions read:
祈願絵馬 = *kigan ema* (prayer votive tablet)
西野神社 = *Nishino Jinja*

This *ema* design is connected to the national team of the Japan Football Association (JFA). It shows two *yatagarasu* (three-legged crows) in the team's uniform that serve as mascots and were designed by the Japanese manga artist *Susumu Matsushita*.

035
Promotion of *ema* of the Japan Football Association. *Narita-san Fukagawa-Fudō-dō* 成田山 深川不動堂. Koto Ward, Tokyo.

036
Miyazaki Jingū Taisai (*Miyazaki* Shrine Grand Festival). Late 20th century. W. 14.5 cm

The Grand Festival shown here is held every year at *Miyazaki Jingū* 宮崎神宮, Miyazaki, Miyazaki Prefecture. The inscription on the right refers to *goshinkō* which means the transfer of the deity's spirit to the *mikoshi* (portable shrine) that will be carried around. The richly decorated horses in the parade are called *shan shan* (after the sound of the bells they wear).

037
Wand with bells 鈴 (*suzu*) for Shinto dance 神楽 (*kagura*). *Ōta Jinja* 大田神社. Kita Ward, Kyoto. Late 20th century. W. 13.8 cm

In ancient times, shaking bells in the *kagura* dance was believed to call for the *kami* to take possession of the dancing *miko* (shrine maiden). The five ribbons represent *goshiki* (the five cardinal colours): green (or blue), purple (or black), red, white and yellow. In traditional East Asian medicine, these five colours are associated with [ML-32]:

- the five elements into which all phenomena can be broken down (wood, water, fire, metal and earth, respectively);
- the five sense organs (eye, ear, tongue, nose and mouth, respectively);
- the five *zang* or *yin* organs: liver, kidney, heart, lung and spleen, respectively);
- the five *fu* or *yang* organs: gallbladder, bladder, small intestine, large intestine and stomach, respectively).

The *zang* and *fu* organs are not anatomical organs in the biomedical sense.

038

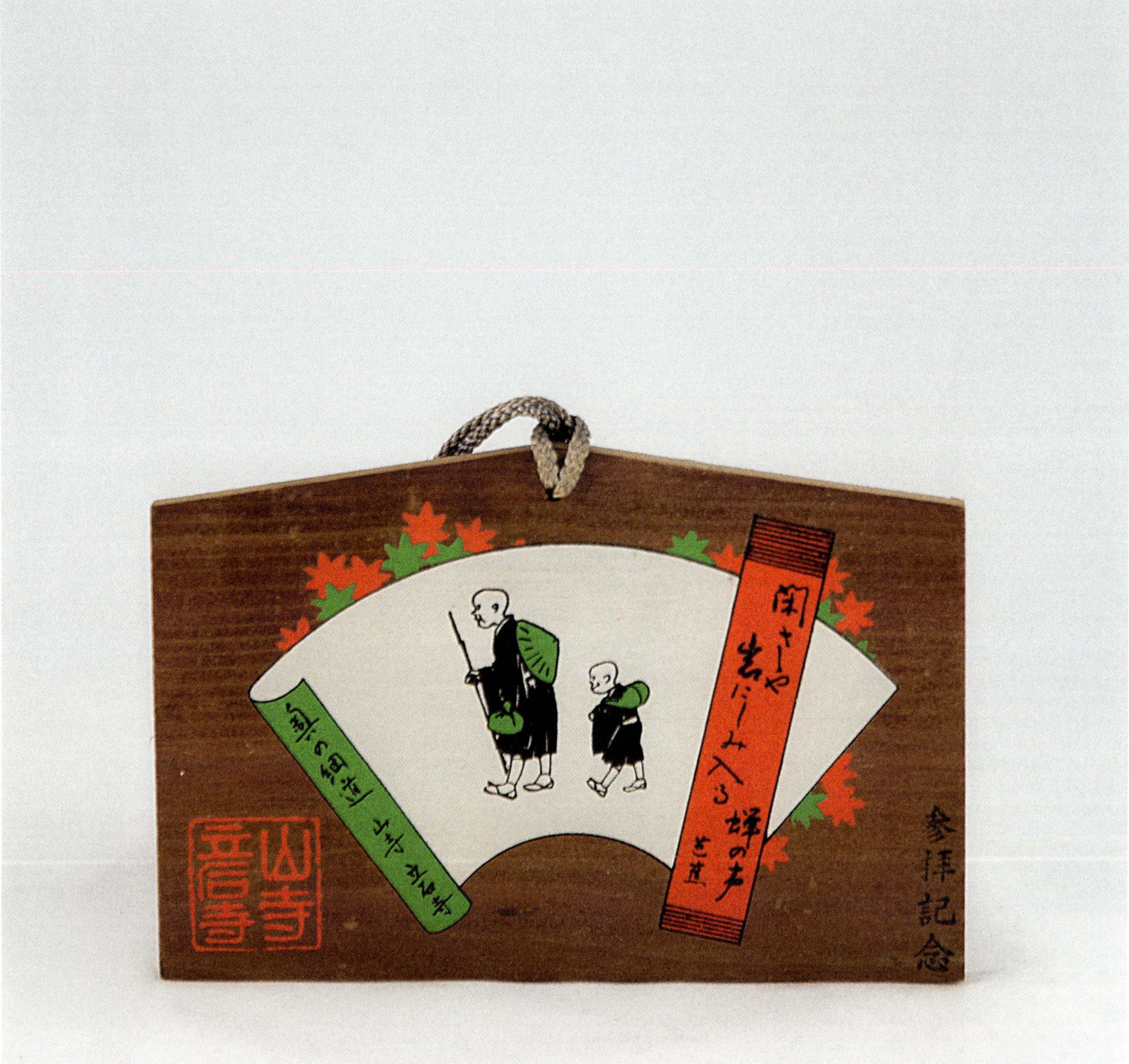
閑さや
岩にしみ入る
蝉の声
芭蕉
山寺
立石寺
参拝記念

039

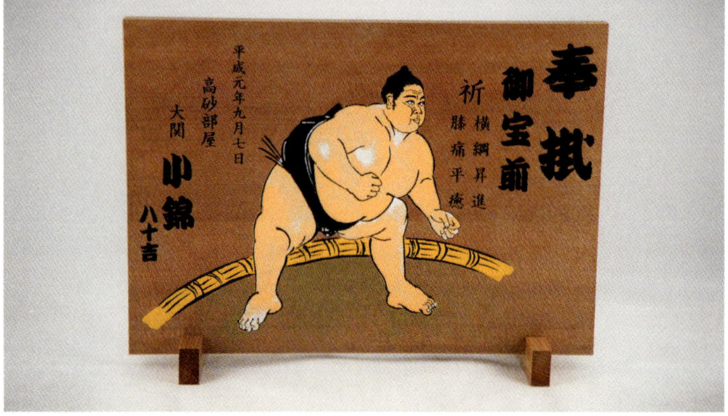
奉納
御宝前
祈
横綱昇進
膝痛平癒
平成元年九月七日
高砂部屋
大関
小錦
八十吉

040

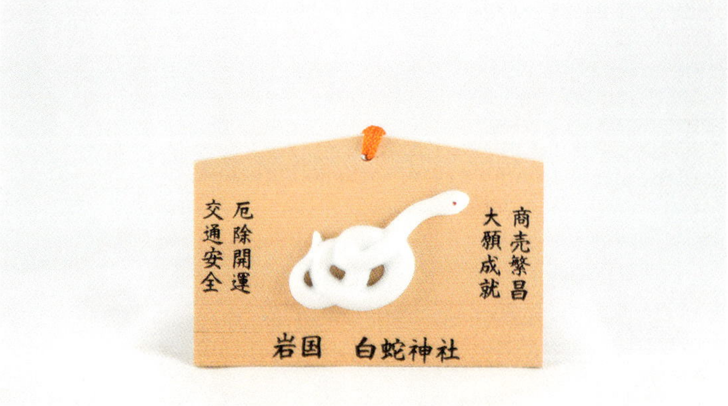
商売繁昌
大願成就
厄除開運
交通安全
岩国　白蛇神社

038
Haiku (Japanese type of poem) *Risshakuji* 立石寺 (also known as *Yamadera* 山寺), Yamagata, Yamagata Prefecture. Late 20th century. W. 13.7 cm

This *ema* portrays two Buddhist travelling monks. The green box on the left identifies the originating temple, whereas the orange box on the right reproduces a famous *haiku* and its 17th century author, the poet *Bashō*. A traditional *haiku* is a very short Japanese poem, which consists of seventeen *on* (sound units), in three groups of five, seven, and five *on* respectively. The haiku on this *ema* reads: *shizukasa ya iwa ni shimiiru semi no koe* (oh in this quietude – seeping into the rock – the voices of cicadas) [GG1-2011/09].

039
Sumo wrestler 相撲 (*sumō*) named *Konishiki Yasokichi*. *Tōjūji* 東充寺 (also known as *Hechima Yakushi* へちま薬師), Higashi Ward, Nagoya. Late 20th century. W. 25.5 cm.

Konishiki Yasokichi was the first non-Japanese sumo wrestler born outside Japan to reach *ōzeki* (the second highest rank in sumo wrestling).

040
Albino Japanese rat snake 白蛇 (*shirohebi*) *Iwakuni Shirohebi Jinja* 岩国白蛇神社
Early 21st century. W. 13.4 cm
The inscriptions read:
商売繁盛 = *shōbai hanjō* (prosperous business)
大願成就 = *daigan jōju* (realization of a great ambition)
岩国白蛇神社 = *Iwakuni Shirohebi Jinja*
厄除開運 = *yakuyoke kaiun* (warding off evil and opening up good luck)
交通安全 = *kōtsū anzen* (traffic safety)
The inscriptions on this single *ema* refer explicitly to a variety of benefits.

041

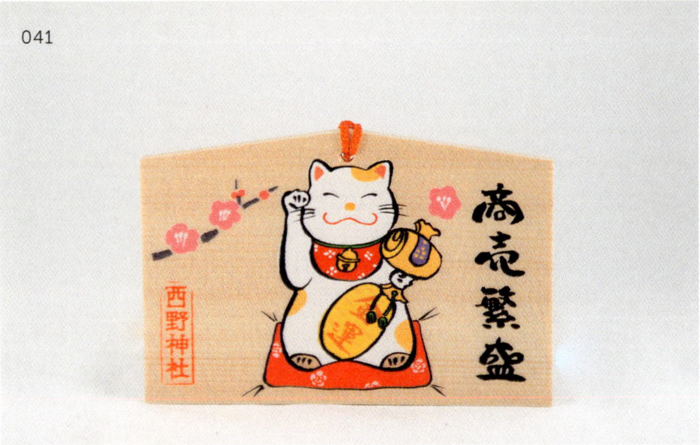

042

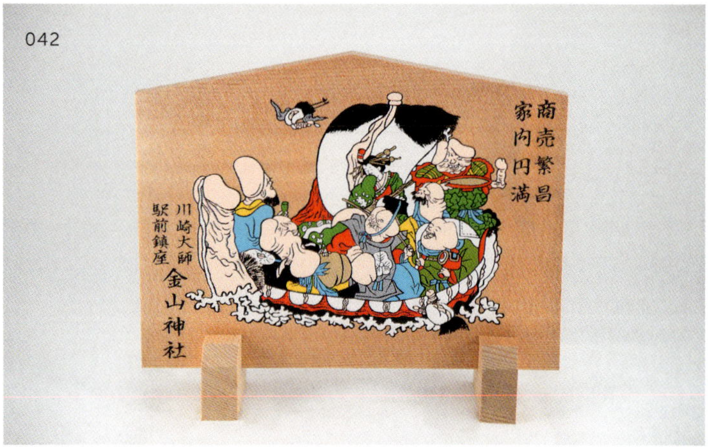

043

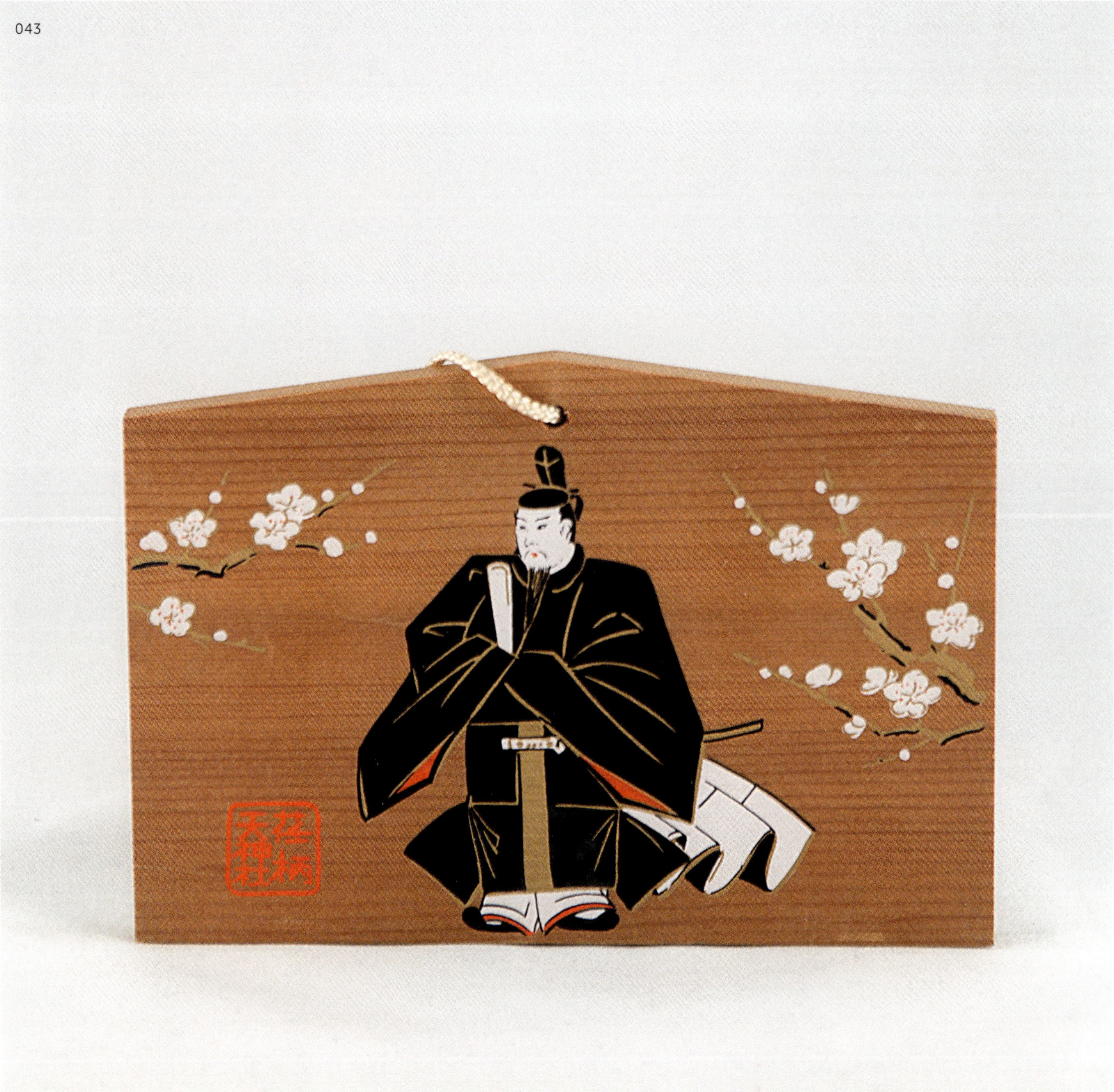

Benefits

By and large, the designs and inscriptions of small *ema* cover the same kinds of *goriyaku* (benefits) as the *mamori* (charms) that are taken home. They are often accommodated in five major categories [IR; RT-45,65,200; GK]:

- *seikatsu no hanei* (prosperity in life)
- *danjo kankei* (male/female relations)
- *sainan yoke* (protection from misfortune)
- *hito no isshō* (human life issues): see part three
- *byōki heiyu* (recovery from illness): see part four.

A few illustrative examples of the first three categories are given below. For more extensive reviews of non-medical types of *ema* the reader is referred to the selected key references on pp.12-13.

Benefits concerning prosperity in life 生活の繁栄 (*seikatsu no hanei*)

- *shōbai hanjō* (business prosperity)
- *jigyō hanei* (flourishing business)
- *kin'un* (monetary fortune)
- *shōbu un* (winning)
- *kaiun* (opening up good luck)
- *shōfuku* (inviting good luck)
- *shogan jōju* (realization of wish)
- *shingan jōju* (realisation of heartfelt wish)
- *gakugyō jōju* (realisation of studies)
- *juken kigan* (prayer for examination)
- *nyūgaku jōju* (realisation of entry into school or university; also expressed as *gōkaku*)
- *gigei jōtatsu* (progress in the arts)

041
Beckoning cat 招き猫 (*maneki neko*). *Nishino Jinja* 西野神社. Sapporo, Hokkaido Prefecture Early 21st century. W. 16.1 cm
The inscriptions read:
商売繁盛 = *shōbai hanjō* (prosperous business)
西野神社 = *Nishino Jinja*

The cat beckons good luck and good business with its upright paw, while holding a lucky mallet and a large *koban* (gold coin used in the Edo period) in its other paw.

042
Kanayama Jinja 金山神社 (in precincts of *Wakamiya Hachimangū* 若宮八幡宮). Kawasaki, Kanagawa Prefecture. Late 20th century or early 21st century. W. 21.0 cm.
The inscriptions read:
商売繁盛 = *shōbai hanjō* (prosperous business)
家内円満 = *kanai enman* (family harmony)
川崎大師駅前鎮座 = *Kawasaki Daishi Ekimae Chinza* (protective shrine in front of Kawasaki Daishi station)
金山神社 = *Kanayama Jinja*

This *ema* portrays the *Shichifukujin* (Seven Gods of Good Fortune) on their treasure ship. They are surrounded by phallic and vaginal symbolism. The same design is painted on the ceiling of the *ema* hall of the shrine. Cf. the entry on phallus on p.75.

043
Sugawara no Michizane 菅原道真. *Egara Tenjinsha* 荏柄天神社. Kamakura, Kanagawa Prefecture. Late 20th century. W. 14.8 cm

Sugawara no Michizane is a famous scholar, poet and politician who lived in the Heian Period. He is now revered as the god of learning *Tenman-Tenjin* (often shortened to *Tenjin*). In this capacity, he can be invoked for success in an entrance examination or academic study.

044

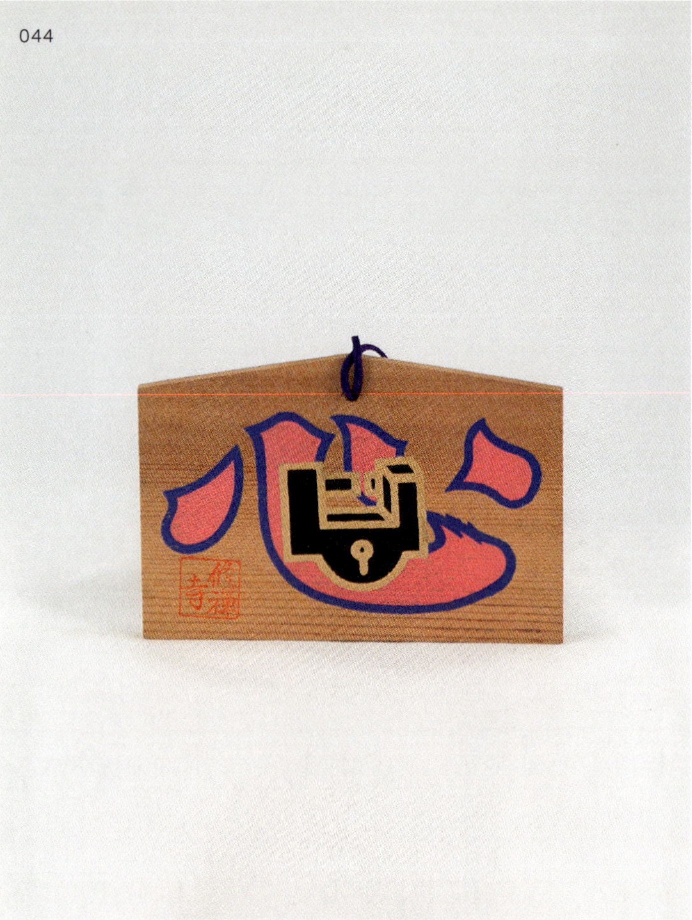

045

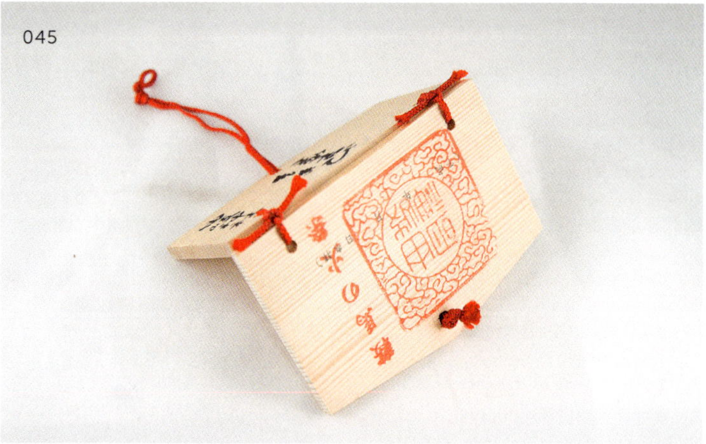

046

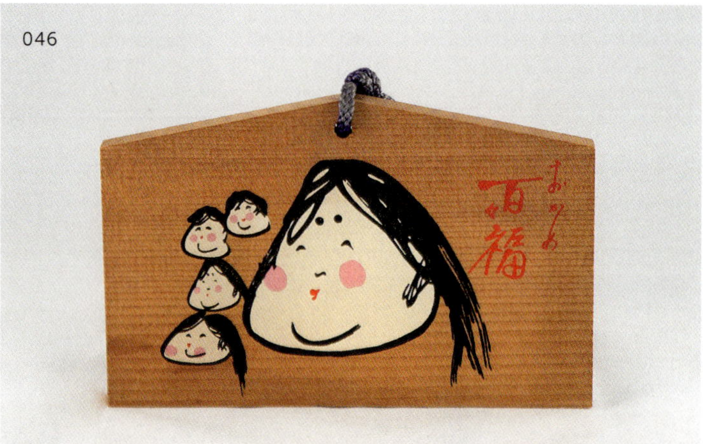

047

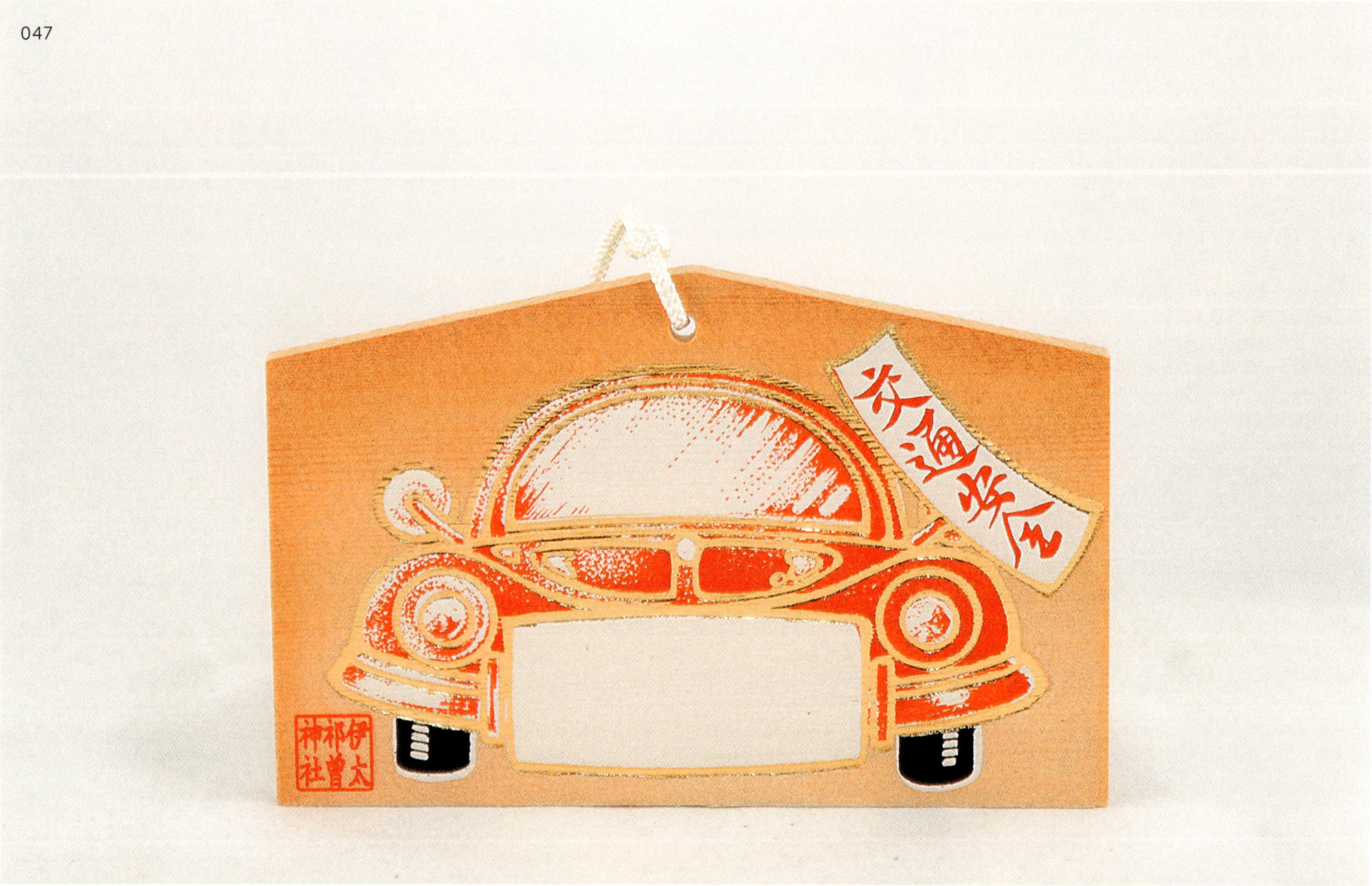

Benefits concerning male/female relations 男女関係 (*danjo kankei*)

- *enmusubi* (joining two people together in love/marriage)
- *ryōen jōju* (realisation of good marriage)
- *enkiri* (separation, divorce)

044
Padlock for the heart 心の鍵 (*kokoro ni kagi*)
Shuzenji 修禅寺. Izu, Shizuoka Prefecture. Late 20th century. W. 13.6 cm

This *ema* design consists of a padlock in front of the kanji 心 = *kokoro* (mind; heart; spirit) to ensure that the heart does not wander in unwanted directions so that marital vows are kept [GG1-2011/09]. For padlock designs see also the section on moderation on p.163.

045
Joined together *ema* 合わせ絵馬 (*awase ema*)
Yuki Jinja 由岐神社. Kurama, Sakyo ward, Kyoto. Late 20th century. W. 12.7 cm
The inscriptions on the front *ema* read:
鞍馬の火祭 = *Kurama no himatsuri* (Kurama Fire Festival)
由岐神社 = *Yuki Jinja*
The inscriptions on the rear *ema* read:
縁結び = *enmusubi* (joining two people together in love/marriage)
由岐神社 = *Yuki Jinja*

This double *ema* is used at *Yuki Jinja* to signify the joining together of two people. Elsewhere this type of *ema* is used to keep secret what is written on the *ema* (cf. the section on contemporary practices on p.21).

Benefits concerning protection from misfortune 災難除け (*sainan yoke*)

- *yakuyoke* (protection from danger)
- *tōnan yoke* (protection from theft)
- *kōtsū anzen* (traffic safety)
- *kanai anzen* (family safety)
- *shinjō anzen* (physical safety)
- *josei shugo* (safeguard for woman/women)
- *kōji anzen* (safety in construction work)
- *hōkō* [protection from unlucky] (direction)
- *kanan yoke* (protection against fires)
- *kaminari yoke* (protection against lightning)
- *akumu tsuihō* (banishment of nightmares)

046
Mask of *Okame* おかめの面 (*Okame no men*)
Senbon Shakadō (also known as *Daihōonji* 大報恩寺). Kamigyo Ward, Kyoto. Late 20th century. W. 17.4 cm
The inscriptions on the front read:
おかめ = *Okame*
万福 = *banpuku* (lit. ten thousand fortunes, i.e. good fortune)
The inscriptions on the reverse read:
家内安全 = *kanai anzen* (family safety)
京 = *Kyō* (short for Kyoto)
おかめ寺 = *Okamedera* (Okame temple)
千本釈迦堂 = *Senbon Shakadō*
開運厄除 = *kaiun yakuyoke* (opening up good luck, preventing misfortune)

There is a sanctuary for *Okame* in the precincts of the temple. According to legend, *Okame* was the wife of the head carpenter building the temple's *hondō* (main hall). After he had made the mistake of making one of the pillars too short, *Okame* solved his problem. She then committed suicide out of fear that her husband would lose face if anyone found out about her help. Her husband carved a mask of her face and attached it to the pillar so that her spirit could see the finished building. Nowadays *Okame* is a symbol that misfortune can become good fortune and *Okame* masks are considered good luck charms.

047
Car 車 (*kuruma*). *Itakiso Jinja* 伊太祁曽神社
Itakiso, Wakayama Prefecture. Early 21st century. W. 15.1 cm
The inscription reads:
交通安全 = *kōtsū anzen* (traffic safety)

This *ema* design offers space to fill in one's personal number plate. A similar design is sold by *Urahoro Jinja* (Urahoro, Tokachi District, Hokkaido Prefecture).

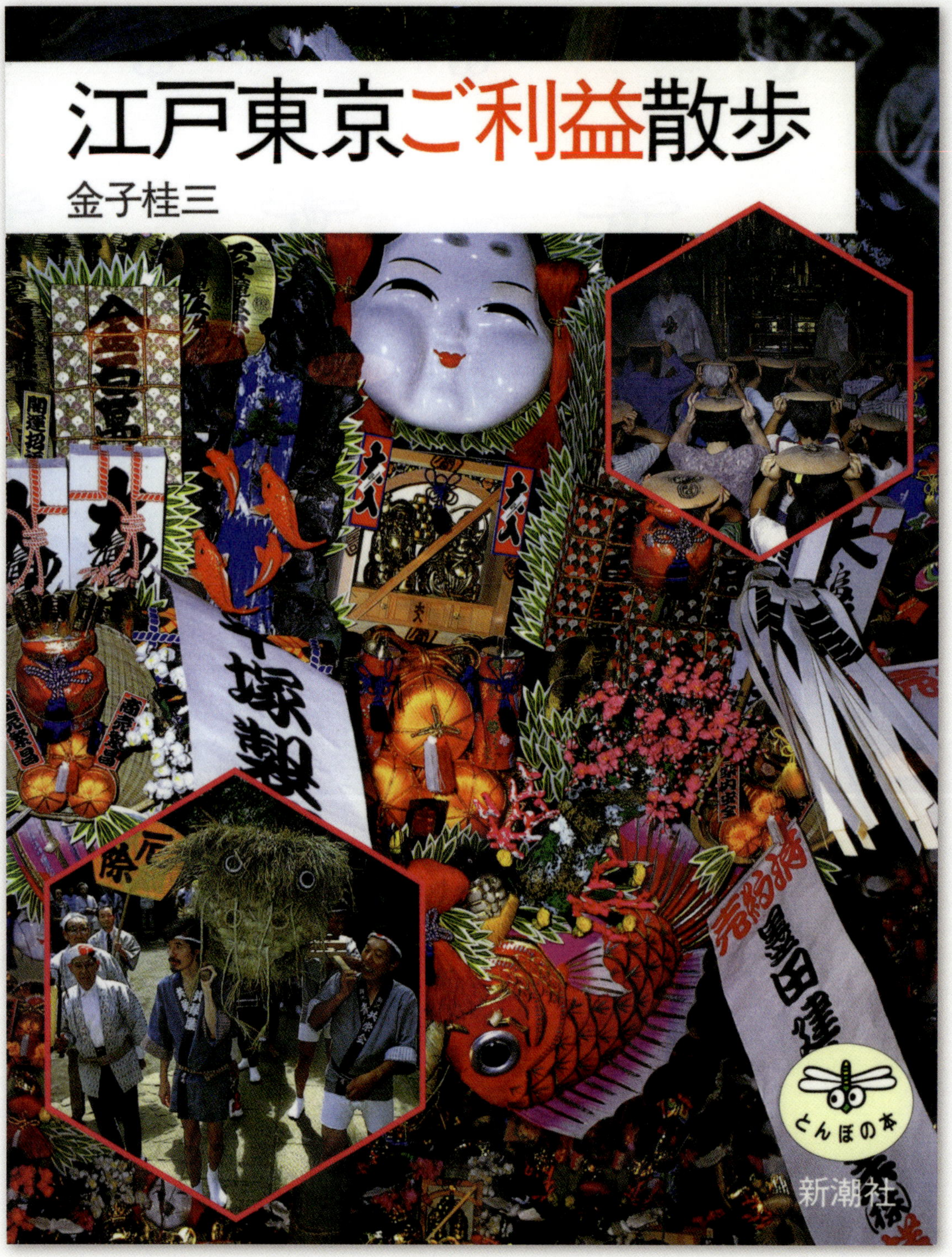
江戸東京ご利益散歩
金子桂三
とんぼの本
新潮社

Table 2
Medical benefits in the categories of *byōki heiyu* (recovery from illness) and *samazama* (various) on www.goriyaku.kotomeguri.com

City (sanctuaries)	Tokyo (53)	Kyoto (41)	Osaka (35)	Nara (18)	Fukuoka (16)	Kobe (17)	Shiga Pref (11)	Total (191)
Purposes								
General	20	11	19	8	9	8	6	81
Epidemics	2	3			1			6
Neoplasms		2	1	2		1		6
Teeth/mouth	5	3	2			2		12
Digestive	1		1					2
Eye	6	4	4	2	2		2	20
Ear	1		1	1				3
Cardiovascular	1	1	1			1		4
Musculoskeletal	3	6	4	2	3	2	1	21
Neurological	2	4	3	1		2	1	13
Mental/behavioural	2	4	3	3		2	1	15
Respiratory	8	4	1		2			15
Skin	4	1	1			1		7
Nutritional/metabolic	1	1	1				1	4
Female	2	2	1			1	1	7
Injuries	1	1						2
Benefits (total)	**59**	**47**	**43**	**19**	**17**	**20**	**13**	**218**

Selection

In the past, there were many guidebooks available in bookshops throughout Japan to describe which *goriyaku* (divine favours) could be found where. These guides generally did not centre on the new religions but only on Shinto shrines and Buddhist temples, that is to say, on the religious institutions of the established religions of Japan [RT-9,239].

Today, these traditional sources are supplemented with or have been replaced by online overviews. The website http://www.goriyaku.kotomeguri.com/ gives a prominent position to 病気平癒 = *byōki heiyu* (recovery from illness). Its start screen focuses on Kyoto but offers links to other major cities further down the webpage (see Table 2). A similar website is http://www.kaiun-goriyaku.com/spots.

048
Printed guide describing the benefits offered by sanctuaries in Tokyo. 江戸東京ご利益散歩 = *Edo Tōkyō goriyaku sanpo Tōkyō* (lit. Tokyo benefits walk). Tokyo: Shinchosha 1999

Reading guide

An English overview of health-related small *ema* has not yet appeared. This void is filled by presenting a large number of contemporary health-related *ema* in this exhibition catalogue. Its core consists of two parts that focus on *hito no isshō* (human life issues) and *byōki no kaifuku* (recovery from illness), respectively. While the former category is surveyed on the basis of illustrative examples, the latter category is reviewed more extensively based on the consulted literature supplemented with searches in Google Images for 絵馬 (*ema*) in combination with numerous Japanese terms for diseases and illnesses [10].

The two central parts (three and four) are preceded by the presentation of *ema* with a health-related subject that are used or may be used for purposes unrelated to health (part two). They are followed by a special part five about *ema* for animal health, after which the book concludes with a final discussion. Since there are already excellent reviews on *ema* in general, the discussion primarily presents a biomedical view on the health-related purposes of *ema*. Since this offers a new perspective on *ema* (even if Japanese sources are taken into consideration), the discussion has been integrally translated into Japanese.

The presentation of the health-related *ema* is structured according to a fixed pattern. The *ema* are first arranged according to their main purpose(s). This arrangement largely follows the so-called *International Classification of Primary Care* (ICPC) [11]. This system allows for the classification of symptoms and complaints from a lay point of view (the so-called "reason for encounter"), whereas the more widely used *International Classification of Diseases* (ICD) is generally based on biomedical diagnoses. Each group of symptoms and complaints starts with a concise biomedical summary. This is often followed by examples where *goriyaku* (divine benefits) for these symptoms and complaints can be found. Hereafter, the *ema* are listed by design. Each *ema* is provided with:

- the name and location of the originating shrine or temple;
- crude estimate of age: early 20th century = 1900-1929; mid-20th century = 1930-1969; late 20th century = 1970-1999; early 21st century: 2000-present
- a specification of its width (excluding the protruding roofs)
- a translation of its inscriptions (with the exception of the red chops because these usually identify the originating sanctuary); the inscriptions are listed from right to left (since this is the Japanese direction of reading texts)
- any further clarification or comment (as needed).

Romanised Japanese words are presented in italics; in accordance with the modified Hepburn system, their long vowels have been transcribed as macrons (e.g., *ō*, *ū*). An exception has been made for geographical names that have been widely adopted into English (e.g., names of major cities and prefectures, such as Hyogo instead of *Hyōgo*).

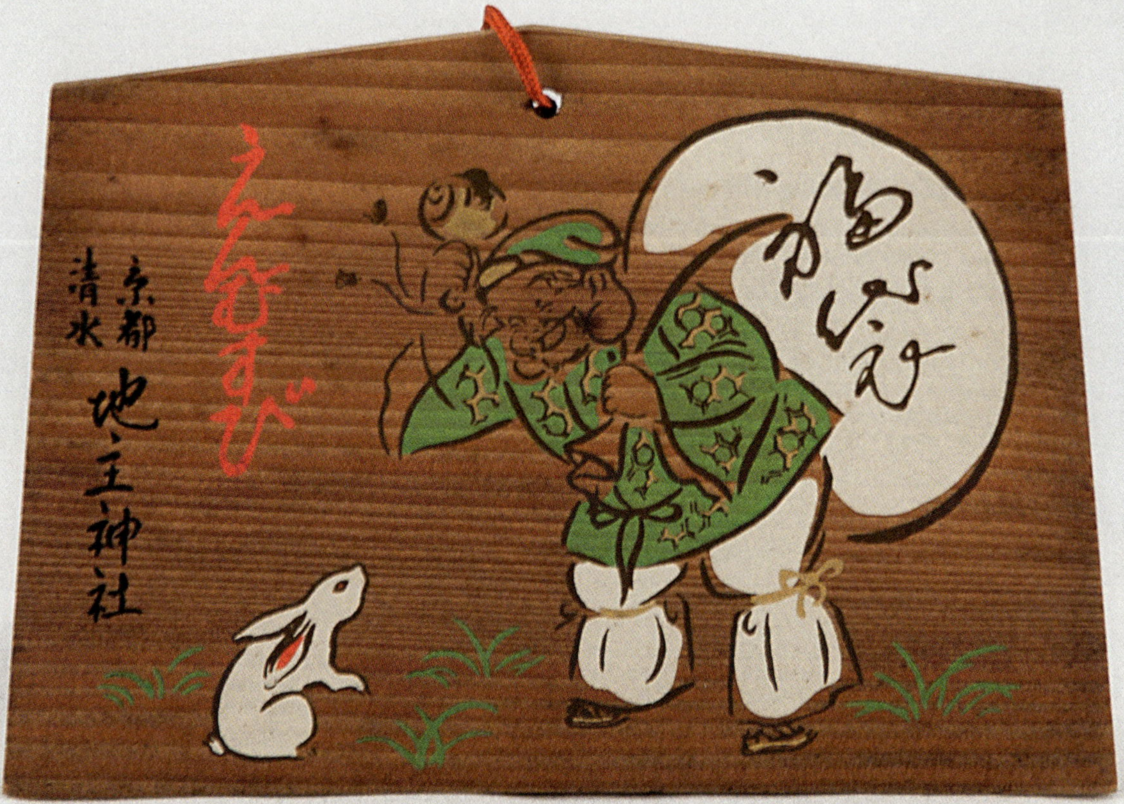
京都
清水
地主神社
えんむすび

2

Health-related images 健康関連画像 (*Kenkō kanren gazō*)

049
Ōkuninushi 大国主 (god of medicine, agriculture and marriage). *Jishu Jinja* 地主神社. Higashiyama Ward, Kyoto. Late 20th century. W. 15.2 cm
The inscriptions read:
えんむすび = *enmusubi* (joining two people together in love/marriage)
京都清水 = *Kyōto Kiyomizu*
地主神社 = *Jishu Jinja*

Jishu Jinja is visited in particular for prayers concerning marriage and love fulfilment. Today the shrine sells an *ema* with a restyled version of the *ema* design shown here (which is estimated to be 30-40 years old). See the entry on *Ōkuninushi* on p.41 for the legendary story portrayed on this *ema* and for other *ema* with *Ōkuninushi*.

Various *ema* bear the image of a deity, festival or ceremony, charm or symbol that is related to health and healing. When such *ema* are intended for a specific human life issue or medical problem, they are reviewed in parts three and four. This part focuses on health-related representations on *ema* that are not meant for a health-related purpose, but have a generic or non-medical aim. For instance, the portrayal of *Ōkuninushi* is a health-related representation, because he is a Shinto deity of medicine and agriculture. However, it does not follow that all *ema* with his image have a health-related purpose, because he is also a deity of marriage and can be invoked for love fulfilment and a good marriage.

050

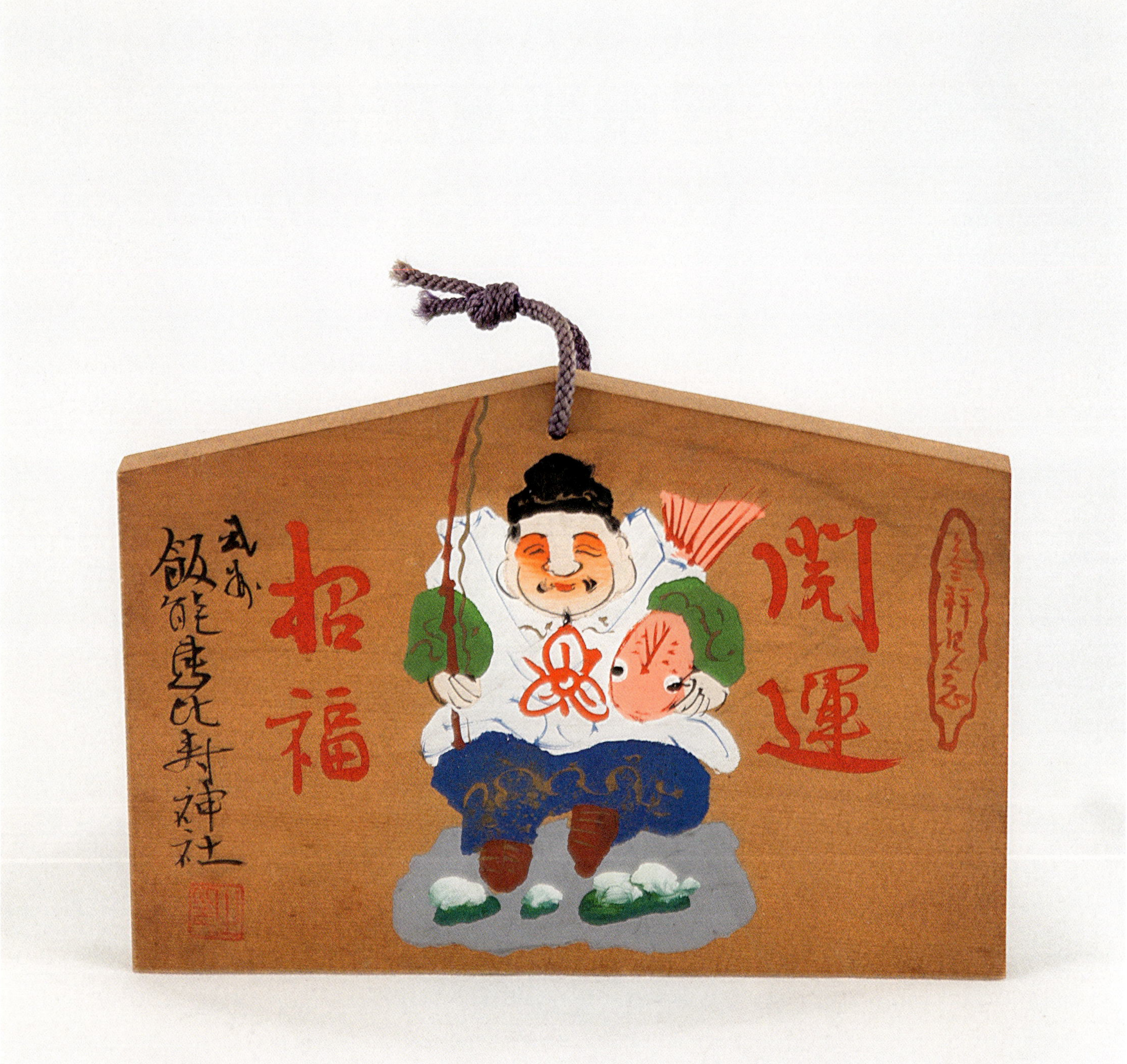

051

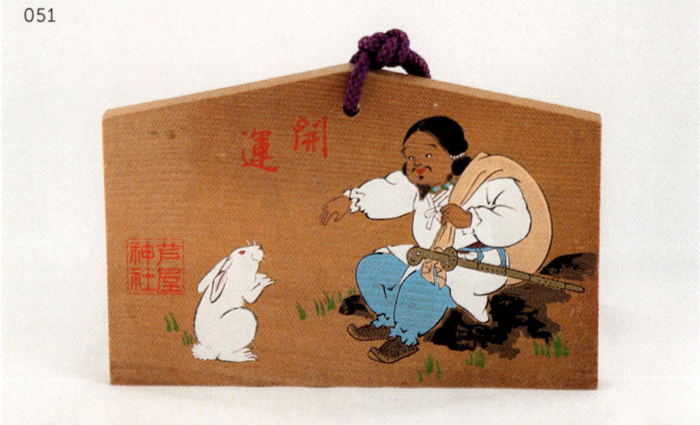

052

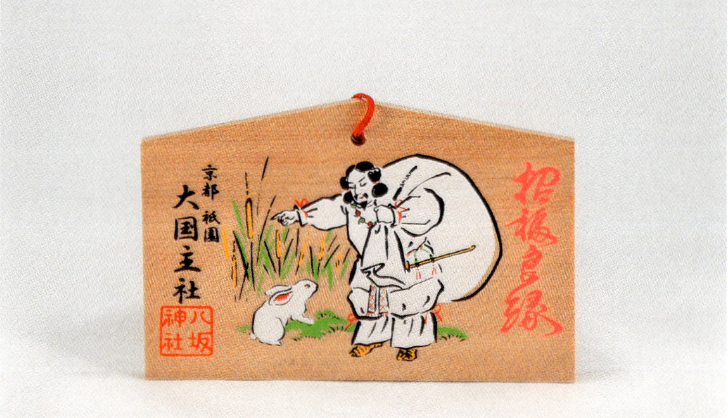

Figures of worship
礼拝の姿
(*Reihai no sugata*)

Shinto figures of worship
神道礼拝の姿
(*Shintō reihai no sugata*)

Background

Shinto deities are designated as *kami, jin, shin, tenjin* (heavenly god), *myōjin* (great god), *sama* (honorific suffix) or *gongen* (avatar, incarnation). These terms not only refer to gods and goddesses, but some of them may also be applied to ancestors and to spirits inhabiting nature (water, rocks, trees, grass, and so on). *Kami* are not necessarily benevolent and many of them have to be appeased to avoid or contain calamities, such as epidemics. Important examples of health-related Shinto deities are listed in Table 3 [EO-150; MS].

Table 3
Shinto deities for illness in general or for a specific type of illness

Reproduced with permission of Cambridge University Press from Ohnuki-Tierney E. Illness and culture in contemporary Japan: an anthropological view 1984 pp.150-151

Deity	Specialisation(s)
Ashide Kōjin (*Kōjin* of the Limbs)	Illnesses of the hip/limbs
Ashiō-sama (Deity of the Lower Limbs)	Illnesses of the hip/limbs
Awashima-sama	Illnesses of women
Hōsoshin (Deity of Smallpox)	Contagious illnesses
Iboishi-sama (Wart-stone Deity)	Illnesses of the face
Idonokami (Deity of the Well)	Illnesses of the eyes
Kawaya-no-Kami (Deity of the Toilet)	Illnesses of the teeth
Kōjin-sama (Deity of the Kitchen)	Illnesses in general
Koshi-no-Kami (Deity of the Hip)	Illnesses of the hip/limbs
Mekuragami (Deity of the Blind)	Illnesses of the eyes
Miminokami (Deity of the Ears)	Illnesses of the ears
Odoku-sama (Deity of Dirt and Poison)	Illnesses of children
Saenokami (Deity of the Boundary)	Illnesses of the ears Illnesses of the hip/limbs
Shiwabuki-sama (Deity of Coughing)	Illnesses of the chest
Tori Daimyōjin (Rooster Daimyōjin)	Illnesses of the throat
Tsuri Tenjin	Illnesses of the stomach

Ema designs

Awashima 粟島

Awashima is invoked for female ailments, for the conception of children and for safe childbirth [KU]. See the entry on dolls (*hina*) on p.193 in part four.

Ebisu 恵比寿

Ebisu is the only god of the *Shichifukujin* (Seven Gods of Good Fortune) who did not come from India or China but originates from Japan itself. He is a god of fishermen and a guardian of the health of small children. In his images he is often holding a rod and a large red sea bream or sea bass. Cf. the entries on *Hiruko* and on *Shichifukujin* (Seven Gods of Good Fortune) below.

050
Originates from an *Ebisu Jinja* 恵比寿神社 (possibly in Hanno, Saitama Prefecture).
Late 20th century. W. 14.4 cm
The large red inscriptions read:
開運= *kaiun* (opening up good luck)
招福 = *shōfuku* (good luck charm)

Hiruko 蛭子

Hiruko is a mythological child who was set adrift in an *ashibune* (reed boat) because he was deformed. This theme is seen on *ema* that are meant to apologise to an aborted foetus (see p.83 in part three). In later times, *Hiruko* was identified with *Ebisu*, one of the *Shichifukujin* (Seven Gods of Good Fortune) [KU].

Ōkuninushi 大国主

Ōkuninushi is a Shinto god of healing, happiness and marriage, who later became *Daikokuten*, one of the *Shichifukujin* (Seven Gods of Good Fortune).

According to mythology, he once travelled with his brothers to compete for the hand of a princess. When his brothers met a skinned hare on a beach, they told it to bathe in the sea which caused a great deal of agony. When *Ōkuninushi* (who was lagging behind) saw this, he advised the hare to bathe in fresh water instead and to cover itself with medicinal *gama* (cattail) flower. After the hare (in reality a deity) had recovered its fluffy coat, it promised *Ōkuninushi* that he would marry the princess [MA-80,228; MS].

051
Ashiya Jinja 芦屋神社, Ashiya, Hyogo Prefecture
Late 20th century. W. 17.5 cm
The inscriptions read:
開運 = *kaiun* (opening up good fortune)
芦屋神社 = *Ashiya Jinja*

052
Ōkuninushisha 大国主社 in precincts of *Yasaka Jinja* 八坂神社 Higashiyama Ward, Kyoto.
Early 21st century. W. 13.8 cm
The inscriptions read:
招福 = *shōfuku* (charm beckoning good fortune)
良縁 = *ryōen* (good match)
京都 祇園 = *Kyōto Gion* (district)
大国主神 = *Ōkuninushisha*

053

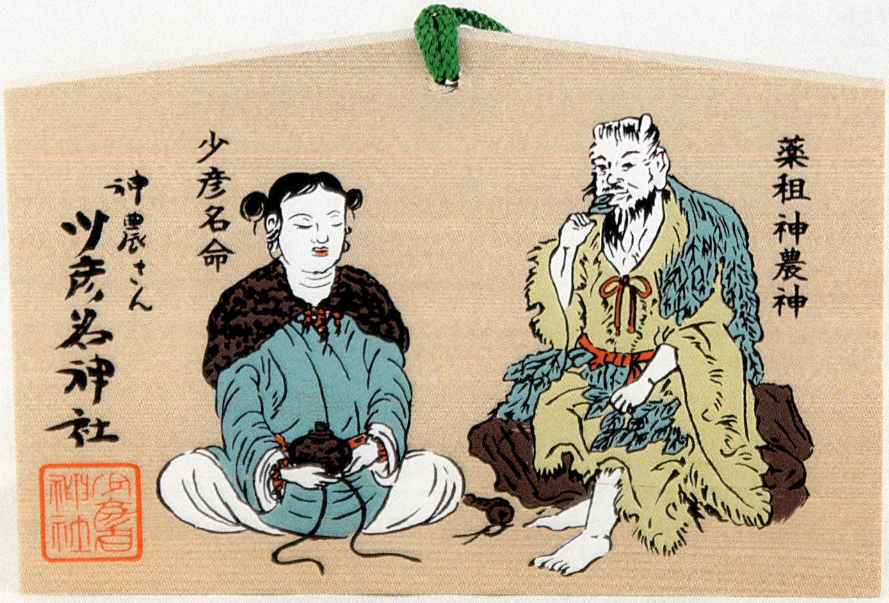

054

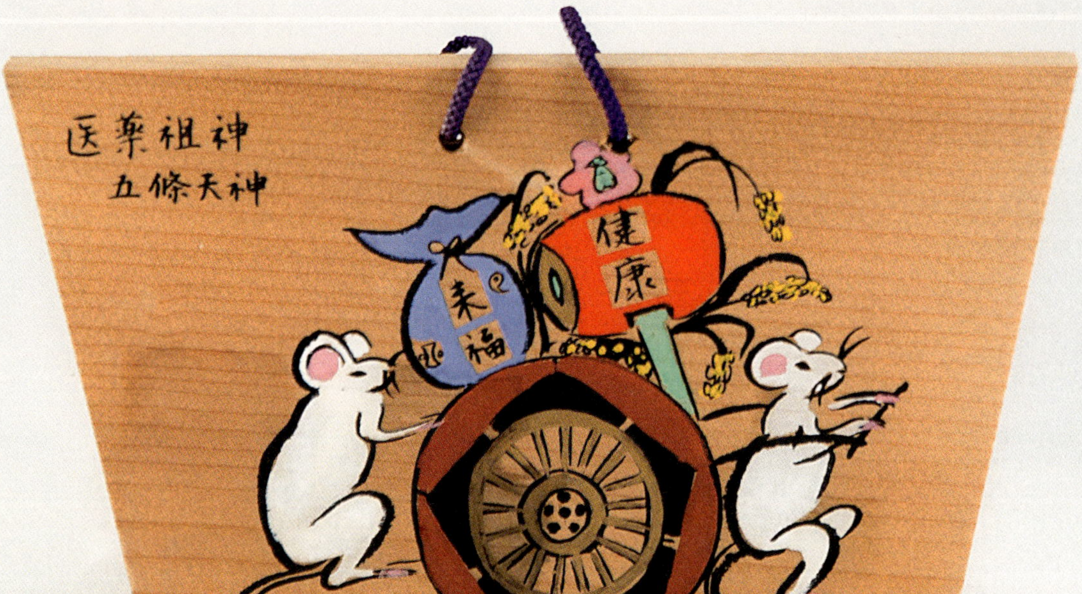

Sukunahikona 少彦名

Sukunahikona (also known as *Sukunabikona, Sukunahikona no kami or Sukunahikona no mikoto*) is a Japanese dwarf deity of healing and sake brewing. He is particularly associated with hot springs and assisted *Ōkuninushi* in creating and solidifying the land.

053
Sukunahikona Jinja 少彦名神社 Chuo Ward, Osaka. Early 21st century. W. 16.0 cm
The inscriptions read:
薬祖神農神 = *yakusojin nōjin* (god of agriculture and ancestral god of medicine)
少彦名命 = *Sukunahikona no mikoto*
神農さん = *Jinnōsan* (deity of agriculture; local honorary name)
少彦名神社 = *Sukunahikona Jinja*

Sukunahikona Jinja is situated in *Doshōmachi*, the old medicine quarter of Osaka. There is a museum of pharmaceutical history in its grounds. The sanctuary enshrines two health-related deities who are depicted together on this *ema*: *Sukunahikona* on the left and *Shinnō* (the Japanese name of *Shennong*, the Chinese god of medicine) on the right. Cf. the entry on *Shinnō* below and the entry on *toraharikо* on p.63.

054
Gojōten Jinja 五條天神社 Taito Ward, Tokyo. Late 20th century. W. 19.3 cm
The inscriptions read:
医薬祖神 = *iyaku soshin* (ancestral deity of medicine)
五條天神 = *Gojōtenjin*

Gojōten Jinja is an *aiden* (shrine building dedicated to two or more deities). It enshrines the god of learning (*Sugawara Michizane*) and two gods of medicine (*Ōkuninushi* and *Sukunahikona*). On the 10th of every month, the shrine organises an *iyaku* (medicine) ceremony where one can pray for *byōki heiyu* (recovery from illness) or *mubyō kenkō* (health free from illness). The Japan Pharmaceutical Association asks the shrine to bless its annual gathering in October.

Tamahime megami 玉姫命女神

Tamahime megami is the daughter of *Ōagata*. She is worshipped at *Ōagata Jinja* as a guardian goddess of women. She can be invoked for female disorders, fertility, and easy delivery. See the entry on *Tamahime megami* on p.195 in part four.

055

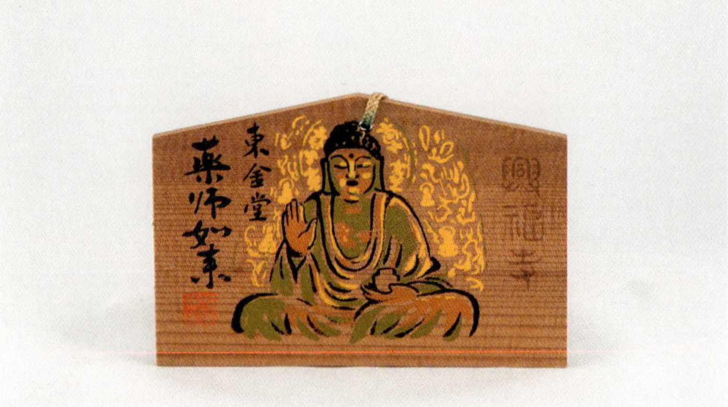

056

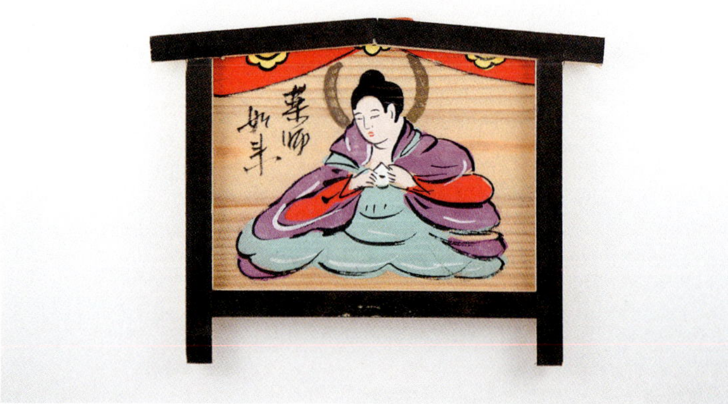

057

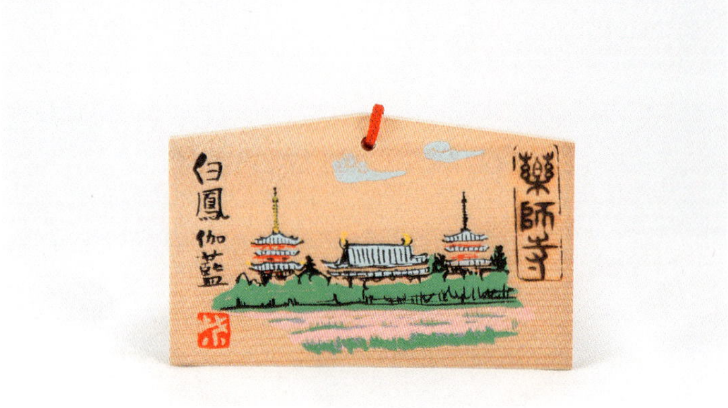

058

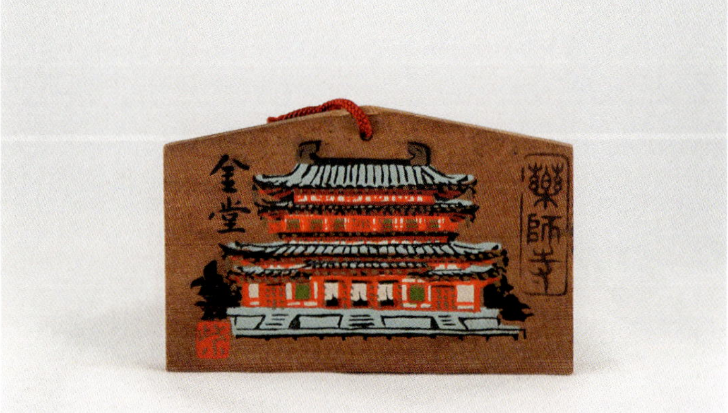

059

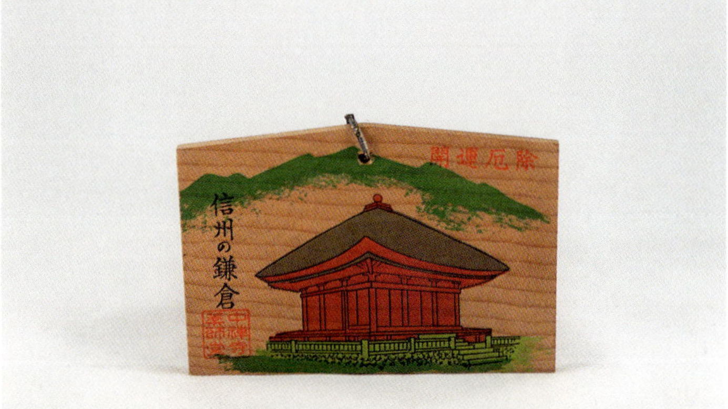

060

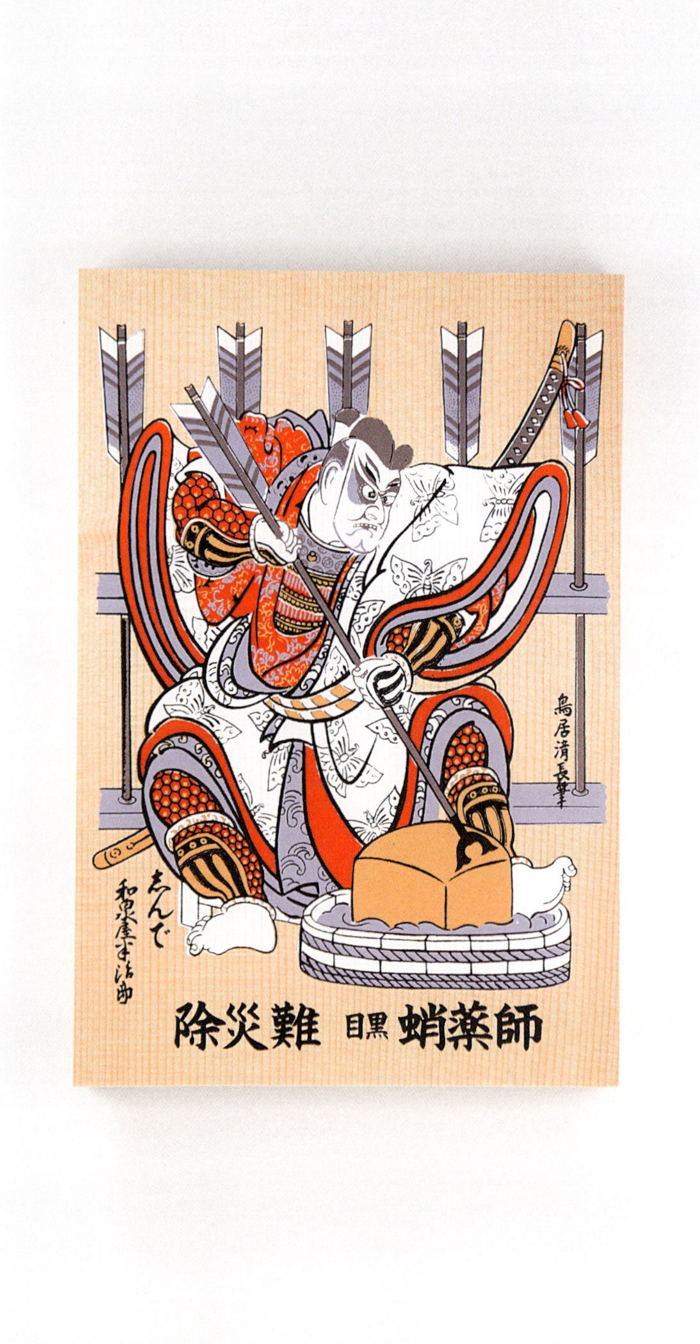

Buddhist figures of worship [1] 仏教徒礼拝の姿 (*Bukkyōto reihai no sugata*)

Background

Most Buddhist figures of worship originated in India (where Buddhism emerged around 500 BC) and are commonly identified by their Sanskrit names. They can be divided into five subcategories that are reproduced here with their Japanese names in italics and their Sanskrit names in brackets [MS]:

- ***Nyorai* (Buddha in Sanskrit) have succeeded in attaining enlightenment. *Mahāyāna* Buddhism (the main form of Buddhism in Japan, China and Korea) recognises many *Nyorai*. Prominent examples are *Amida Nyorai* (Buddha of Infinite Light and Life) and *Yakushi Nyorai* (Medicine Buddha).**
- ***Bosatsu* (Bodhisattva in Sanskrit) have almost reached enlightenment and will certainly become Buddha, but they have temporarily renounced this final transition to remain on earth in various guises to help living beings to achieve salvation. *Jizō Bosatsu* and *Kannon Bosatsu* belong to this group. Both deities have numerous manifestations, many of which are specialised in healing (see Table 4 on p.47 and Table 5 on p.49).**
- ***Myō-ō* (Vidyaraja in Sanskrit) are a group of warlike figures headed by the ferocious *Fudō Myō-ō*.**
- ***Tenbu* (Deva in Sanskrit) are divine protectors of Buddhist Law. Three of the *Shichifukujin* or Seven Gods of Good Fortune (*Benzaiten, Bishamonten* and *Daikokuten*) were originally Deva in the Hindu pantheon of India.**
- **Other Buddhist sacred entities such as venerated sect founders or monks and combinatory Shinto/Buddhist deities.**

Ema designs

Yakushi Nyorai 薬師如来 *(Medicine Buddha, Buddha of Healing)*

According to Buddhist doctrine, one dwells in suffering, so long as *nirvana* (perfect enlightenment) has not been achieved. The ideal is that one will not suffer again through further rebirth. Illness is caused by ignorance or delusion. The task of *Yakushi Nyorai* (Bhaisajyaguru in Sanskrit) is not to tell people exactly what to do when they are ill, but to inspire them to search for and to apply the right therapeutic approach. This requires treatment of the whole person, especially his or her mental state, and not just a particular physical ailment. When Buddhism spread eastward, it assimilated many indigenous beliefs and practices that were considered helpful in attaining enlightenment. When it arrived in Japan in the 6th century A.D., it was also influenced by local practices and beliefs that later coalesced into what became the Shinto tradition. As the pragmatic Japanese were interested in healing practices, the Medicine Buddha quickly became revered for his power to heal earthly suffering and illness [2].

Although *Yakushi Nyorai* can be addressed for illnesses in general, some temples enshrining this Buddha recommend him especially for a particular type of illness (see the sections on eye illnesses and skin illnesses in part four).

055
Kōfukuji 興福寺 Nara, Nara Prefecture.
Late 20th century. W. 13.6 cm
The inscriptions read:
興福寺 = *Kōfukuji*
東金堂 = *Tōkondō* (one of the main halls)
薬師如来 = *Yakushi Nyorai*

056
Hand-painted reproduction for a Japanese club of *ema* collectors called *Nihon Ema Tomo no Kai* (Friends of Japanese Ema Society). No.295. Late 20th century. W. 17.9 cm. The original *ema* design came from *Ryūkakuji* (Sakae, Chiba Prefecture).

Temples housing Yakushi Nyorai

Several temples in Nara (*Hōryūji, Yakushiji, Gankoji, Kōfukuji*, and *Tōshōdaiji*) accommodate statues of *Yakushi Nyorai* from the 7th or 8th century. Most of them are holding a small medicine jar (*yakko*) in the left hand while making a 'fear not' gesture with the right hand. However, the statue in the *kondō* (main hall) of *Yakushiji* does not show a medicine jar and is seated on a medicine box instead. It is flanked by two assistant figures: *Nikkō Bosatsu* (Sunlight *Bosatsu*) on the right and *Gekkō Bosatsu* (Moonlight *Bosatsu*) on the left [MS; 3].

057
Yakushiji 薬師寺 Nara, Nara Prefecture.
Early 21st century. W. 13.6 cm
The inscriptions read:
薬師寺 = *Yakushiji*
白鳳伽藍 = *Hakuhō Garan* (Phoenix hall)

058
Kondō (main hall) of *Yakushiji* 薬師寺. Nara, Nara Prefecture. Late 20th century. W. 13.6 cm
The inscriptions read:
薬師寺 = *Yakushiji*
金堂 = *Kondō* (Main Hall)

The main hall of the temple houses the statues of *Yakushi Nyorai* and two attendant Bodhisattvas.

059
Chūzenji Yakushidō 中禅寺薬師堂
Ueda, Nagano Prefecture. Late 20th century. W. 12.7 cm
The inscriptions read:
開運厄除 = *kaiun yakuyoke* (opening up good luck/ warding off evil)
信州の鎌倉 = *Shinshū no Kamakura*

Takoyakushi 蛸薬師

In several temples in Japan, the *tako* (octopus) is a symbol of *Yakushi Nyorai* (Medicine Buddha), and *Takoyakushi* is worshipped for good health and recovery from illness.

060
Takoyakushi Jōjūin 蛸薬師 成就院, Meguro Ward, Tokyo. Early 21st century. W. 17.2 cm
The inscriptions read:
蛸薬師 = *Takoyakushi*
目黒 = *Meguro*
除災難 = *sainanyoke* (to abolish calamity)

Takoyakushi Jōjūin enshrines a statue of three legendary *tako* (octopuses) carrying *Yaskushi Nyorai* (Medicine Buddha) (cf. the entry on octopus on p.183 in part four). This unusually large *ema* is meant for *sainanyoke* (to abolish calamity) and *geinō jōtatsu* (progress in accomplishments) [IH1-240; RT-249].

061

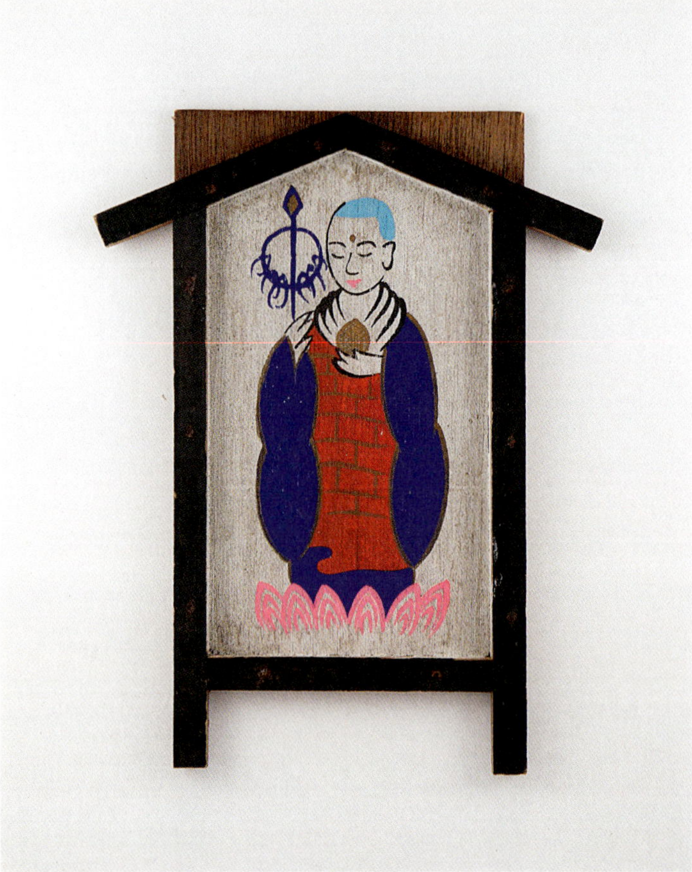

062

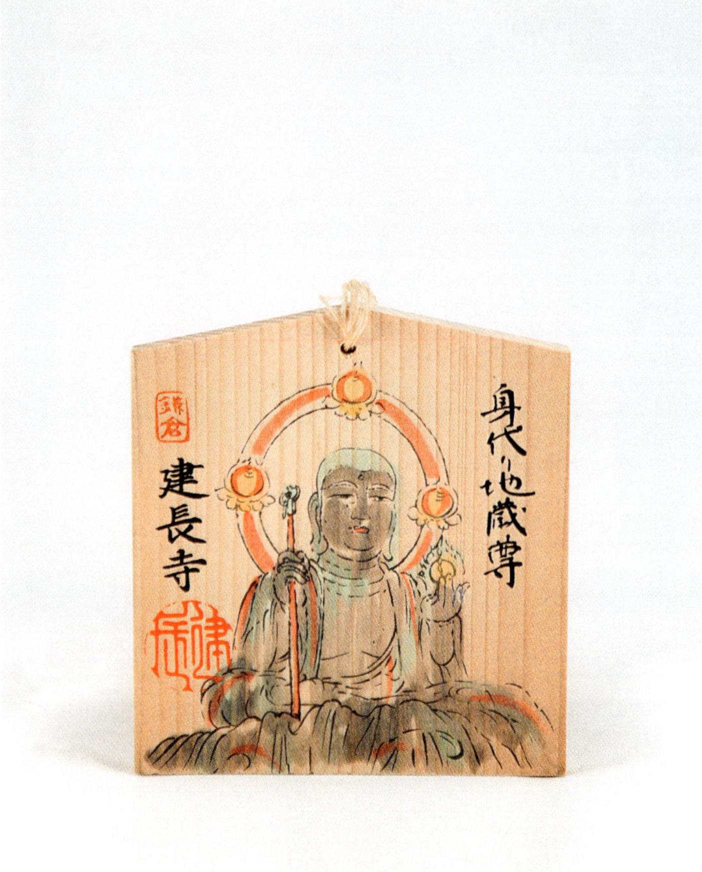

063

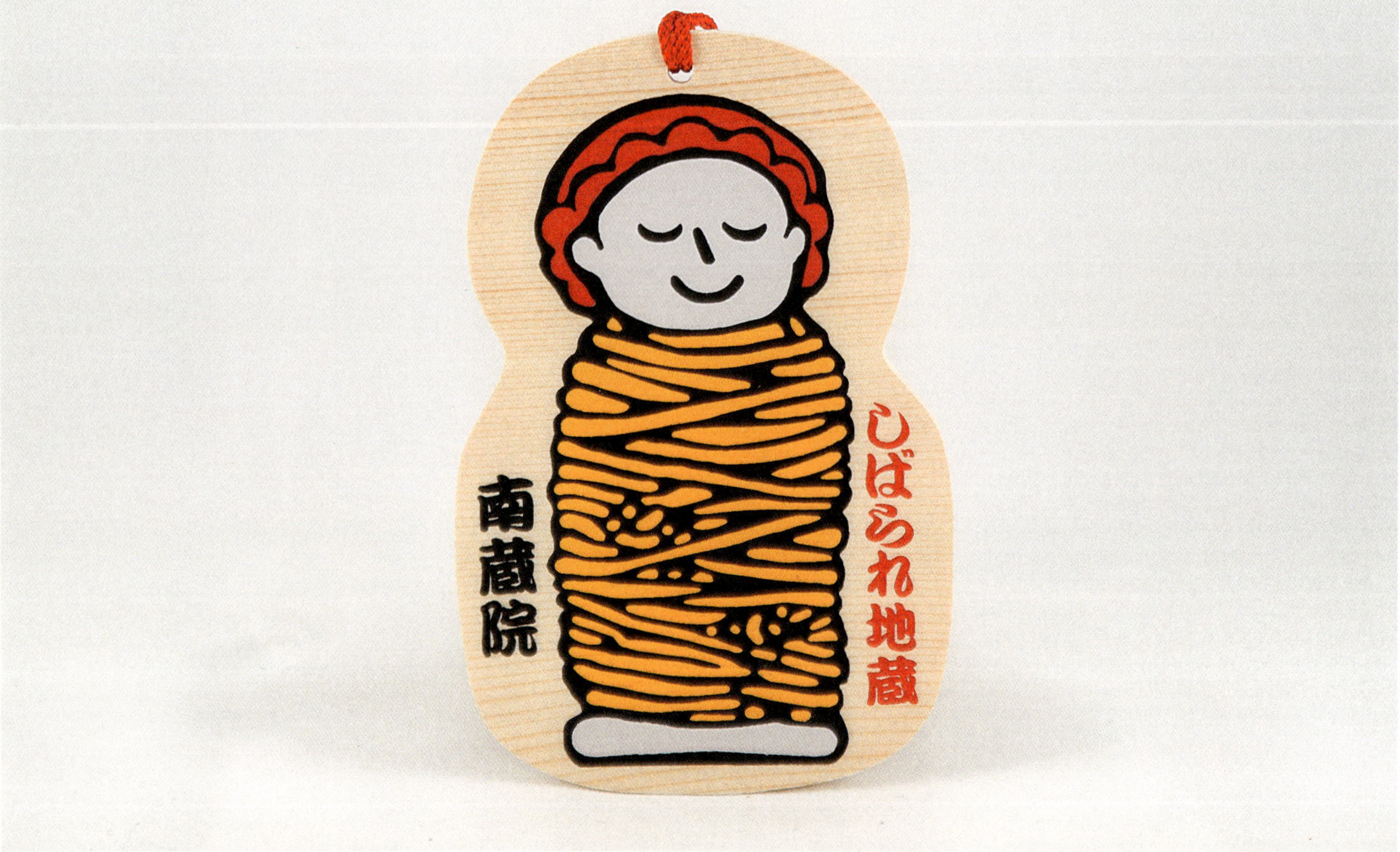

Jizō 地蔵

Jizō is a patron of children, expectant mothers, firemen, travellers and pilgrims. He eases suffering and helps the faithful to reach *Amida*'s western paradise (where inhabitants are no longer trapped in the six states of desire and karmic rebirth). He appears in numerous forms, many of which can be invoked for medical reasons (Table 4) or human life issues. For instance, *ema* with an image of *Jizō* originating from *Jizōdō* (*Jizō* halls) in Saitama Prefecture and elsewhere have been associated with benefits concerning *yonaki* (crying at night), *neshōben* (bed-wetting) and *kannomushi* (short-temperedness) [IH2-60].

His customary symbols are a wish-granting jewel (*hōjunotama*) and a six-ring staff (*shakujō*). The latter symbolises that he does not reside in Buddhist Heaven but remains active to assist all who are still trapped in the six realms of existence and have not yet achieved enlightenment. When he wears a red bib, this may reflect the Japanese folk belief that red is the colour for expelling demons and illness [MS].

061

Jizōson 地蔵尊. Origin unknown. Mid-20th century. W. 11.2 cm

062

Migawari Jizō 身代り地蔵 (Substitute *Jizō*)
Kenchōji 建長寺. Kamakura, Kanagawa Prefecture. Late 20th century. W. 11.6 cm
The inscriptions read:
身代り地蔵尊 = *Migawari Jizōson* (Substitute *Jizō*)
建長寺 = *Kenchōji*

If someone is suffering or is threatened by ill fortune, *Migawari Jizō* (Substitute *Jizō*) acts as a substitute. His spiritual force absorbs or deflects any negative force or bad luck, and thereby opens the way to good fortune [RT-46; MS].

063

Shibarare Jizō しばられ地蔵 (Rope-Tied *Jizō*)
Nanzōin 南蔵院. Katsushika Ward, Tokyo. Early 21st century. W. 8.9 cm
The inscriptions read:
しばられ地蔵 = *Shibarare Jizō*
南蔵院 = *Nanzōin*

This is a new *ema* design that has recently replaced a classical type of *ema* that also depicted a statue of *Shibarare Jizō* [TS-18].

According to legend, a store clerk transporting kimono cloth stopped to rest near a *Jizō* statue and dozed off. When he woke up, his goods were gone. The investigating magistrate ordered the arrest of the *Jizō* statue and had it bound with ropes, because it had failed to protect the clerk. When many spectators came to see the roped statue, he fined each of them a roll of cloth for trespassing. Among the rolls he received, one belonged to the clerk and thereby led to the thieves. Today, *Shibarare Jizō* (Rope-Tied *Jizō*) is believed to grant various wishes (including better health and protection from robbery or evil). Someone who makes a wish, binds the *Jizō* with a rope, which is untied again after the wish has come true.

Manifestation	Specialisation(s)
Agonashi Jizō (*Jizō* Without Chin)	For illnesses of the mouth and for toothache
Ameyami Jizō (Rain-Stopping *Jizō*)	For illnesses of the eye
An Jizō	For illnesses of the skin
Arai Jizō (Rough *Jizō*)	For illnesses in general
Ashi Jizō	For illnesses of the legs/feet
Bokefūji Jizō	For the prevention of senility
Gankake Jizō (Prayer *Jizō*)	For illnesses of the throat
Hanakake Jizō (Noseless *Jizō*)	For illnesses in general
Hechima Jizō (Sponge Gourd *Jizō*)	For respiratory illnesses (cough, asthma)
Hōroku Jizō (Earthenware Pan *Jizō*)	For illnesses of the head/neck
Kamihari Jizō (Paper-Pasted *Jizō*)	For boils or other illnesses
Kinomoto Jizō	For illnesses of the eye
Koduki Jizō	For cough
Kubi Jizō (Head/neck *Jizō*)	For illnesses of the head/neck
Kuginuki Jizō (Nail Pulling *Jizō*)	For the relief of pain; for illnesses in general
Migawari Jizō (Substitute *Jizō*)	For illnesses in general
Mimi Jizō (*Jizō* of the Ears)	For illnesses of the ear
Miwa Jizō	For toothache
Mochiage Jizō (Lifting *Jizō*)	For illnesses of the face
Nabekaburi Jizō (Pot-Capped *Jizō*)	For illnesses of the eye
Naderu Jizō (Rubbing *Jizō*)	For illnesses in general
Nurikobe Jizō	For illnesses of the teeth
Onegai Jizō (Wish *Jizō*)	For illnesses in general
O-Keshō Jizō (Makeup *Jizō*)	For illnesses in general
Sekidome Jizō (Cough-Stopping *Jizō*)	For cough
Shibari Jizō (Roped *Jizō*)	For illnesses of the chest and other respiratory organs; illnesses of the stomach; illnesses in general
Shio Jizō (Salt *Jizō*)	For illnesses of the teeth; for the removal of warts
Shiokake Jizō (*Jizō* amidst salt)	For *odeki* (boils)
Tako Jizō (Octopus *Jizō*)	For *dacchō* (abdominal hernia); for illnesses in general
Tawashi Jizō (Kitchen-Brush *Jizō*)	For rheumatism [GS-311]
Togenuki Jizō (Splinter-Pulling *Jizō*)	For illnesses in general
Wagata Jizō (Wheel-Track *Jizō*)	For the health of horses and cattle (inter alia)

Table 4 Manifestations of *Jizō* for illness in general or for a specific type of illness [4]

064

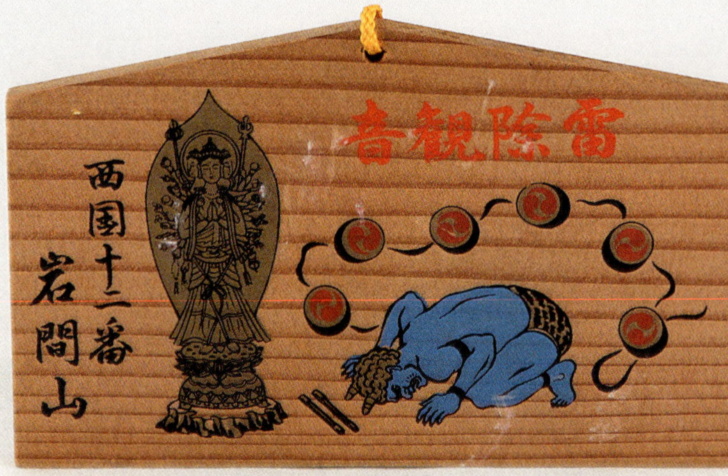

雷除観音
西国十二番
岩間山

065

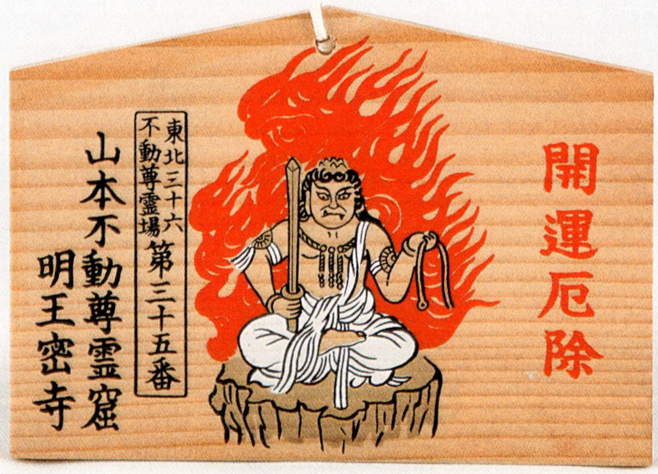

開運厄除
東北三十六不動尊霊場第三十五番
山本不動尊霊窟
明王密寺

066

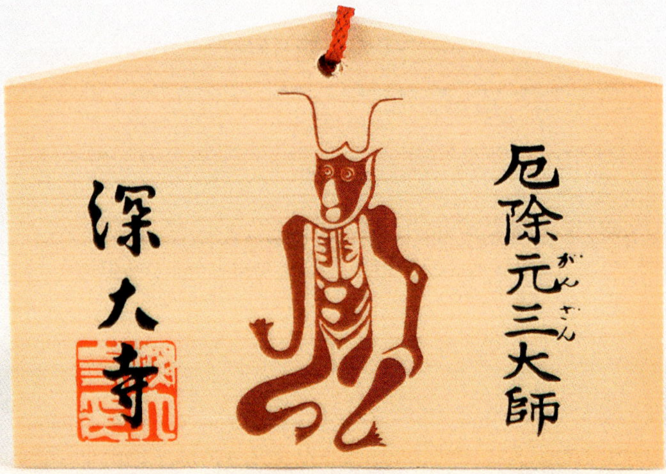

厄除元三大師
深大寺

Kannon 観音

Kannon is the widely beloved Bodhisattva of mercy and compassion, the Japanese equivalent of the Chinese figure of worship *Guanyin*. In the past, *Kannon* was often shown as male but nowadays *Kannon* is often portrayed as female. *Kannon* appears in countless manifestations to assist with all manner of earthly petitions and to protect all those trapped in the six realms of karmic rebirth.
See Table 5 for manifestations of *Kannon* for illness in general or for a specific type of illness [MS]. When an *ema* with *Kannon* serves a specific medical or human life issue, it is dealt with in a later section reviewing that particular issue (parts three and four).

064
Senju Kannon 千手觀音 (Thousand-Armed *Kannon*). *Iwamasan Shōhōji* 岩間山正法寺. Otsu, Shiga Prefecture. Late 20th century. W. 14.5 cm
The inscriptions read:
雷隠観音 = *Kaminariyoke Kannon* (Thunder-averting *Kannon*)
第十二番 = *daijūniban* (number twelve, i.e., on the Saikoku pilgrimage)
岩間山 = *Iwamasan*

Kannon is worshipped here by a blue horned *Raijin* (god of thunder) with six drums hovering over him. This suggests that *Kannon* is portrayed on this *ema* as a protector against thunder, which impression is confirmed by one of the inscriptions.

Today, the main benefit offered by the temple is *boke fūji* (prevention of senility). There is a special statue of *Boke Fūji Kannon* in the precincts and the temple also offers *hōro ku kyū* (baking pan moxibustion) for *boke fūji*. The temple is the 12th one on the Saikoku pilgrimage.

Fudō Myō-ō 不動明王

Ema representing *Fudō Myō-ō* (Ācala in Sanskrit) have been used for numerous purposes, including protection against evil spirits and fire calamity, prosperous business and traffic safety. *Fudō* may also feature on *ema* for cancer or for leg/feet problems (see p.123 and p.151 in part four) [TS-18; IH2-18].

065
Yamamoto Fudōson 山本不動尊. Tanagura, Fukushima Prefecture. Late 20th century. W. 13.0 cm
The inscriptions read:
開運 = *kaiun* (opening up good luck)
厄除 = *yakuyoke* (warding off evil)
東北三十六不動尊霊場 = *Tōhoku sanjūroku Fudōson reijō* (*Tōhoku* thirty-six *Fudōson* sacred ground)

Manifestation	Specialisation(s)
Batō Kannon (Horse-Headed *Kannon*)	For the health of horses and cattle
Bokefūji Kannon	For the prevention of senility
Jūichimen Kannon (Eleven-Headed *Kannon*)	For illnesses in general
Nyoirin Kannon	For the illnesses of women (inter alia)
Senju Kannon (Thousand-Armed *Kannon*)	For illnesses of the eye; for illnesses in general
Yōryū Kannon (Willow *Kannon*)	For the prevention/cure of headaches and other illnesses

Table 5 Manifestations of *Kannon* for illness in general or for a specific type of illness [MS]

第三十五番 = *daisanjūgoban* (number thirty-five)
山本不動尊霊窪 = *Yamamoto Fudōson reikubo* (sacred cave)
明王密寺 = *Myō-ō Mitsuji*

Enma 閻魔

Enma belongs to the *Tenbu* (Deva in Sanskrit). He is the king of the underworld and main judge of the dead (deciding whether someone has been good or bad). At *Genkakuji* (Bunkyo Ward, Tokyo), a statue of him known as *Konnyaku Enma* can be petitioned for a cure for an eye problem (see p.133 in part four) [RT-250; MS].

Ganzan Daishi 元三大師

Ganzan Daishi is the honorific title bestowed posthumously on the Tendai priest *Ryōgen*, who lived around 1000 A.D. Upon his death he did not depart to the Pure Land but remained as protector of Mount Hiei (where the first outpost of Japanese Tendai Buddhism was founded). His reputation centred on his power in *yakuyoke* (warding off evil). In the past, amulets with his image were widely used (e.g., fastened above entrances) to ward off malevolent spirits, to avert natural disasters and to cure illness [5].

066
Jindaiji 深大寺. Chofu, Tokyo Metropolis. Early 21st century. W. 13.0 cm
The inscriptions read:
厄除け元三大師 = *Yakuyoke Ganzan Daishi*
深大寺 = *Jindaiji*

067

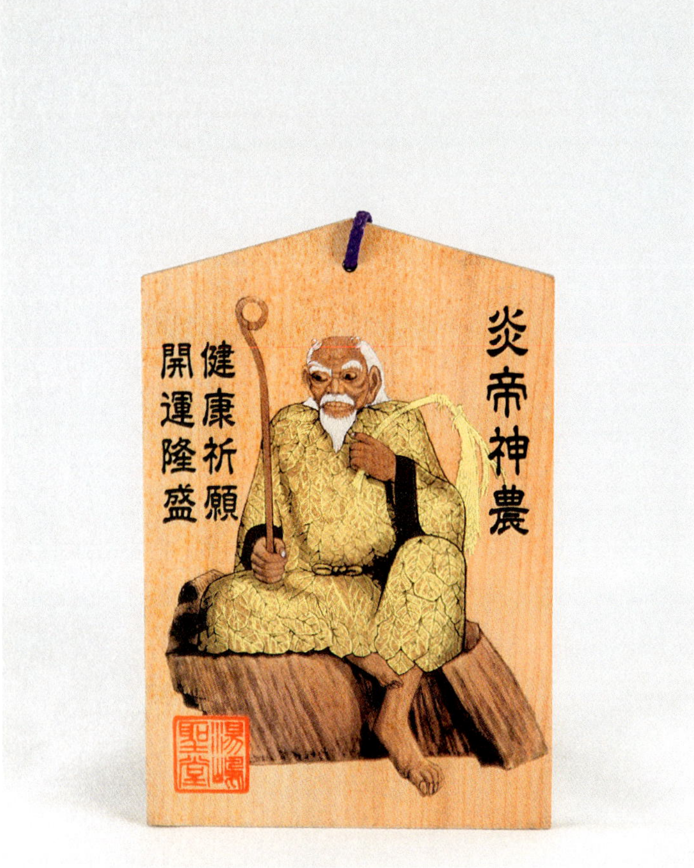

068

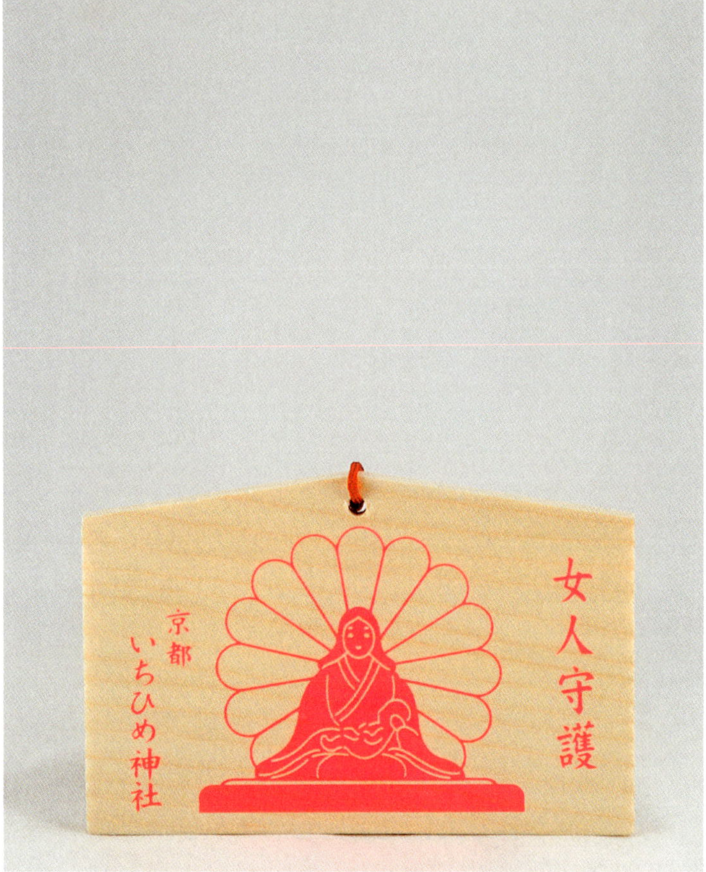

069

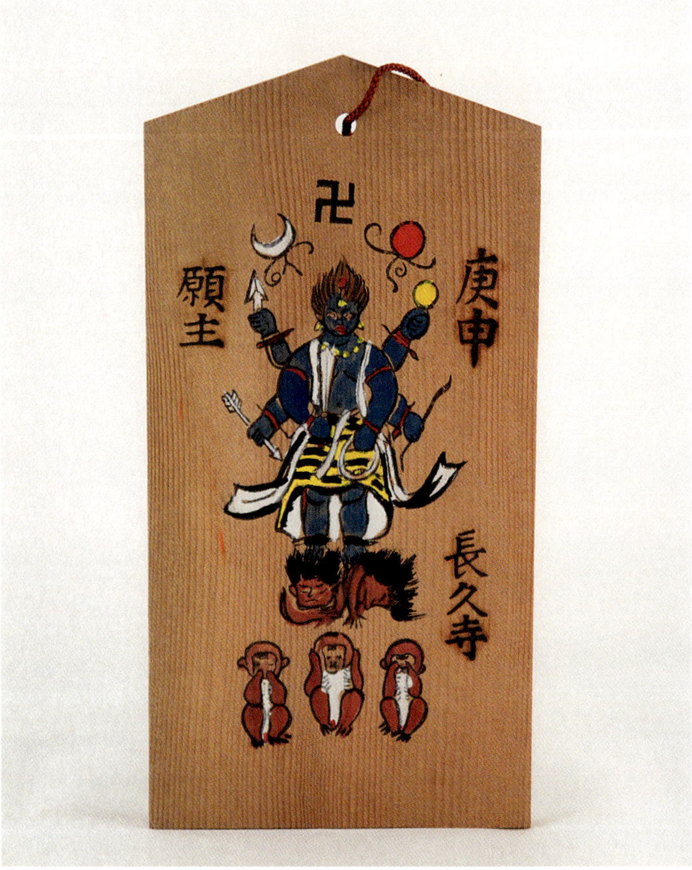

070

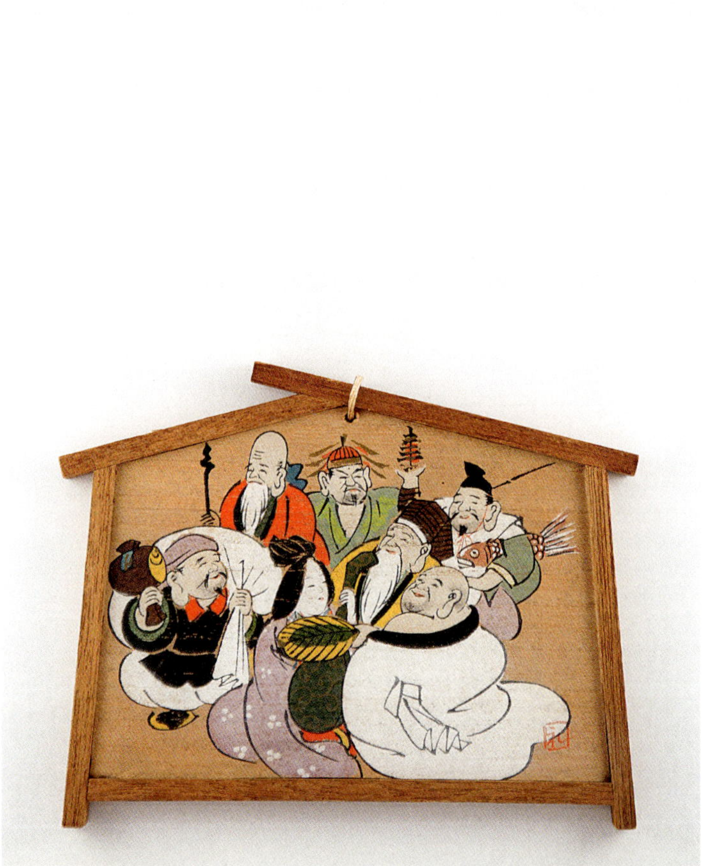

Other figures of worship 他の礼拝の姿 (*tano reihai no sugata*)

Background

Other health-related figures of worship in Japan often originate from the Chinese Taoist tradition. Examples are *Shinnō* (the Chinese god of agriculture and medicine), *Shōmen-Kongō* (who is worshipped by followers of the *Kōshin* faith), and three of the seven *Shichi-fukujin* deities (*Fukurokuju, Hotei, Jurōjin*) [MS]. Although Taoism never developed into an institutionalised religion in Japan, it has heavily influenced folk beliefs there. It would be misleading, however, to equate such Japanese beliefs with Chinese Taoism because the original Chinese system was thoroughly transformed and incorporated into the broader Japanese religious traditions, with elements of Taoist thought and practice, along with its deities, being subsumed within Japanese Shinto and Buddhism [EO-149].

Ema designs

Shinnō 神農

Shinnō is the Japanese name of the Chinese god of agriculture and medicine, *Shennong* (literally Divine Farmer). He is easily recognisable by the characteristic cloak of leaves he is wearing. As *Shennong* discovered the medicinal properties of herbs by testing them on himself, he is often portrayed as holding or chewing a plant stem or leaf [6]. See also the entry on the Shinto deity *Sukunahikona-no-Mikoto*.

067

Yushima Seidō 湯島聖堂. Bunkyo Ward, Tokyo. Early 21st century. W. 11.1 cm

The inscriptions read:

炎帝神農 = *Honō Tei Shinnō* (Blazing God *Shinnō*)

健康祈願 = *kenkō kigan* (prayer for health)

開運隆盛 = *kaiun ryūsei* (better fortune and prosperity)

湯島聖堂 = *Yushima Seidō*

Nyonin shugo 女人守護

Nyonin shugo (guardian of women) could be a Shinto deity but could also be a folk deity without formal Shinto connection. The benefits of *Nyonin shugo* include *nyonin yakuyoke* (warding off evil from women), *ryōen* (good match for marriage), *kosazuke* (child bestowed), and *anzan* (easy delivery).

068

Ichihime Jinja 市姫神社. Shimogyo Ward, Kyoto. Early 21st century. W. 15.0 cm

The inscriptions read:

女人厄除 = *nyonin yakuyoke* (warding off evil from women)

京都いちひめ神社 = *Kyōto Ichihime Jinja*

This *ema* design depicts a female with a child on her lap.

Shōmen-Kongō 青面金剛

Shōmen-Kongō is the main health-related deity in Japanese Taoism. He is sometimes said to have been a demon who originally inflicted illnesses but who became a protector against illness after being conquered by Buddha's army.

Shōmen-Kongō is the main deity of the *Kōshin* faith. According to this faith, everyone has three small insect-like creatures inside his/her body (called *Sanshi*) which keep track of his/her good and bad deeds. Every 60 days, on the night of *Kōshin*, these *Sanshi* will leave the body while the person is sleeping, and report to the Heavenly God about his/her deeds. As a result, the Heavenly God may decide to make bad people ill or to shorten their lives. Believers in *Kōshin*, who have reason to fear this, will stay awake during the night of *Kōshin*. They hold a ritual vigil called *Kōshinmachi* to prevent the *Sanshi* leaving their body and to ask *Shōmen-Kongō* (who is believed to eat the *Sanshi*) for protection.

069

Chōkyūji 長久寺. Nagoya, Aichi Prefecture. Late 20th century. W. 12.0 cm

The inscriptions read:

庚申 = *Kōshin*

長久寺 = *Chōkyūji*

願主 = *ganshu* (petitioner)

Shōmen-Kongō is represented here as a blue-faced warrior-like deity standing over an *oni* (evil spirit) to symbolise his ability to protect against illness. According to the *Kōshin* belief, the three monkeys shown beneath him can prevent the *Sanshi* from reporting to the Heavenly God by not seeing, speaking or hearing about bad deeds. The swastika in the upper centre is widely used in the world as a symbol of prosperity and good fortune. For Buddhists in India, it symbolises the Buddha's feet or footprints.

The three monkeys are also regularly found on *ema* without the *Kōshin* deity *Shōmen-Kongō*. They are known collectively as *Sanzaru* and individually as *Iwazaru* (speak no evil monkey), *Kikazaru* (hear no evil monkey) and *Mizaru* (see no evil monkey) [MS].

Shichifukujin 七福神 (*Seven Gods of Good Fortune*)

Only one of the *Shichifukujin* stems from the Japanese Shinto tradition (*Ebisu*). Three gods were originally Deva from India (*Benzaiten, Bishamonten, Daikokuten*) and the remaining three have come from the Chinese Taoist-Buddhist tradition (*Fukurokuju, Hotei, Jurōjin*).

At one time or another, health-related connotations have been attributed to most of the *Shichifukujin*: *Hotei* has been associated with good health, *Jurōjin* and *Fukurokuju* have been connected to longevity, *Ebisu* has been considered as a guardian of the health of small children and *Bishamonten* as a healer of illness [MS].

070

Origin unclear. Mid-20th century. W. 18.5 cm

Starting from the top middle and going clockwise: *Bishamonten* (with a pagoda) as god of warriors, wealth, good fortune; *Ebisu* (with a fishing rod and sea bream) as god of fishermen and prosperity; *Jurōjin* (with a long white beard) as god of longevity; *Hotei* (with a fan) as god of happiness; *Benzaiten* (with a lute) as goddess of music, fine arts, beauty; *Daikokuten* (with a treasure sack and magic mallet) as god of the earth, agriculture, wealth, and the kitchen; and *Fukurokuju* (with a high forehead and a cane) as god of wealth and longevity [MS].

071

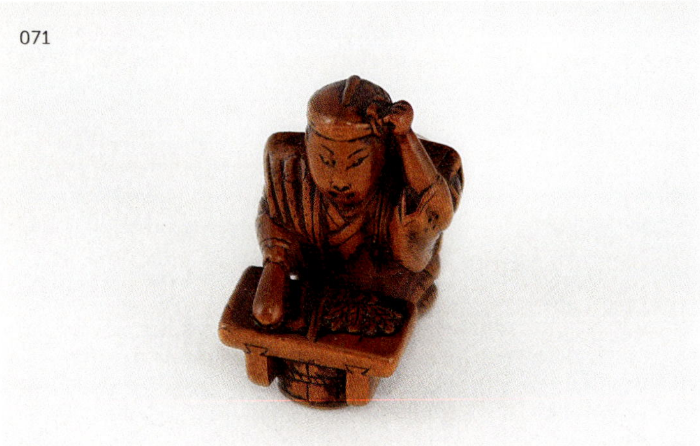

072

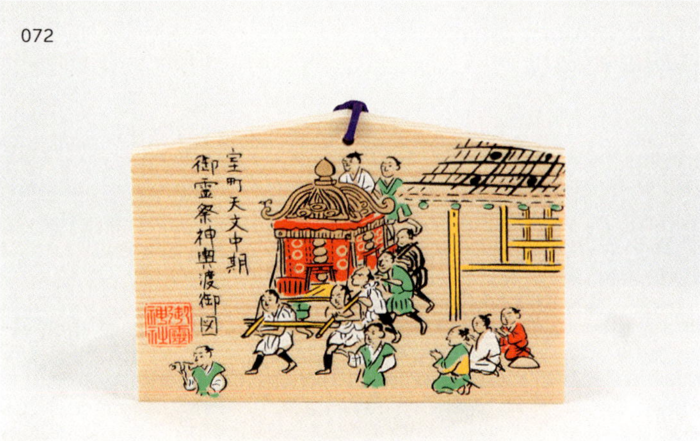

073

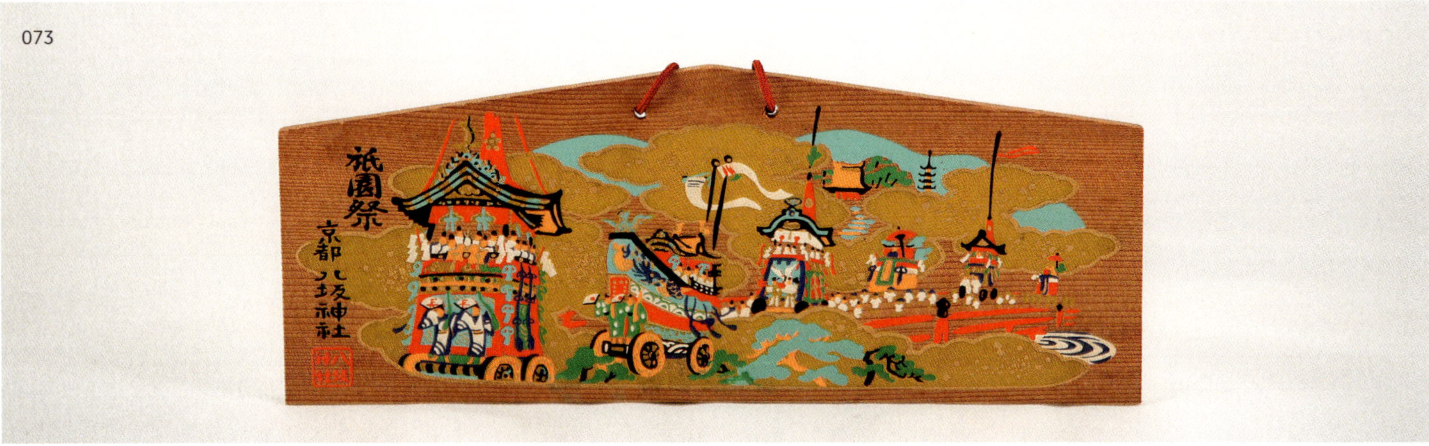

074

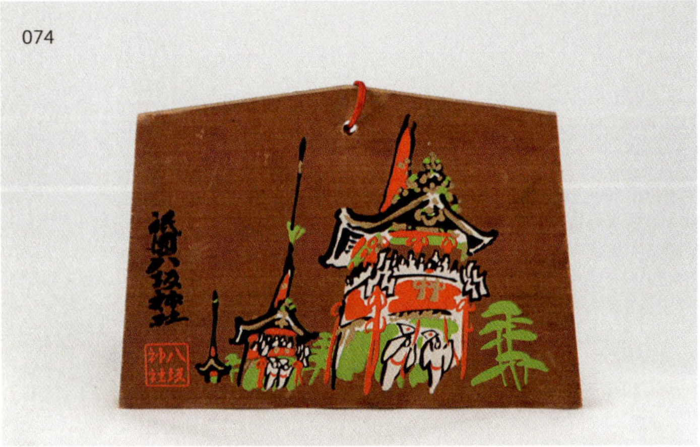

075

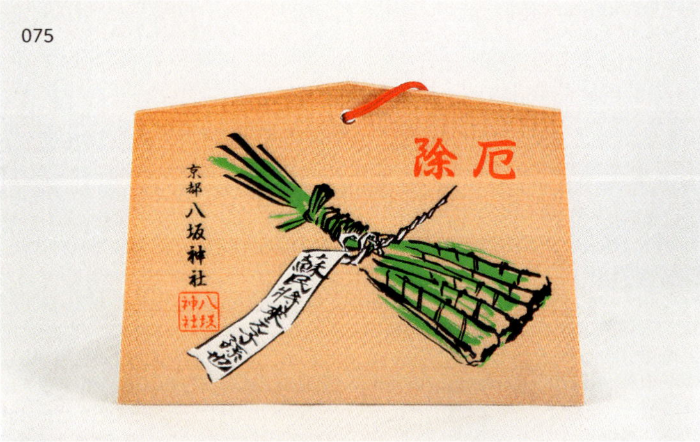

076

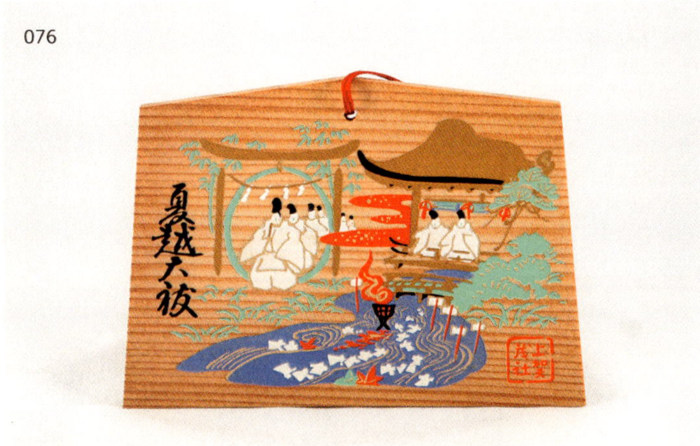

077

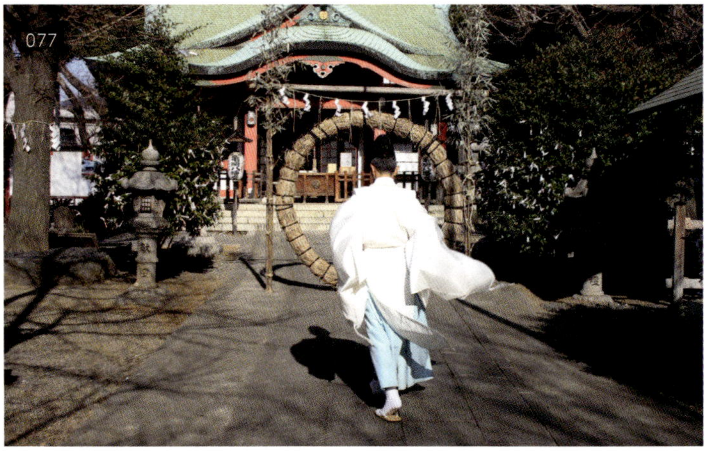

Festivals 祭 (*matsuri*)

Background

Japan is famous for its numerous *matsuri* (festivals) and other annual festivities. Some are nationwide celebrations but many more are organised on a more local scale. Several were originally staged to pray for a health-related purpose, such as the aversion of an epidemic or to seek future good health. Examples of these will be presented in this section, in so far as they are reproduced on *ema* and are not aimed at a specific medical or lifecycle problem. The latter will be discussed in relevant later sections, e.g., *Hina Matsuri* (Dolls Festival) in the section on women's illnesses in part four. *Matsuri* that originated in order to pray for protection from epidemics, but that have now evolved into spectacles for good health in general are included here [1].

071
Festival of Seven Herbs 七草の節句 (*Nanakusa no sekku*). Wooden netsuke. First half 19th century. H. 3.1 cm

This netsuke portrays a step in the Festival of Seven Herbs by showing how the head of the family is chopping seven different herbs on the evening of 6 January. The next morning, everyone would eat rice gruel cooked with the seven chopped herbs so that evil spirits and illnesses would be warded off in the new year.

Ema designs

Goryō Festival 御霊祭 *(Goryō Matsuri)* and *Gion Festival* 祇園祭 *(Gion Matsuri)*

The societal impact of epidemic diseases in ancient days is still visible in certain *matsuri* (festivals) that are performed each year. Their origin goes back to the Heian period (794-1185), when the inhabitants of *Heian-kyō* (then the capital and now Kyoto) started to appease evil spirits with shrines and festivals. Disasters such as epidemics, floods, fires and earthquakes were especially attributed to malevolent *goryō* (lit. spirits of deceased persons) particularly if they had died unhappily and therefore bore grudges against the living. During an epidemic in 863, a festival was held in the Imperial gardens of Kyoto and temporary shrines were erected for six of the most feared *goryō* (later increased to eight). These spirits were permanently enshrined at Kyoto's two *Goryō* shrines. A few years later (in 869), *Gion Jinja* (later called *Yasaka Jinja*) organised its first *Gion Matsuri* (*Gion* Festival) in an attempt to free the city of an epidemic that was attributed to the rampaging deity *Gozu Tennō*. A century later the festival became an annual affair, suggesting the growing endemicity of infectious disease [WF; 2].

072
Parade at *Goryō* Festival. *Goryō Jinja* 御霊神社
Kamigyo Ward, Kyoto. Early 21st century.
W. 14.0 cm
The inscriptions read:
室町天文中期 = *Muromachi Tenbun chūki* (middle of the *Muromachi Tenbun* period 1532-1555)
御霊祭神輿渡御図 = *Goryō matsuri mikoshitogyo zu* (picture of *Goryō* festival and the carrying of portable shrines)
御霊神社 = *Goryō Jinja* (also known as *Kamigoryō Jinja*)

073
Parade at *Gion* Festival. *Yasaka Jinja* 八坂神社
Higashiyama Ward, Kyoto. Early 21st century.
W. 25.0 cm
The inscriptions read:
祇園祭 = *Gion matsuri*
京都八坂神社 = *Kyōto Yasaka Jinja*

074
Parade at *Gion* Festival. *Yasaka Jinja* 八坂神社
Higashiyama Ward, Kyoto. Late 20th century.
W. 15.4 cm
The inscriptions read:
祇園八坂神社 = *Gion Yasaka Jinja*
八坂神社 = *Yasaka Jinja*

075
Nagoshi-sai rite at *Gion* Festival. *Yasaka Jinja* 八坂神社. Higashiyama Ward, Kyoto. Early 21st century. W. 15.3 cm
The inscriptions read:
厄除 = *yakuyoke* (warding off evil)
京都八坂神社 = *Kyōto Yasaka Jinja*

The closing event of *Gion Matsuri* at *Yasaka Jinja* is the *Nagoshi-sai* rite at its subshrine *Ekijin-sha*, which enshrines *Susanoo-no-mikoto*. On this occasion, *Yasaka Jinja* sells charms in the shape of a *chimaki* (cake wrapped in bamboo leaves). These talismans have *chigaya* (cogon grass) inside and are often provided with the text "we are descendants of *Somin Shōrai*". They can be hung on the door of one's home for *yakuyoke* (warding off evil) until the next year. Cf. the entry on *Somin Shōrai* on p.65.

076
Summer purification rite 夏越の祓 (*Nagoshi-no-harae*). *Kamigamo Jinja* 上賀茂神社.
Kita Ward, Kyoto. Late 20th century. W. 15.4 cm
The inscription on the left reads:
夏越の祓 = *Nagoshi-no-harae*

The *Nagoshi-no-harae* rite at *Kamigamo Jinja* is similar to the *Nagoshi-sai* rite at *Yasaka Jinja*. Participants pass through a large *chinowa* (ring of cogon grass) to be purified and to be protected from misfortune.

077
A Shinto priest walking towards a similar *chinowa* (ring of cogon grass) at *Ichigaya Kamegaoka Hachimangū* (Shinjuku Ward, Tokyo).

078

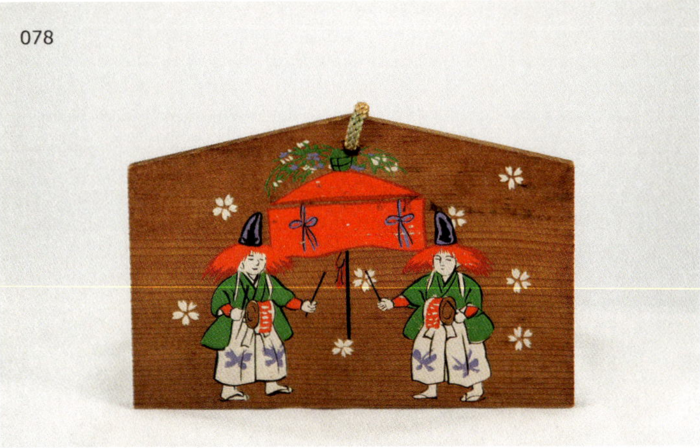

079

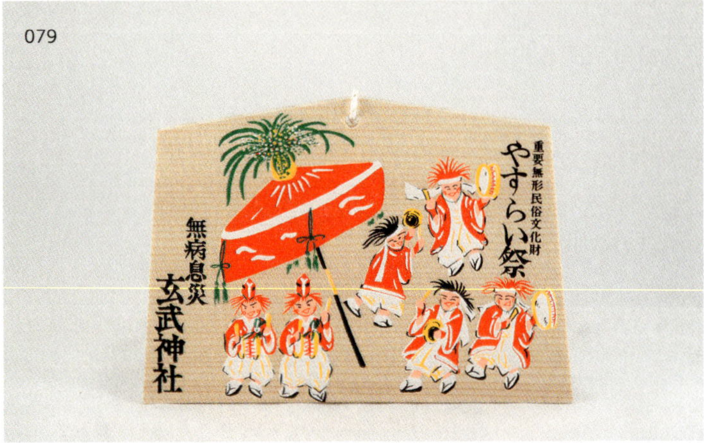

080

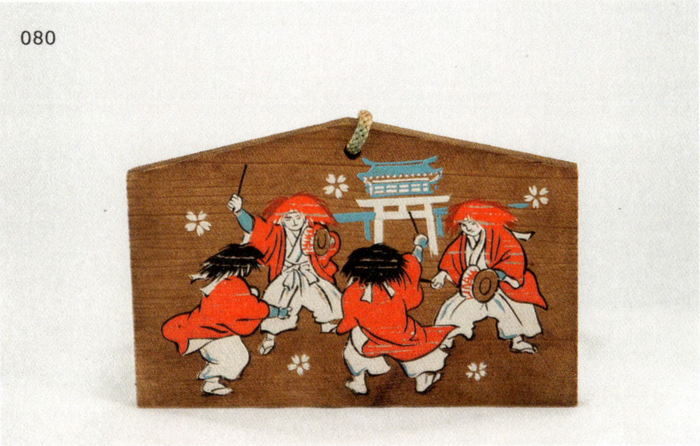

081

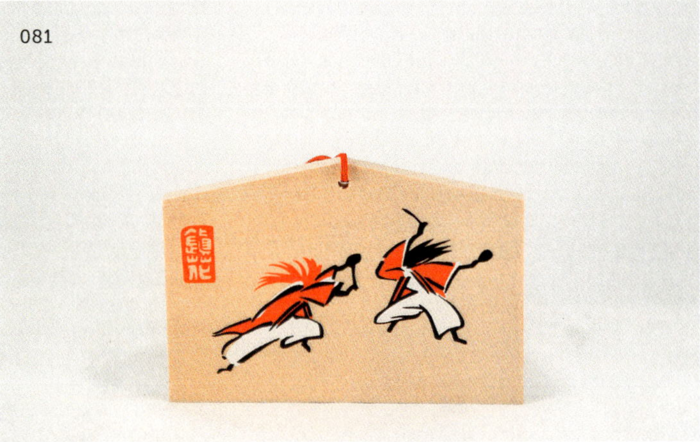

082

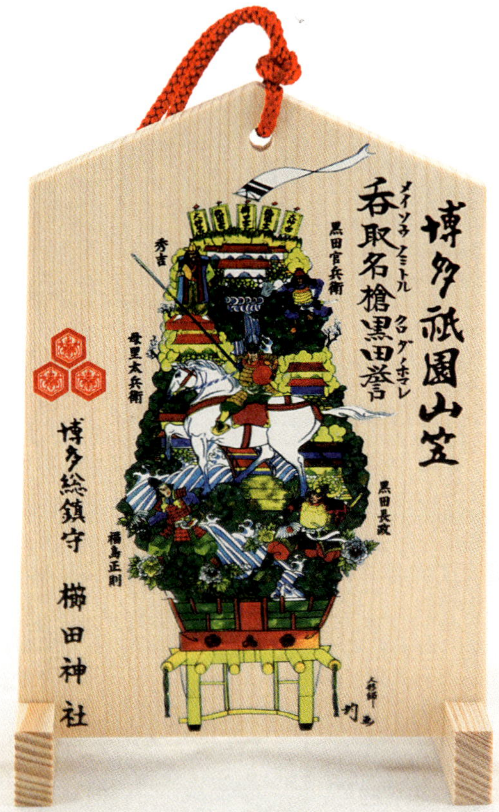

Yasurai Festival やすらい祭 *(Yasurai Matsuri)*

Another epidemic-based festival is the *Yasurai* Festival that is organised jointly by three shrines in Kyoto (*Imamiya Jinja*, *Genbu Jinja* and *Kawakami Daijingū*). It features dancers with red or black wigs representing *oni* (demons) and the taking of shelter from evil under big red umbrellas (which will give good health in the coming year). In ancient Japan, blossoming cherry trees (especially those with branches drooping to the ground) connected the land of the living with the land of the dead. Cherry blossom petals scattered by the wind were associated with storms caused by the *goryō* (spirits of the angry dead). As these *goryō* brought misfortune and disaster, a number of rituals existed for their pacification. Festival dances called *yasurai hana* (quieting blossoms) were performed to exorcise evil spirits known as *ekijin*, who were believed to spread epidemics at the same time, when the flower petals of the cherry blossom were scattered [3].

078
Imamiya Jinja 今宮神社. Kita Ward, Kyoto.
Late 20th century. W. 17.3 cm
An inscription on the reverse reads:
紫野今宮 = *Murasakino* (place name) *Imamiya*

079
Genbu Jinja 玄武神社. Kita Ward, Kyoto.
Early 21st century. W. 17.0 cm
The inscriptions read:
重要無形民俗文化財 = *jūyō mukei minzoku bunkazai* (important intangible folk cultural asset)
やすらい祭 = *Yasurai matsuri* (*Yasurai* festival)
無病息災 = *mubyō sokusai* (good health)
玄武神社 = *Genbu Jinja*

080
Imamiya Jinja 今宮神社. Kita Ward, Kyoto.
Late 20th century. W. 17.5 cm
An inscription on the reverse reads:
紫野今宮 = *Murasakino* (place name) *Imamiya*

081
Imamiya Jinja 今宮神社. Kita Ward, Kyoto.
Early 21st century. W. 14.0 cm
The inscription reads:
今宮神社 = *Imamiya Jinja*

Hakata Gion Yamakasa 博多祇園山笠

The *Hakata Gion Yamakasa* Festival takes place in Hakata (former name of Fukuoka in northern Kyushu) and is hosted by *Kushida Jinja* which enshrines the deity *Gion*. The festival is said to have started in the 13th century, when a Buddhist priest helped victims of a plague in Hakata by sprinkling holy water on the street. The festival is famous for its *yamakasa* (floats), which come in two types:

- 10 meter high *kazariyama*, which are placed for display on street corners;
- 5 meter high *kakiyama*, which are carried by men running through the streets of Hakata Ward with the float on their shoulders.

Ema with the picture of a *yamakasa* were associated with *ekibyō taisan* (dispersal of plagues) and *gokokuhōjō* (abundant harvest) [IH2-25; NM-Z22654].

082
Kushida Jinja 櫛田神社. Hakata Ward, Fukuoka.
Early 21st century. W. 12.5 cm
The inscription on the far right reads:
博多祇園山笠= *Hakata Gion Yamakasa* (Hakata Gion float)
The inscriptions on the far left read:
博多総鎮守 = *Hakata Sōchinju* (all the guardian deities of Hakata)
櫛田神社 = *Kushida Jinja*

This contemporary *ema* portrays a *yamakasa*, but its reverse is so densely written that there is no room for writing a wish. It is therefore a souvenir rather than a real votive tablet.

083

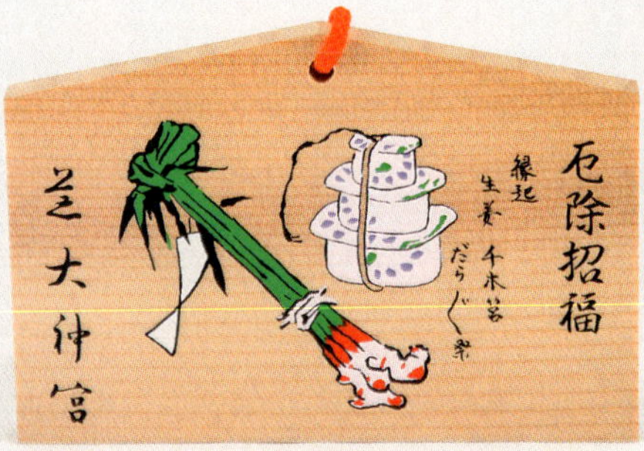

084

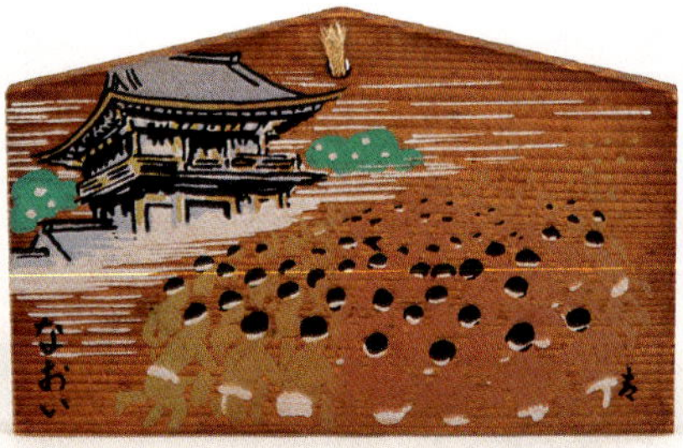

085

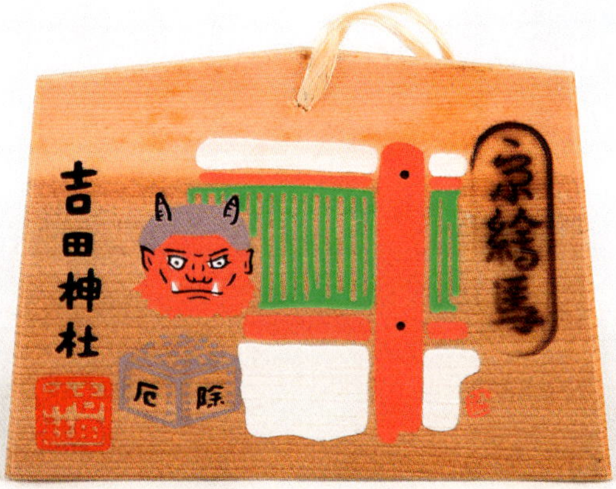

086

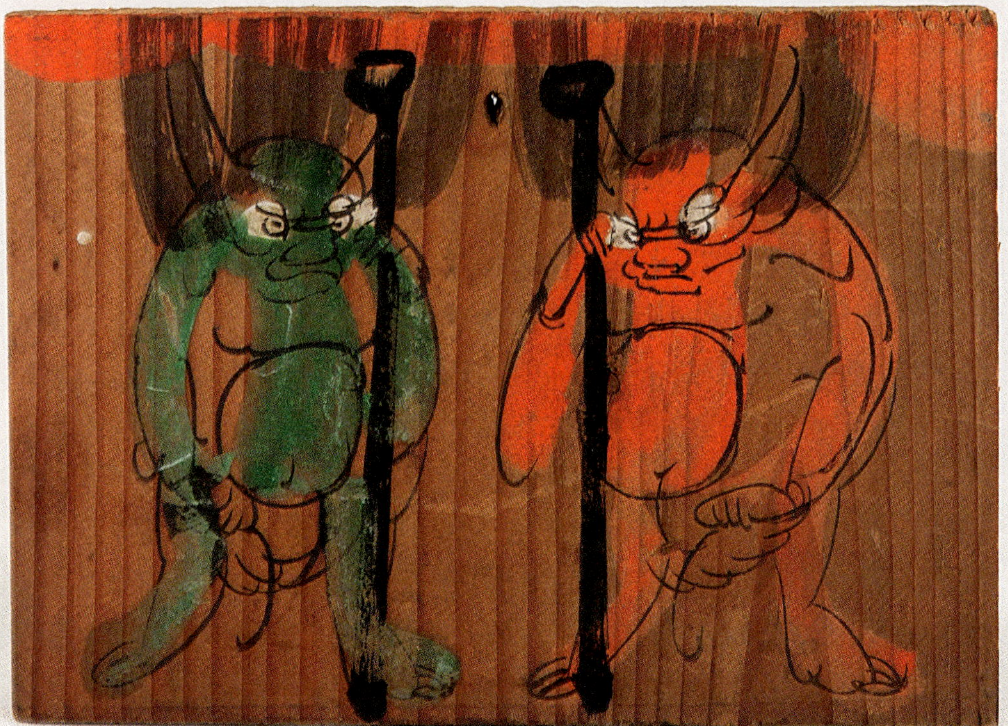

Ginger Festival 生姜祭 *(Shōga Matsuri)*

Each year in September, *Shiba Daijingū* (Minato Ward, Tokyo) holds a Ginger Festival, which dates back to the Edo Period. It is particularly known for the selling of fresh *shōga* (ginger) and a protective charm called *chigibako* (set of boxes tied together). Eating the ginger will protect one from catching *kaze* (the common cold), while acquiring a *chigibako* is said to bring about a good relationship. In the Edo period, females would purchase this charm in order to enlarge their wardrobe, based on the pun that *chigi* could refer to a thousand pieces of clothing [GG1-2011/11].

083
Shiba Daijingū 芝大神宮. Minato Ward, Tokyo. Early 21st century. W. 15.3 cm
The inscriptions read:
厄除招福 = *yakuyoke shōfuku* (good luck charm for warding off evil)
縁起 = *engi* (foundation story of shrine/temple)
生姜 = *shōga* (ginger)
千木筥 = *chigibako* (set of boxes)
だらだら祭 = *Daradarasai* (alternative name for the Ginger Festival)
芝大神宮 = *Shiba Daijingū*

Hadaka Festival はだか祭り *(Hadaka Matsuri)*

The *Hadaka* Festival (also known as *Naoi-shinji*) finds its origin in the age of plagues. It goes back to 767 AD, when the governor of Owari Province (presently Aichi Prefecture) visited *Kōnomiya Jinja* to drive away evil spirits and calamities, after the Emperor had ordered invocations to dispel a plague. Today the festival is performed to get rid of bad luck and to bring about good luck and good harvests.

The central person in the festival is a naked man called *Shin-Otoko*, who symbolically absorbs evil and calamities. The other participants (wearing only loincloths) chase him because touching him will take all bad luck away. There are many forms of *Hadaka matsuri* all over Japan that also contain the theme of defying the cold, as they often occur in the snow.

084
Owari Ōkunitama Jinja 尾張大國霊神社 (also known as *Kōnomiya Jinja*). Inazawa, Aichi Prefecture. Late 20th century. W. 14.2 cm
The inscription reads なおい = *Naoi*

Setsubun 節分

Setsubun is associated with the Lunar New Year. On February 3 (the day before the beginning of spring according to the pre-modern calendar), it is celebrated at shrines and temples all over Japan. The main ceremony is called *mamemaki* (bean scattering). It involves the throwing of roasted soybeans called *fukumame* (good fortune beans) at masked persons representing *oni* (demons) while crying *oni wa soto – fuku wa uchi* (demons out – good fortune in). The purpose of this is to drive out the illness-bringing spirits of the past year and to bring in good luck for the year to come. Afterwards, one should eat the same number of beans as one's age for a year of good health [KU].

085
Yoshida Jinja 吉田神社. Sakyo Ward, Kyoto. Late 20th century. W. 12.1 cm
The inscriptions read:
京絵馬 = *kyō ema* (imperial capital – especially Kyoto – votive tablet)
吉田神社 = *Yoshida Jinja*
The inscription on the box with beans reads:
厄除 = *yakuyoke* (warding off evil)

086
Red demon 赤鬼 (*akaoni*) and blue demon 青鬼 (*aooni*) at *Setsubun*. *Kijin Jinja* 鬼鎮神社. Ranzan, Saitama Prefecture. Mid-20th century. W. 14.3 cm

Setsubun at *Kijin Jinja* is different from the ceremony at most other sanctuaries. Instead of casting the *oni* (demons) out, they are invited in by crying *fuku wa uchi – oni wa uchi – akuma soto* (good fortune in – demons in – devils out).

This *ema* was used for *akuryō taisan* (dispersal of evil spirits). It was taken home as a *fuda* (charm) and prayed to every day. People in the community served by the shrine traditionally attach it to the entrance of their houses to ward off evil and to prevent fire [TS-20; IH2-77; GG1-2011/10].

087

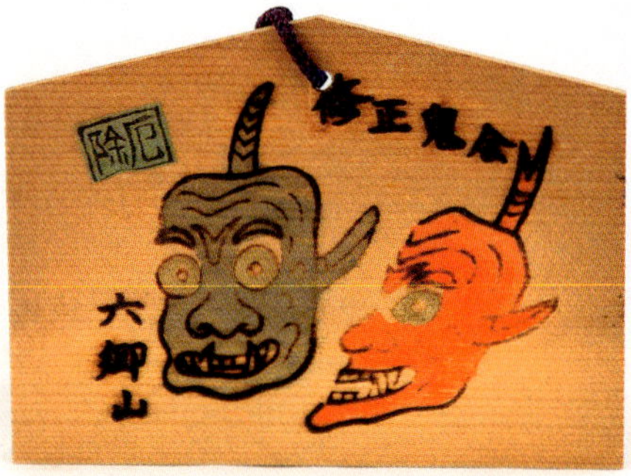

089

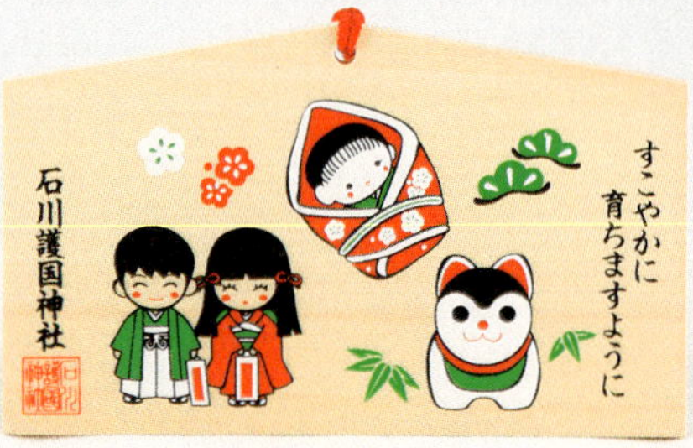

088

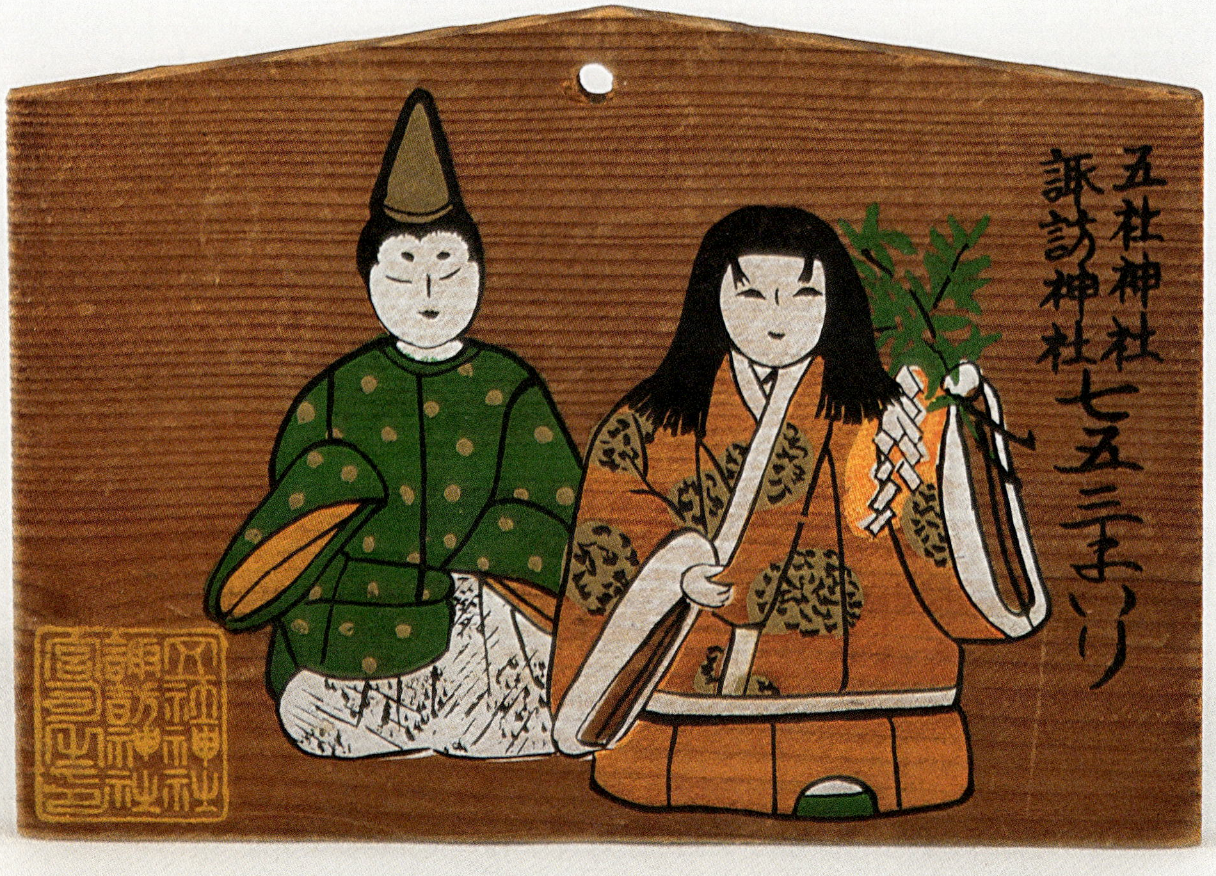

Shujōonie 修正鬼会

At *Rokugō Manzan* (Oita Prefecture), the festival on the occasion of the Lunar New Year is called *Shujōonie*. Two masked priests representing an *akaoni* (red demon) and a *kurooni* (black demon) perform various activities while carrying burning torches to bring in *kanai anzen* (family safety), *gokokuhōjō* (abundant harvest), and *mubyōsokusai* (sound health).

087

Rokugō Manzan 六郷満山. Kunisaki Peninsula, Oita Prefecture. Late 20th century (dated 1972 by original owner). W. 15.2 cm

The inscriptions read:
修正鬼会 = *Shujōonie*
厄除 = *yakuyoke* (warding off evil)
六郷山 = *Rokugōsan* (Rokugo Mountain)

Shichigosan 七五三

Shichigosan (literally seven-five-three) is an annual festival, on which three- and seven-year-old girls as well as three- and five-year-old boys (consistent with the belief that these odd numbers are lucky) are dressed up in formal clothes and brought to a nearby shrine or temple for ritual purification and to pray for their healthy growth and prosperous future. After the ceremony, the child is given *chitose ame* (thousand year candy) in an elongated bag adorned with cranes and turtles that symbolize longevity [JM-528].

088

Gosha Jinja 五社神社 / *Suwa Jinja* 諏訪神社
Hamamatsu, Shizuoka Prefecture. Late 20th century. W. 12.6 cm

The inscriptions read:
五社神社 = *Gosha Jinja*
諏訪神社 = *Suwa Jinja*
七五三まいり = *shichigosan mairi* (visit)

The girl on the right is holding a *sakaki* (branch of evergreen) decorated with a *shide* (white zigzag paper).

089

Ishikawa Gokoku Jinja 石川護國神社
Kanazawa, Ishikawa Prefecture. Early 21st century. W. 14.9 cm

The inscriptions read:
すこやかに育ちますように = *sukoyaka ni sodachimasu yō ni* (may you grow up healthy)
石川護國神社 = *Ishikawa Gokoku Jinja*

Shichigosan is shown on the left. The charm on the right is a papier-mâché toy dog called *inuhariko*. Since dogs are the symbol of good health and since puppies grow rapidly and are always active, such toy dogs have been presented to newborn babies since ancient days as a charm for healthy growth. This happens particularly on the occasion of the first visit to the shrine (*miyamairi*) which is a traditional Japanese rite of passage for newborns.

090

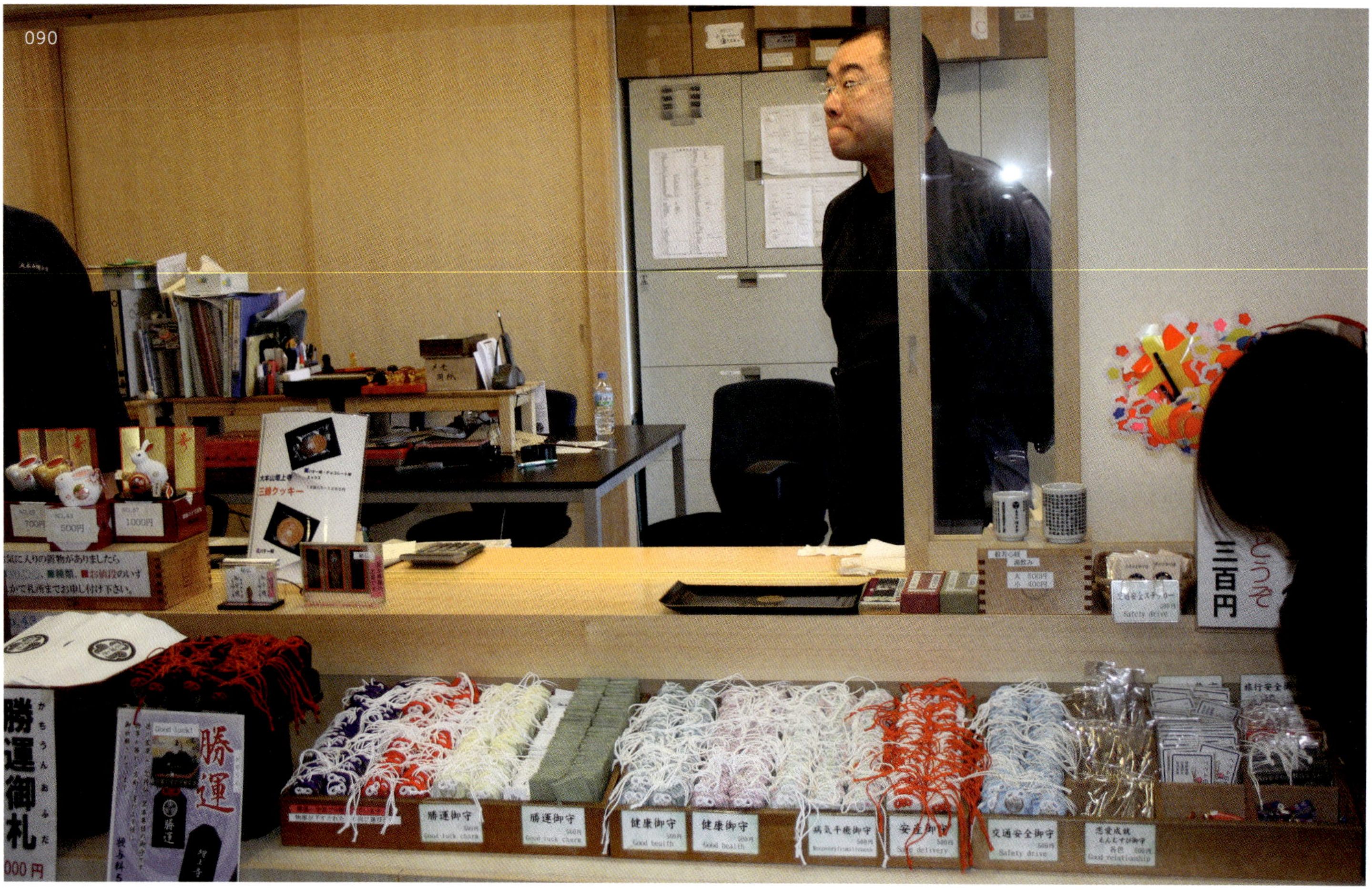

093

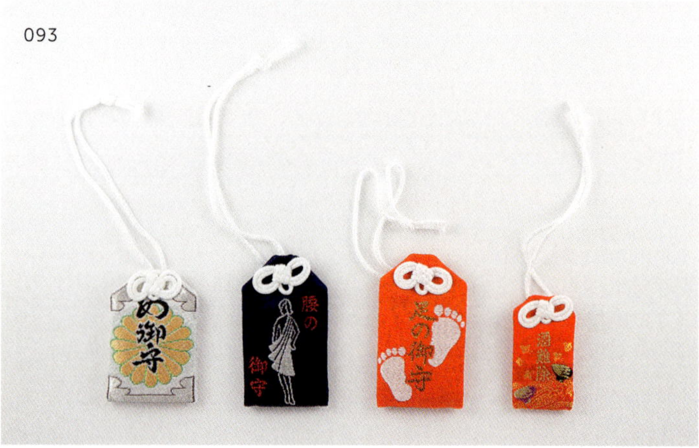

092

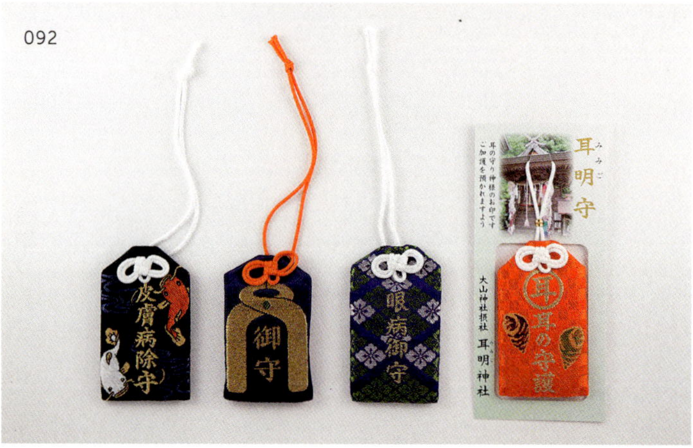

091

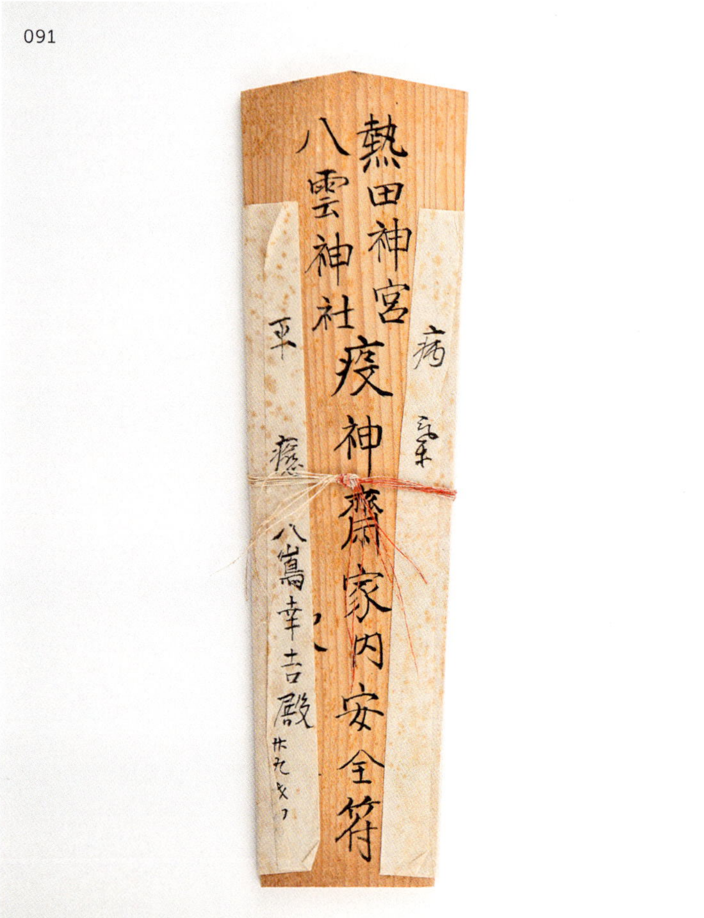

Charms
守り
(*mamori*)

Background

Worshippers can not only buy *ema* (votive tablets) at shrines and temples to leave a personal prayer or wish there, but they can also purchase various kinds of charms, amulets or talismans that are meant to be taken home. The ethnological literature has sometimes contrasted amulets as objects protecting against harm versus talismans as objects bringing good luck. However, this is an impractical differentiation, since the literature also defines amulets and talismans in other ways, which makes the use of these terms potentially confusing. Instead of reproducing them here, "charm" will be used as a general label. English-Japanese dictionaries offer various Japanese terms for the concept of charm. As suggested by Table 6, charm, talisman and amulet are often used in translations in a more or less interchangeable way. However, certain Japanese types (*mamori*, *mayoke*, *kuwabarakuwabara*) are primarily associated with *yakuyoke* (warding off evil), while certain other types (*engimono*, *omajinai*, *shōfuku*) commonly deal with *kaiun* (opening up good luck) [RT-46,67; 1].

Two ubiquitous types of charm that cover the whole range of *goriyaku* (divine favours) are *fuda* and *mamori*. Japanese people commonly refer to both using the honorific *o* (honourable) in front of the term, so frequently they are referred to as *ofuda* and *omamori*.

Fuda usually consist of a paper wrapped around a thin piece of wood in the shape of a pentangle with long sides that is inscribed with religious texts (which include the name of the sanctuary and the deity enshrined there).

Mamori consist of a paper carrying a prayer or some other form of religious inscription, invocation or sacred text in a small rectangular bag usually made of brocade or comparable material. Both types are considered to be a *bunshin* (offshoot) or *kesshin* (manifestation) of the spiritual force of the figure of worship that is enshrined at the sanctuary from which they originate. When they are acquired from a manufacturing company, they are merely objects. A ritual is required (usually involving placing them before a deity or buddha and invoking prayers) to ensure that the *bunshin* (spirit) of the deity or buddha enters them. They can be differentiated not only by their outward appearance, but also by looking at the beneficiaries of their action: *fuda* protect or bring fortune to a location (such as a house and its occupants) while *mamori* protect the individual person wearing or carrying them [RT-46,67].

Another major category of charms is collectively known as *omocha* or folk toys. Although this translation suggests otherwise, these objects do not have a practical function of playthings for children. Originally, most of them were charms for the blessing and protection of children as well as adults and material expressions of certain holy places and their tutelary deities. Although they have kept such connotations to some degree, they are now primarily regarded as collectibles and souvenirs today [2].

Term	English translation(s)
engimono (縁起物 · 縁起もの)	talisman; lucky charm
fu (符)	charm; talisman; amulet; sign
fuda (札)	token; ticket; charm; talisman
gofu · *gofū* (護符 · 御符 · 御封)	talisman; amulet; charm
jufu (呪符)	amulet; charm
jumon (呪文 · じゅ文)	spell; charm; incantation; magic word
kuwabarakuwabara (桑原桑原)	charm to ward off lightning and misfortune
mamori (守り · 護り)	protection; defence; amulet; charm; talisman
mamoribukuro (守り袋)	small pouch containing a paper charm or talisman
mamorifuda (守り札)	paper charm or talisman
mayoke (魔除け)	charm against evil spirits; talisman; amulet
omajinai (お呪い · 御呪い)	good luck charm
omamori (お守り · 御守り · お守 · 御守)	charm; amulet
shinpu (神符)	amulet; charm
shōfuku (招福)	good luck charm; something that encourages or invites good luck
reifu (霊符)	charm; amulet; talisman
ujikofuda (氏子札)	charm for shrine visitors

Table 6 Japanese terms for the English concept of "charm" [Based on http://tangorin.com/general/]

090
Mamori (charms) for sale at *Zōjōji* 増上寺, Minato Ward, Tokyo.

091
Health-related *fuda* (charm). Wood and paper. Mid-20th century. L. 30.1 cm
The inscriptions on top read:
熱田神宮 = *Atsuta Jingū* (Nagoya, Aichi Prefecture)
八雲神社 = *Yakumo Jinja* (Yakumo, Hokkaido Prefecture)
Used for 病氣平癒 = *byōki heiyu* (recovery from illness) and for 家内安全 = *kanai anzen* (household safety)

092–093
When a *mamori* (charm) for illness comes from a shrine or temple that also issues one or more *ema* for the same illness, the *mamori* and *ema* often have similar designs. The examples shown here were all collected in the 21st century.

092 from right to left:
- *Mimigo Jinja* 耳明神社, Onomichi, Hiroshima Prefecture. Design of turban shells (*sazae*) for ear illnesses. See p.141 for corresponding *ema*
- *Shiba Daijingū* 芝大神宮, Minato Ward, Tokyo. For eye illnesses
- *Shakuzōji* 石像寺, Kamigyo Ward, Kyoto Design of pincers (*kuginuki*) for pulling out pain and illness. See p.113 for corresponding *ema*
- *Yōhai Jinja* 遥拝神社, Yatsushiro, Kumamoto Prefecture. Design of catfish (*namazu*) for skin illnesses. See p.179 for corresponding *ema*

093 from right to left
- *Kinomiya Jinja* 来宮神社, Atami, Shizuoka Prefecture. Design of sake cups (*sakazuki*) for moderation in drinking (*sesshu*). See p.165 for *ema* with comparable designs
- *Goō Jinja* 護王神社, Kamigyo Ward, Kyoto Design of feet (*ashi*) for illnesses of the feet See p.147 for corresponding *ema*
- *Goō Jinja* 護王神社, Kamigyo Ward, Kyoto. Design of *bakku* (back) for illnesses of the loins.
- *Yusanji* 油山寺, Fukuroi, Shizuoka Prefecture For eye illnesses. See p.137 for corresponding *ema*

094

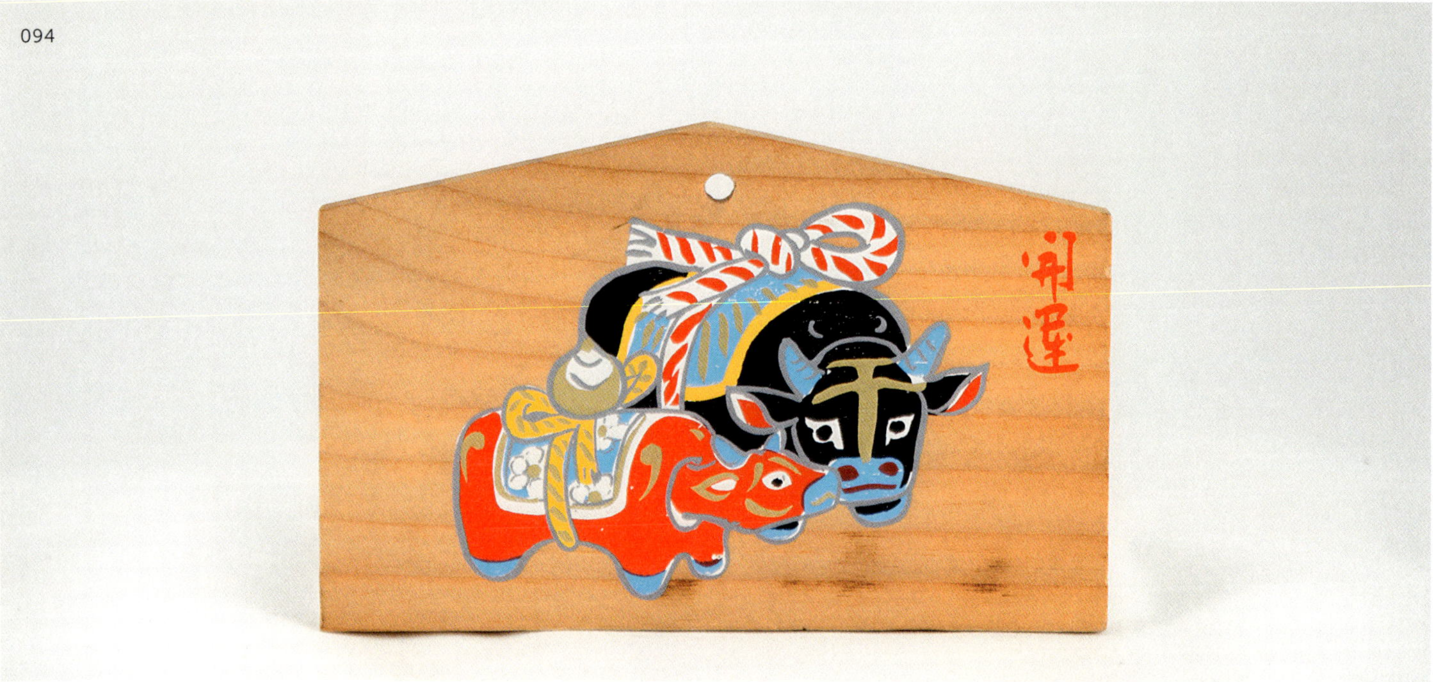

095

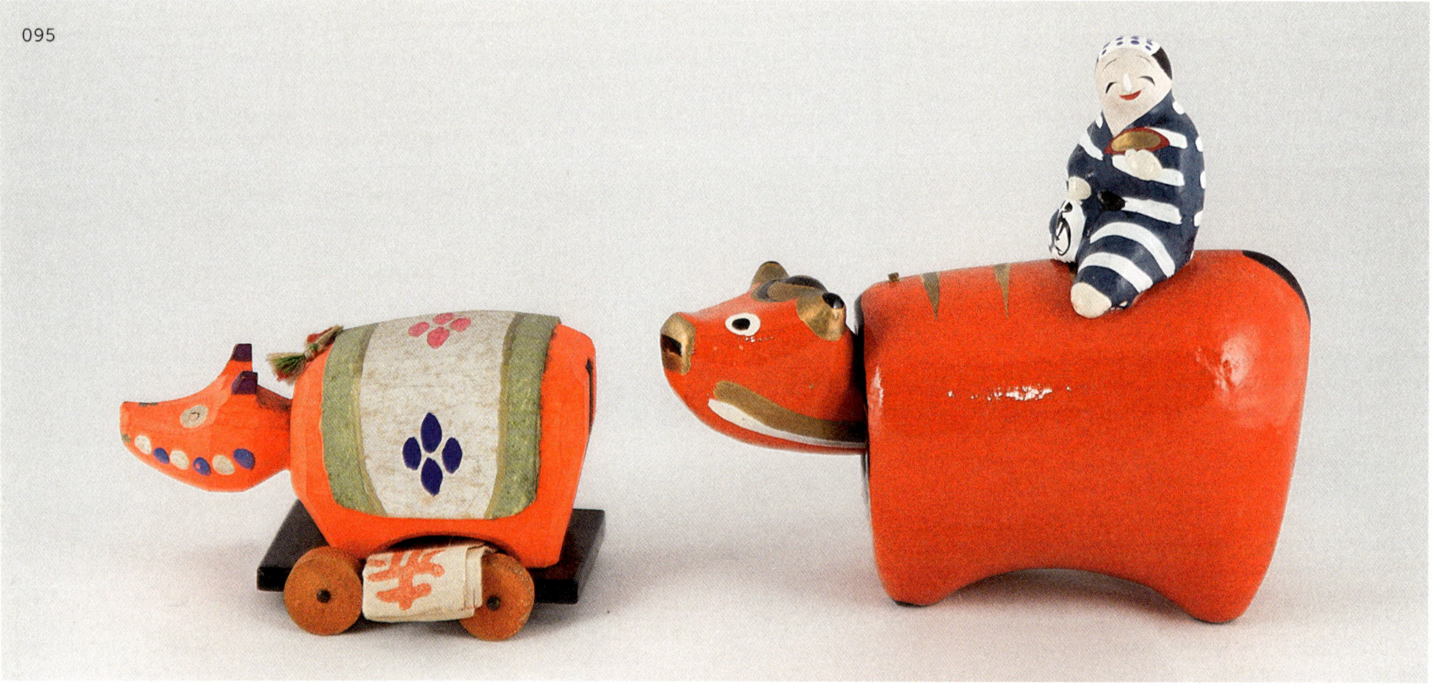

096

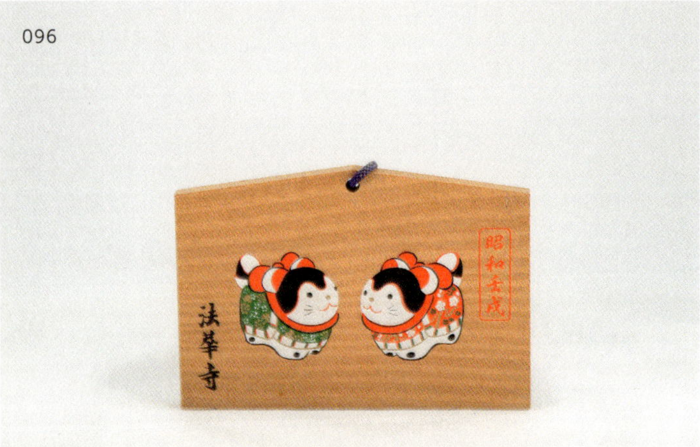

097

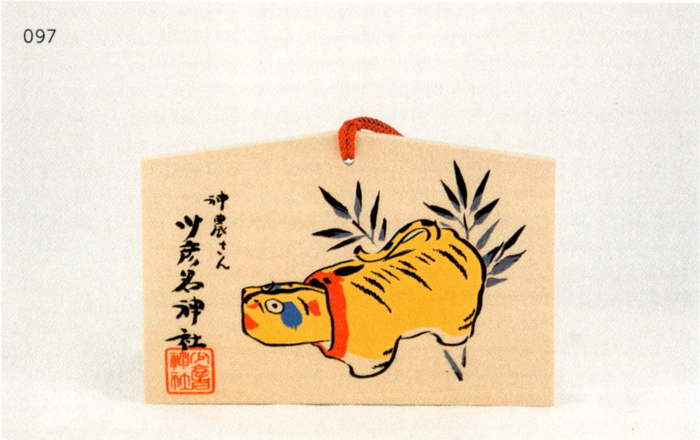

Ema designs

It is beyond the scope of this publication to review the Japanese charms that are directly or indirectly related to health or healing [e.g. GG1-2011/07]. Below, the focus is on some of the charms that have been reproduced on *ema* and that are used for health-related purposes in general. Examples of charms for specific human life issues or specific medical problems will be presented in parts three and four.

Red cow 赤べこ (*akabeko*)

Akabeko are folk toys in the form of a red cow that generally originate from Fukushima Prefecture. According to folk belief, the colour red expels demons and illness. After it had been noticed that children with an *akabeko* toy were not affected by smallpox, this type of toy became valued as an amulet against illness. It is looked upon as an omen of good luck and prosperity and is given as a gift on auspicious occasions such as New Year.

094
Ema showing red cow folk toy (*akabeko*) and black cow folk toy (*kurobeko*). Late 20th century. W. 17.6 cm

095
Akabeko folk toys made of papier-mâché (right) and wood (left). Late 20th century. L. 13 cm and 9 cm

Papier-mâché dog 犬張子 (*inuhariko*)

Since dogs are the symbol of good health and since puppies grow rapidly and are always active, toy dogs have been presented to newborn babies since ancient days as a charm for healthy growth. This happens particularly at the first visit to the shrine (*Hatsu Miyamairi*) which is a traditional rite of passage for newborns in Japan. Since female dogs can give birth to many puppies and are believed to suffer no pain in delivery, these toys also became charms for mothers for an easy delivery and for bearing many healthy children [JM-528].

096
Hokkeji 法華寺. Nara, Nara Prefecture. Late 20th century. W. 14.0 cm
The inscriptions read:
昭和壬戊 = *Shōwa jin bo* (9th and 5th calendar sign)
法華寺 = *Hokkeji*

Papier-mâché tiger 虎張子 (*torahariko*)

097
Sukunahikona Jinja 少彦名神社. Chuo Ward, Osaka. Early 21st century. W. 16.2 cm
The inscriptions read:
神農さん = *Jinnōsan* (deity of agriculture; local honorary name)
少彦名神社 = *Sukunahikona Jinja*

Sukunahikona Jinja is situated in *Doshōmachi*, the old medicine quarter of Osaka. Papier-mâché tigers have been a popular symbol of the shrine ever since Osaka suffered from an outbreak of cholera in the early 19th century. The people made such tiger figures and prayed for their health at the shrine, while pharmacists sold pills containing ground tiger skull. Cf. the entry on *Sukunahikona* on p.43.

098

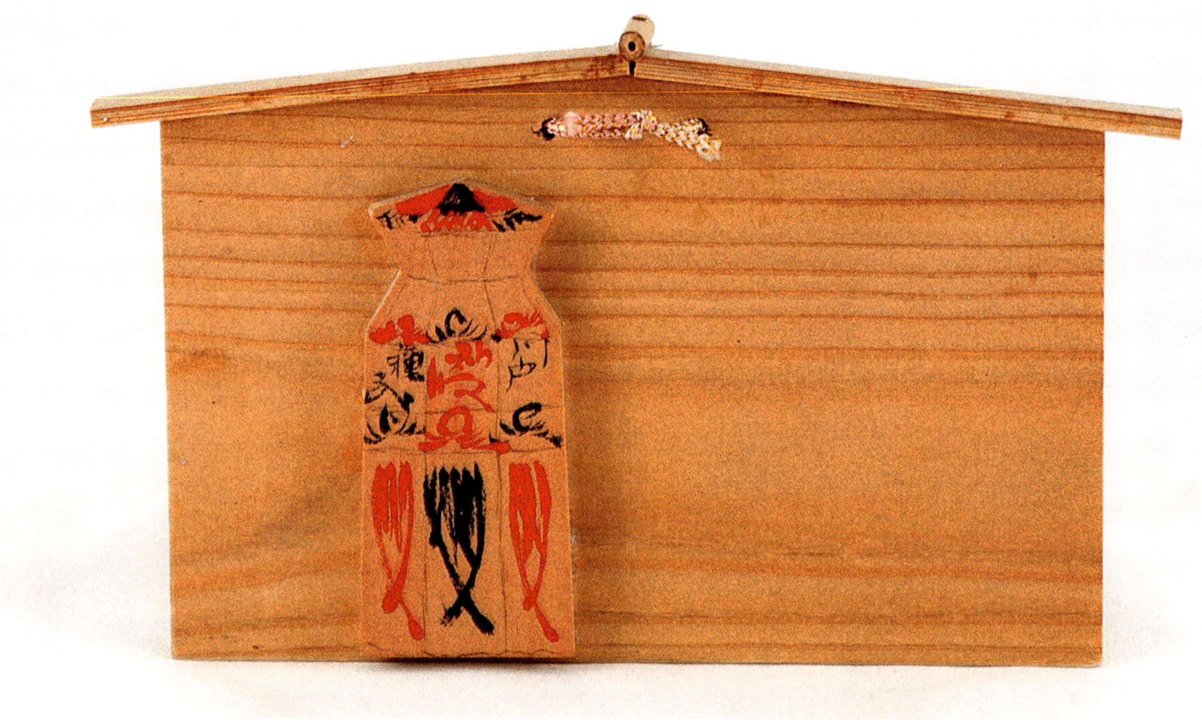

099

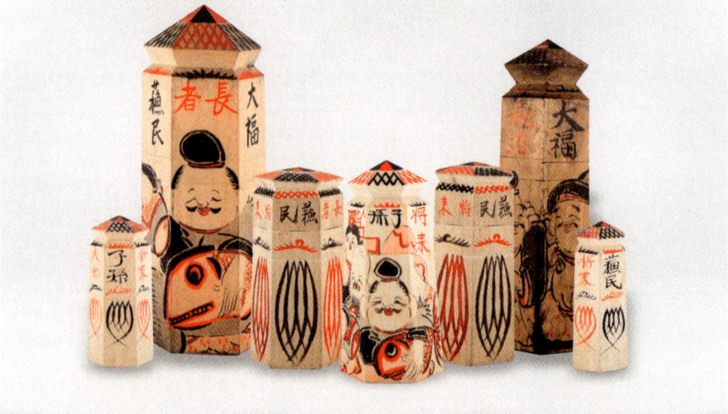

100

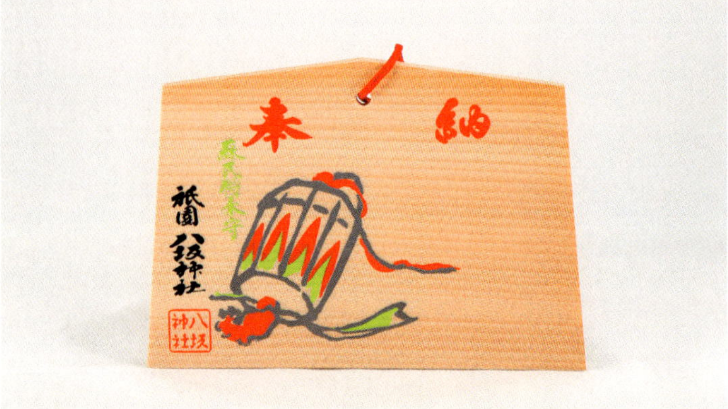

101

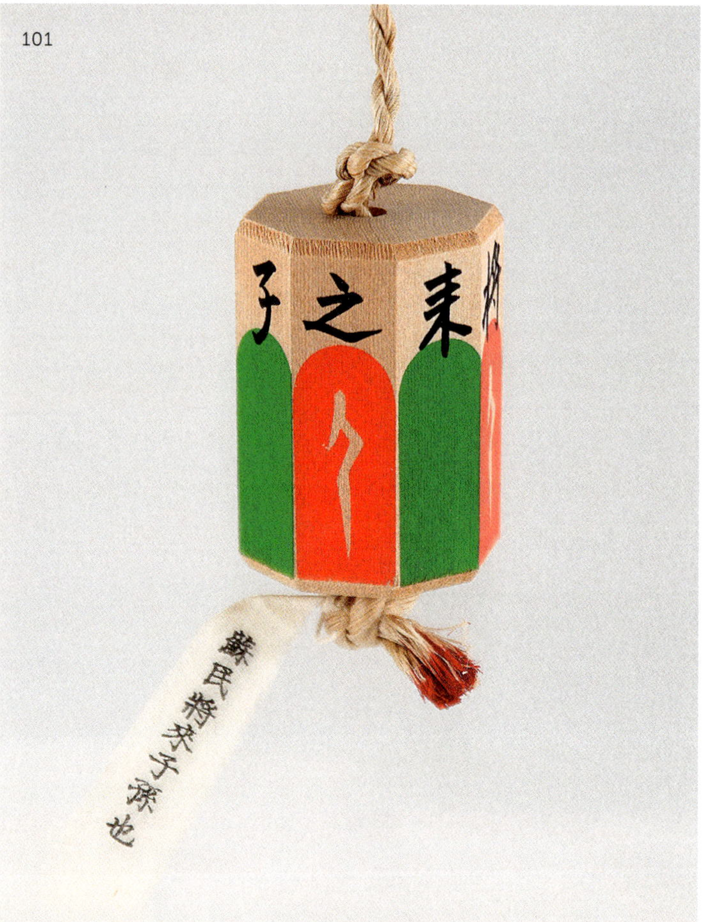

Somin Shōrai 蘇民将来

Several Japanese shrines and temples sell wooden *Somin Shōrai* charms for good luck and especially for good health and the prevention of epidemics. The underlying legendary story is that the Shinto deity *Susanoo-no-mikoto* once sought a resting place after travelling had made him tired. He came upon two brothers, a wealthy one (*Kotan Shōrai*) and a poor one (*Somin Shōrai*). While the former refused to lodge him, the latter welcomed him and shared what he had. The deity repaid his kindness by presenting *Somin* with a ring made of *chigaya* (cogon grass). Wearing this ring around his waist would ward off epidemics. By doing the same and by declaring that they were descendants of *Somin Shōrai*, his offspring would enjoy similar patronage.

The charms are mostly pillar-shaped, hexagonal or octagonal talismans made of the willow tree. Kanji found on such charms include: 蘇民 = *Somin*; 蘇民将来 = *Somin Shōrai*; 子孫 = *shison* = descendants, posterity; 大福 = *daifuku* (great fortune, good luck); 長者 = *chōja* (one's superior; one's senior). Small amulets may be used as charms for children to wear while larger pieces may be offered at an altar. The most famous source of *Somin Shōrai* charms is an annual market at *Shinano Kokubunji*, Nagano Prefecture, where two different types are sold: the regular type and the so-called *e-Somin* (painted with figural images and motifs). The former type is cut by nearby farmers and decorated with symbols and letters by the temple staff. The *e-Somin* type is made by families of parishioners, each of which has its own unique design, such as treasure ships, *Daruma* or the *Shichifukujin* (Seven Gods of Good Fortune) [GG1-2011/09].

Other sanctuaries that sell or have sold *ema* with *Somin Shōrai* charms are *Shinano Kokubunji* (Ueda, Nagano Prefecture) and *Owari Tsushima Jinja*, Tsushima, Aichi Prefecture (not illustrated here).

098
Takedera 竹寺. Minami, Saitama Prefecture. Early 21st century. W. 14.8 cm

099
Somin Shōrai charms. Early to late 20th century. H. 8.9 to 24.1 cm

100
Yasaka Jinja 八坂神社. Higashiyama Ward, Kyoto. Early 21st century. W. 15.2 cm
The inscriptions read:
祇園八坂神社 = *Gion Yasaka Jinja*
八坂神社 = *Yasaka Jinja*

101
Somin Shōrai charm. *Yasaka Jinja* 八坂神社 Higashiyama Ward, Kyoto. Early 21st century. H. 7.0 cm (without string)

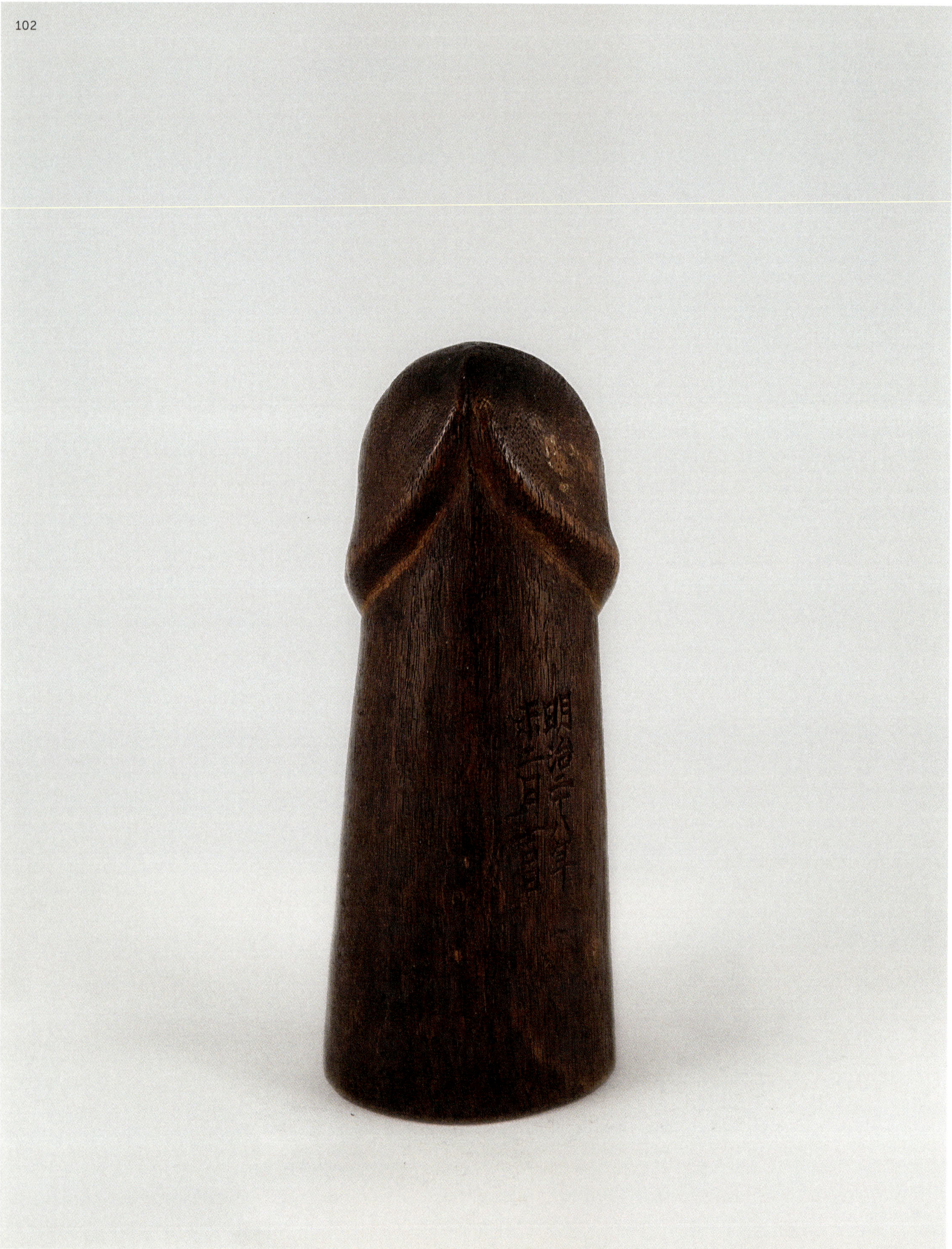

3

Human life
人の一生
(*Hito no isshō*)

102
Wooden effigy of a phallus. Late 19th century.
H. 12.5 cm
The inscriptions read:
明治二十八 = *Meiji ni jū hachi* (Meiji 28 = 1895)
十二月 = *jūni gatsu* (12th month = December)
吉日 = *kichinichi* (lucky day)

This explicit sign of virility and fertility may have served as a votive, a souvenir, a lucky charm (*engimono*) or an object of worship. As such, it may have been connected with praying for *gokokuhōjō* (abundant harvests), *shōbai hanjō* (prosperous business) or *kodakara* (the treasure that is children) [KM-126; 1].

A health-related category of *goriyaku* (benefits) that the Japanese treat separately from *byōki heiyu* (recovery from illness) is that of *hito no isshō* (human life). Its issues range from *kodakara* (the treasure that is children), *anzan* (easy delivery), *junyū* (breastfeeding) and *kosodate* (child rearing) to wishes for *chōju* (longevity) and *pokkuri* (a sudden painless death). Wishes concerning *kenkō* (health in general) and *mizuko* (which literally means water child and refers to an aborted, stillborn or miscarried foetus) are also included.
As these human life issues are less strictly medical than recovery from illness, only a modest selection of *ema* for these purposes is represented here.

103

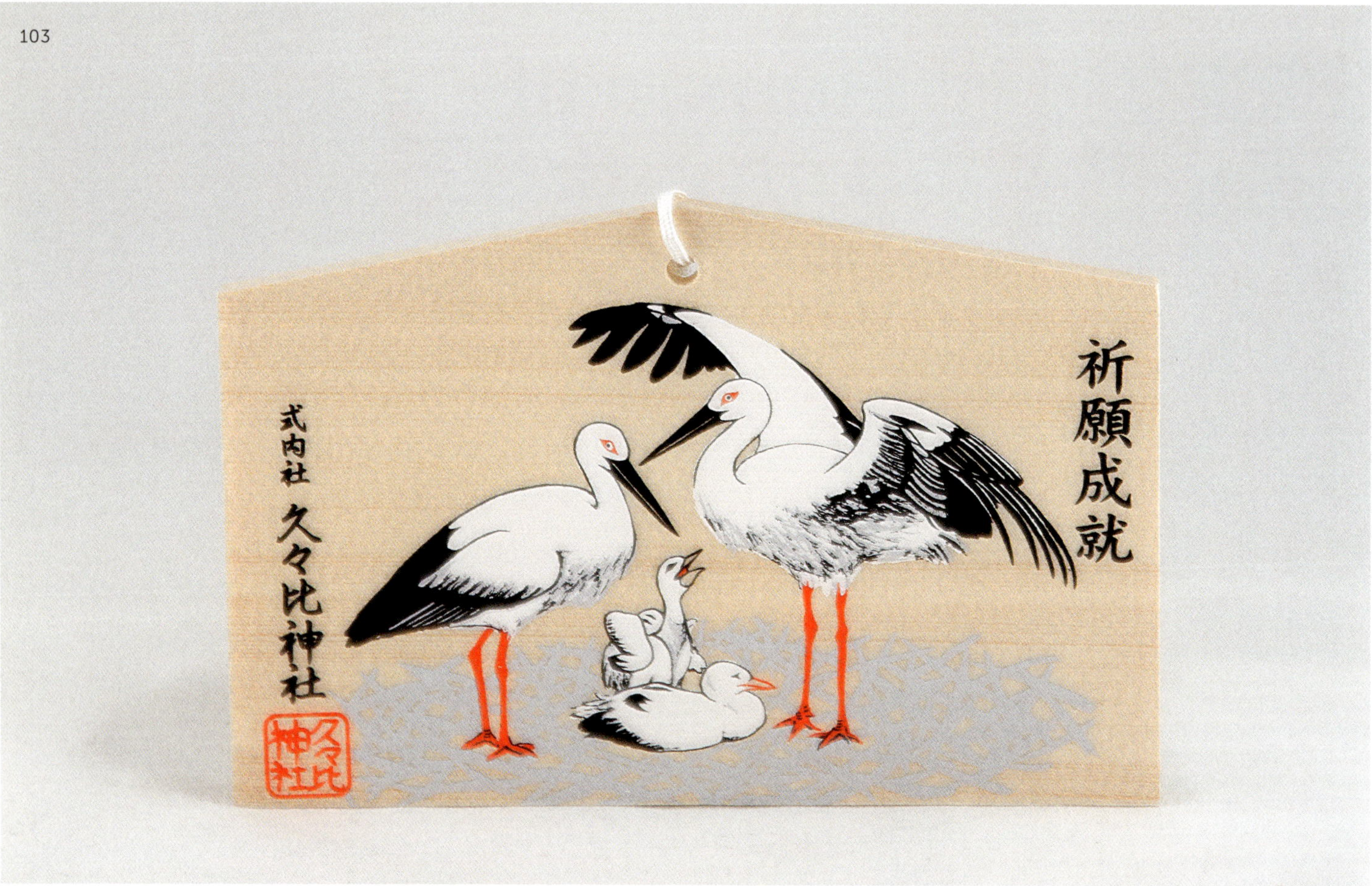

104

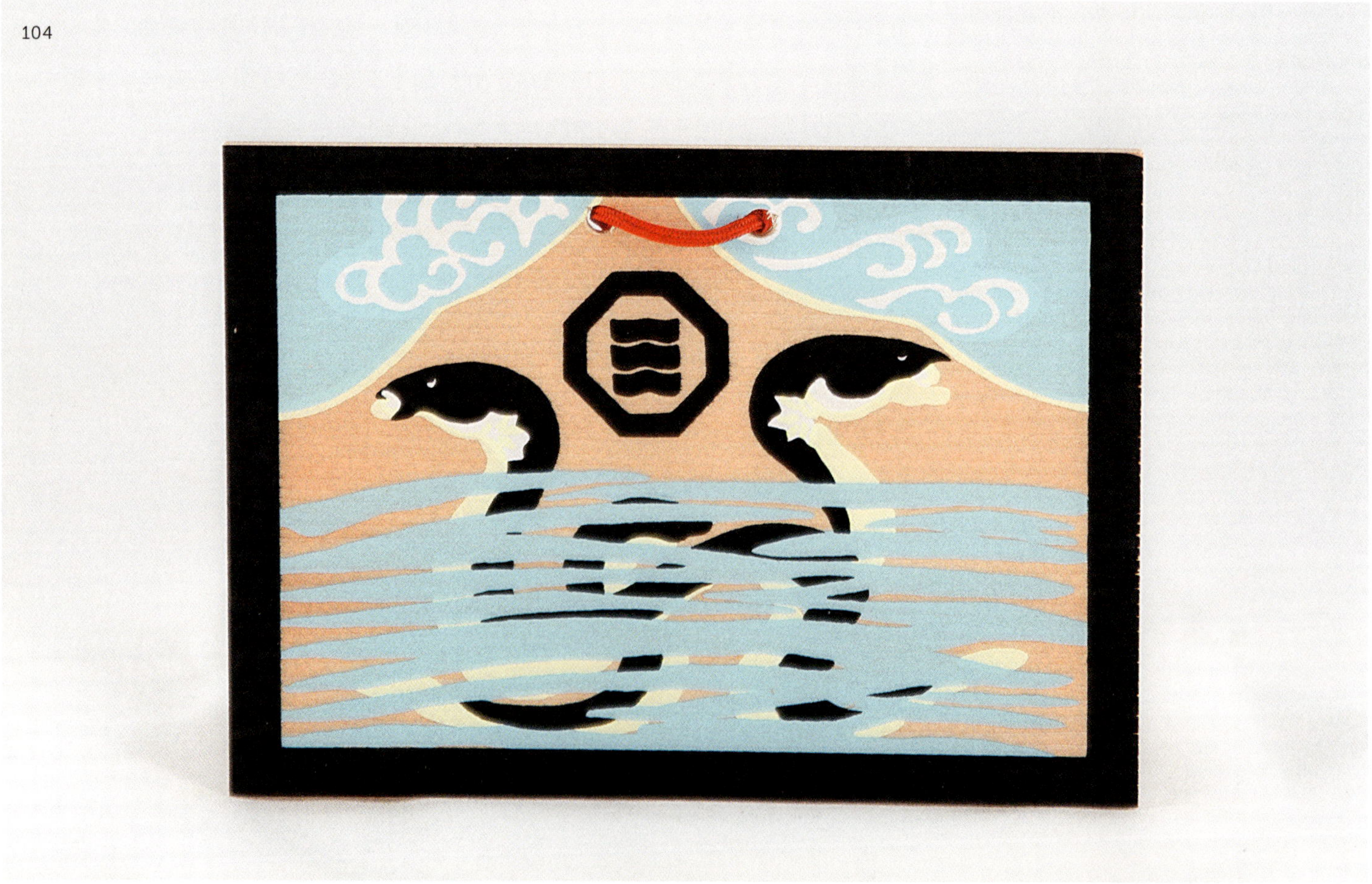

The treasure that is children 子宝 (*kodakara*)

Background

Prayers for *kodakara* (the treasure that is children) or *kosazuke* (to be blessed with a child) relate to the desire to have children and to issues surrounding fertility (*ninyōnō*) and infertility (*funinshō*).

A common measure of fertility is the so-called total fertility rate (TFR), which represents the average number of children that would be born per woman if all women lived to the end of their childbearing years and bore children according to the current age-specific fertility rate at each age. As the TFR refers to births per woman, it is a more direct measure of the level of fertility than the crude birth rate. In theory, the TFR could become as high as 35 births per woman, but the highest value that has actually been observed anywhere in the world is 10.9 [2]. In Japan, the TFR has gradually decreased from 5.10 in 1925 to 1.41 in 2012, in spite of the new biomedical treatments for infertility that became possible in the second half of the 20th century. It has been suggested that 10-15% of the current Japanese population in the reproductive age may consist of individuals with potential fertility problems. Among the many reasons are primarily lifestyle factors (such as late marriage, late childbearing, psychological stress, increased smoking rates among young women, and weight abnormalities). Medical reasons include gynaecologic disorders and sexually transmitted diseases (such as chlamydia) [SY15; 3]. Fear of the future also played a role in the late 20th century.

More likely than not, fertility issues made a substantial contribution to the stagnation of the Japanese population growth in the 18th and early 19th centuries. It has been suggested that the more relevant underlying causes included the absence of spouses due to *dekasegi* (temporary migration for labour) and *seibyō* (venereal diseases) [4].

Ema designs

Oriental stork 鸛 *(kōnotori)*

103
Kukuhi Jinja 久々比神社. Toyoka, Hyogo Prefecture. Early 21st century. W. 15.5 cm
The inscriptions read:
祈願成就 = *kigan jōju* (prayer for fulfilment of all wishes)
式内社 = *shikinaisha* (shrine registered in set of ancient governmental regulations)
久々比神社= *Kukuhi Jinja*

Eels 鰻 *(unagi)*

The *ema* design of two *unagi* (eels) can be used for *kosazuke kigan* (prayer for being blessed with a child) and for marital harmony [FS-18; TS-6; IH2-46; NM-Z22713].

104
Mishima Jinja 三嶋神社. Higashiyama Ward, Kyoto. Early 21st century. W. 15.5 cm

Mishima Jinja also sells an *ema* with three eels for easy delivery and abundant offspring (see p.87).

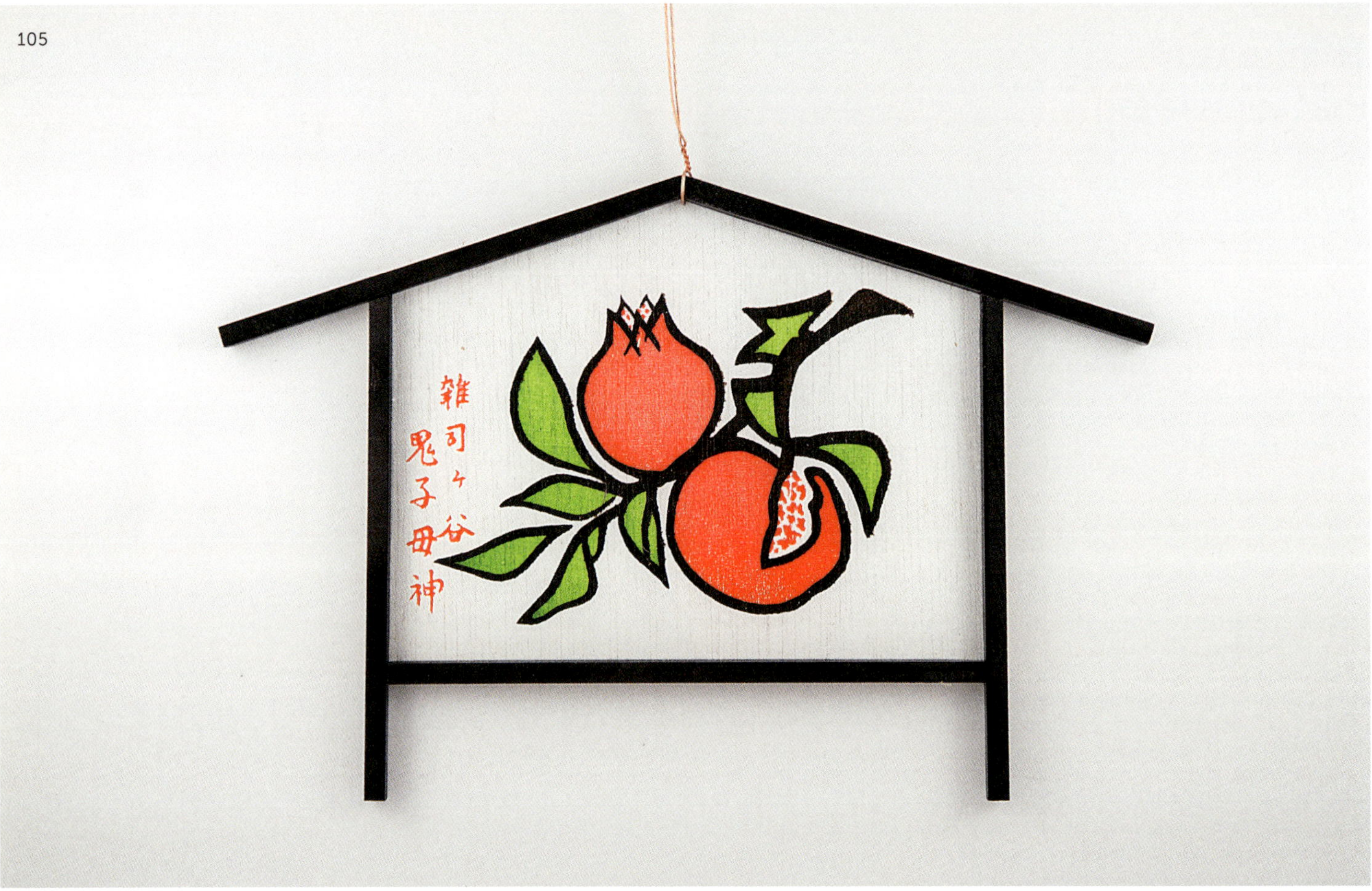

105

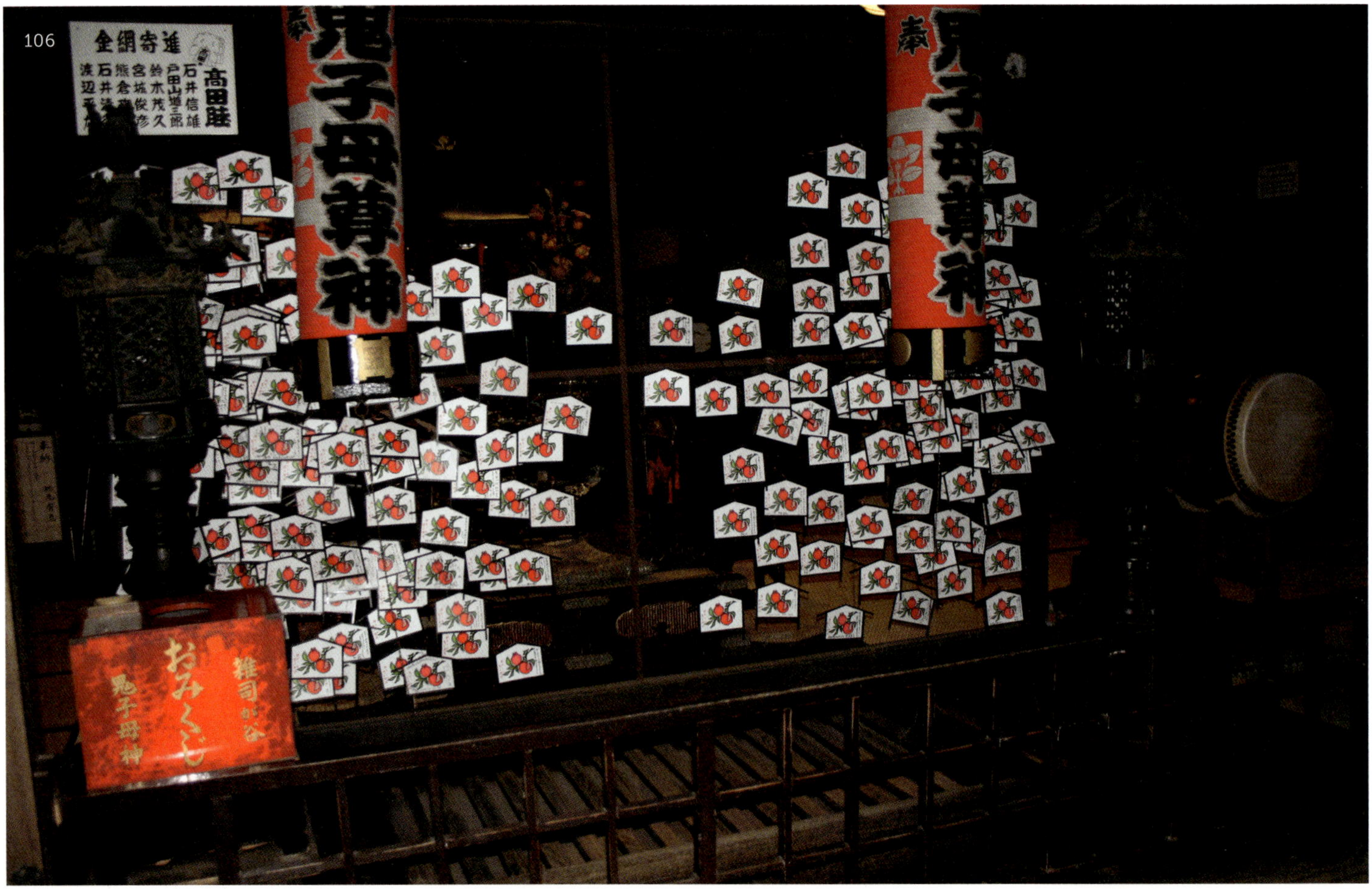

106

Pomegranate 石榴 *(zakuro)*

As the *zakuro* (pomegranate) has many seeds, this *ema* design is intended for *kodakara* (the treasure that is children) and for *anzan* (easy delivery) [TS-9; IH2-48,50].

105
Kishimojindō 鬼子母神堂. Toshima Ward, Tokyo. Hand-painted *ema*. Early 21st century. W. 18.1 cm
The inscriptions read:
雑司ケ谷 = *Zōshigaya*
鬼子母神 = *Kishimojin* (neighbourhood in Toshima Ward)

Kishimojin is a female deity of children and childbirth, who is often portrayed with a child in her arms or holding a branch or fruit of the pomegranate in her hand.
Another *ema* design with a pomegranate is offered by *Konzōji* (Zentsji, Kagawa Prefecture).

106
Zakuro (pomegranate) *ema* at *Kishimojindō* (Toshima Ward, Tokyo).

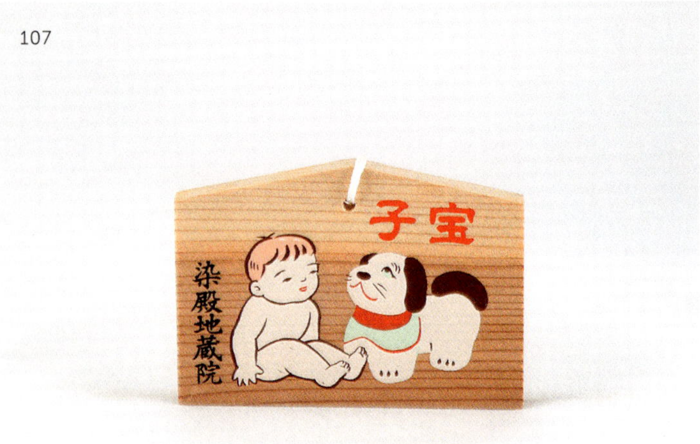

107

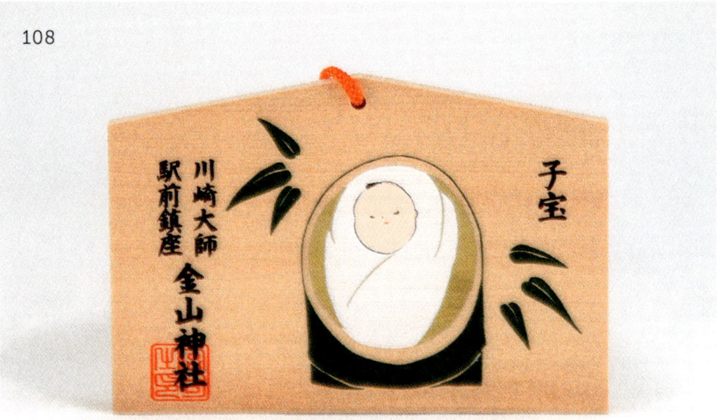

108

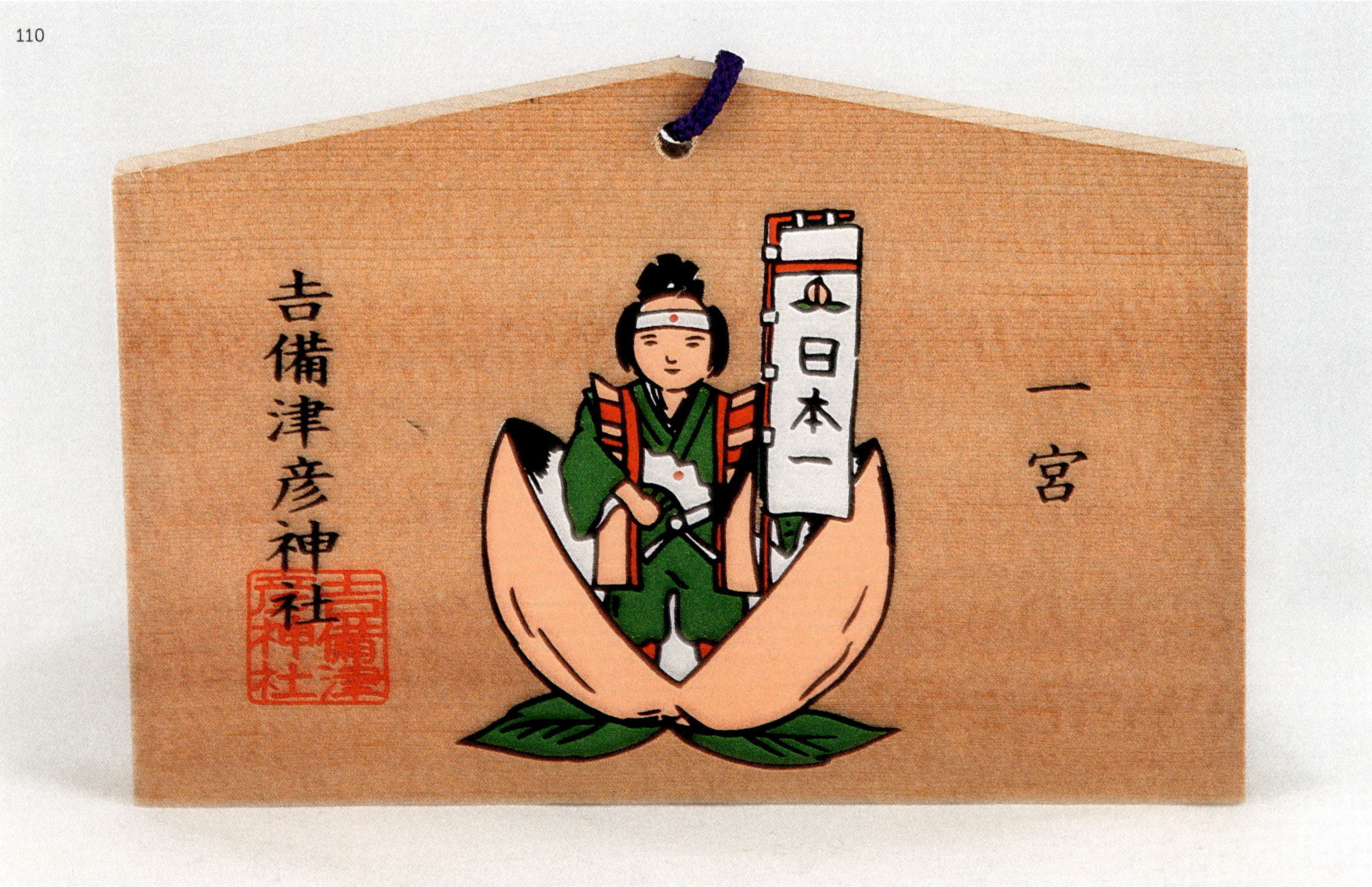

110

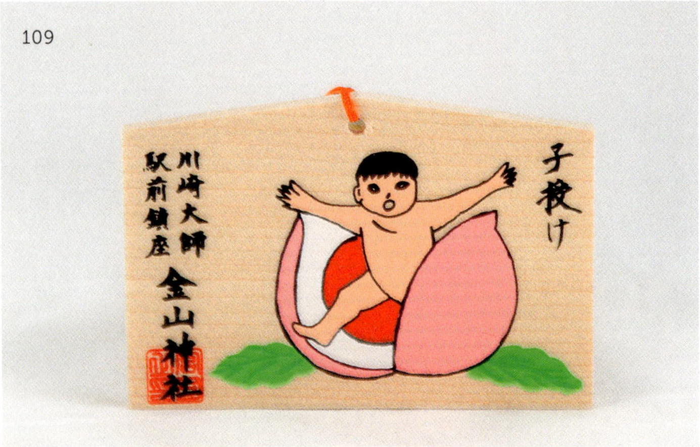

109

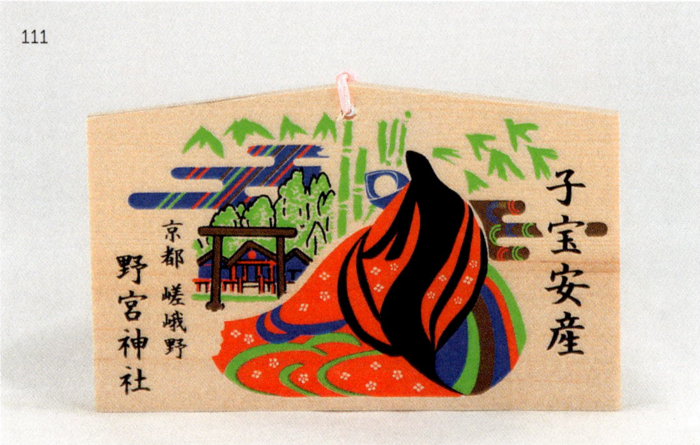

111

Infant and dog 乳児と犬 *(nyūji to inu)*

Ema portraying an *inu* (dog) do not always represent this animal as a zodiac sign, but can also relate to *kodakara* (the treasure that is children) or *anzan kigan* (prayer for easy childbirth), when they are inscribed as such. The association is that dogs give birth easily [GG2-2013/04; EO-183].

107
Somedono Jizōin 染殿地蔵院. Nakaygyo Ward, Kyoto. Late 20th century. W. 9.1 cm
The inscriptions read:
子宝 = *kodakara* (the treasure that is children)
染殿地蔵院 = *Somedono Jizōin*

Princess Kaguya かぐや姫 *(Kaguya Hime) and Peach Boy* 桃太郎 *(Momotarō)*

These figures occur in popular Japanese folk legends and stories in which childless people are blessed by the gods with the gift of children who magically appear and bring them blessings. The implication is that the children are a reward for having led good lives.

Kaguya Hime (Princess *Kaguya*) was discovered as a baby inside the stalk of a bamboo plant by an old childless bamboo cutter. *Momotarō* (Peach Boy) came to earth inside a giant peach, which was found floating down a river by an old childless woman. When she and her husband opened the peach to eat it, they discovered the child, who explained that he had been sent by heaven to be their son.

108
Princess *Kaguya* かぐや姫 (*Kaguya Hime*) *Kanayama Jinja* 金山神社 (in precincts of *Wakamiya Hachimangū*), Kawasaki, Kanagawa Prefecture. Early 21st century. W. 12.9 cm
The inscriptions read:
子宝 = *kodakara* (the treasure that is children)
川崎大師 駅前鎮座 = *Kawasaki Daishi ekimae chinza* (enshrined near *Kawasaki Daishi* station)
金山神社 = *Kanayama Jinja*

109
Peach Boy 桃太郎 (*Momotarō*). *Kanayama Jinja* 金山神社 (in precincts of *Wakamiya Hachimangū*), Kawasaki, Kanagawa Prefecture. Early 21st century. W. 12.5 cm
The inscriptions read:
子授け= *kosazuke* (to be blessed with a child)
川崎大師 駅前鎮座 = *Kawasaki Daishi ekimae chinza* (enshrined near *Kawasaki Daishi* station)
金山神社 = *Kanayama Jinja*

110
Peach Boy 桃太郎 (*Momotarō*). *Kibitsuhiko Jinja* 吉備津彦神社. Okayama, Okayama Prefecture. Late 20th century. W. 15.0 cm
The inscriptions read:
一宮 = *Ichinomiya* (location of shrine)
日本一 (on banner) = *nihon-ichi* (Japan's number one)
吉備津彦神社 = *Kibitsuhiko Jinja*

This *ema* is most probably intended to ask for *kosazuke* (to be blessed with a child). It shows the emergence of *Momotarō* from his peach (cf. the previous *ema*). The fan in his right hand and his headband are decorated with the red sun of the Japanese flag.

Worship with baby 赤子との参拝 *(akago to no sanpai)*

111
Nonomiya Jinja 野宮神社. Sagano Ward, Kyoto Early 21st century. W. 14.0 cm
The inscriptions read:
子宝 = *kodakara* (the treasure that is children)
安産 = *anzan* (easy delivery)
京都 嵯峨野 = *Kyōto Sagano*
野宮神社 = *Nonomiya Jinja*

The *ema* displays a female dressed in a *jūnihitoe* (twelve-layered ceremonial kimono worn by court ladies). She is sitting in front of a *torii* (shrine gate) while holding a baby.

The shrine is famous as one of the scenes of the *Genji Monogatari*, a classic masterwork of Japanese literature attributed to a noblewoman from the 11th century.

112

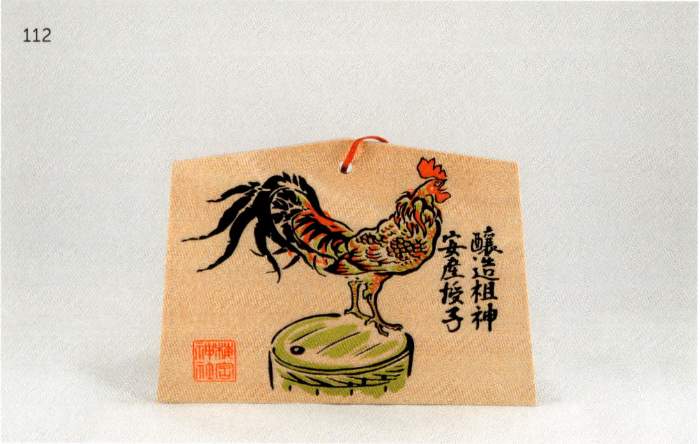

113

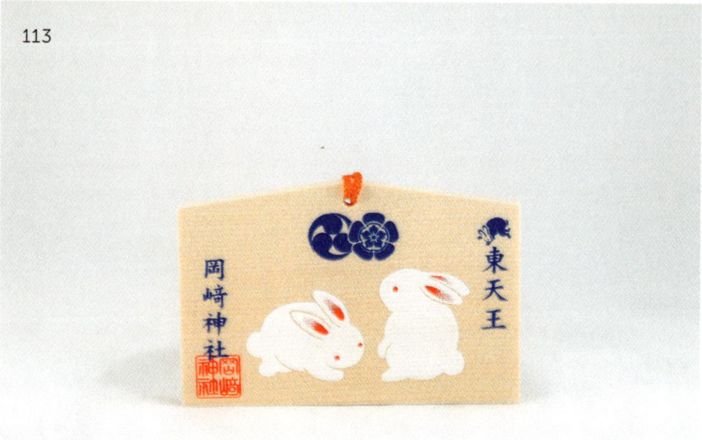

114

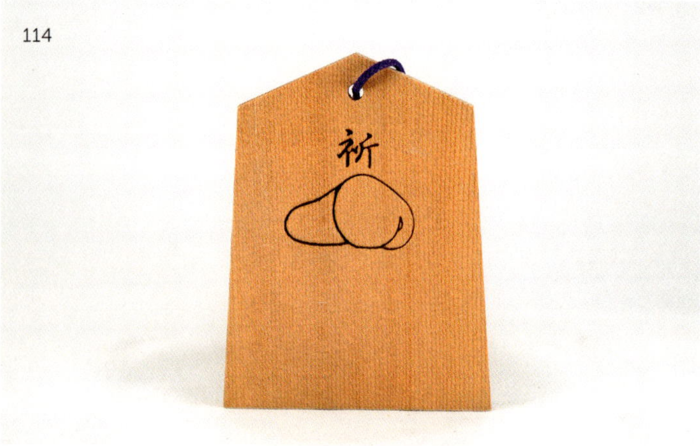

116

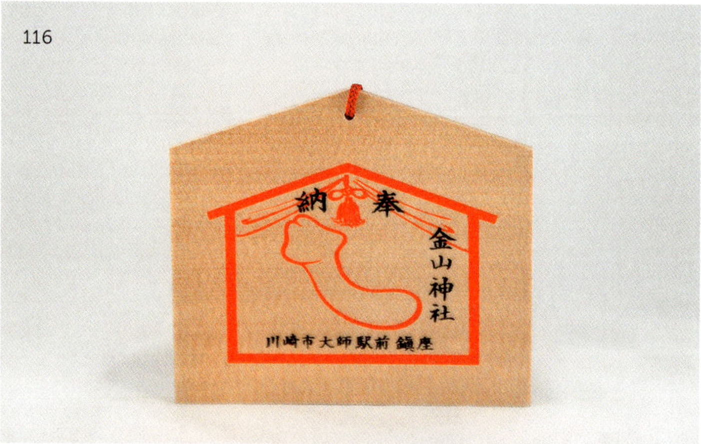

115

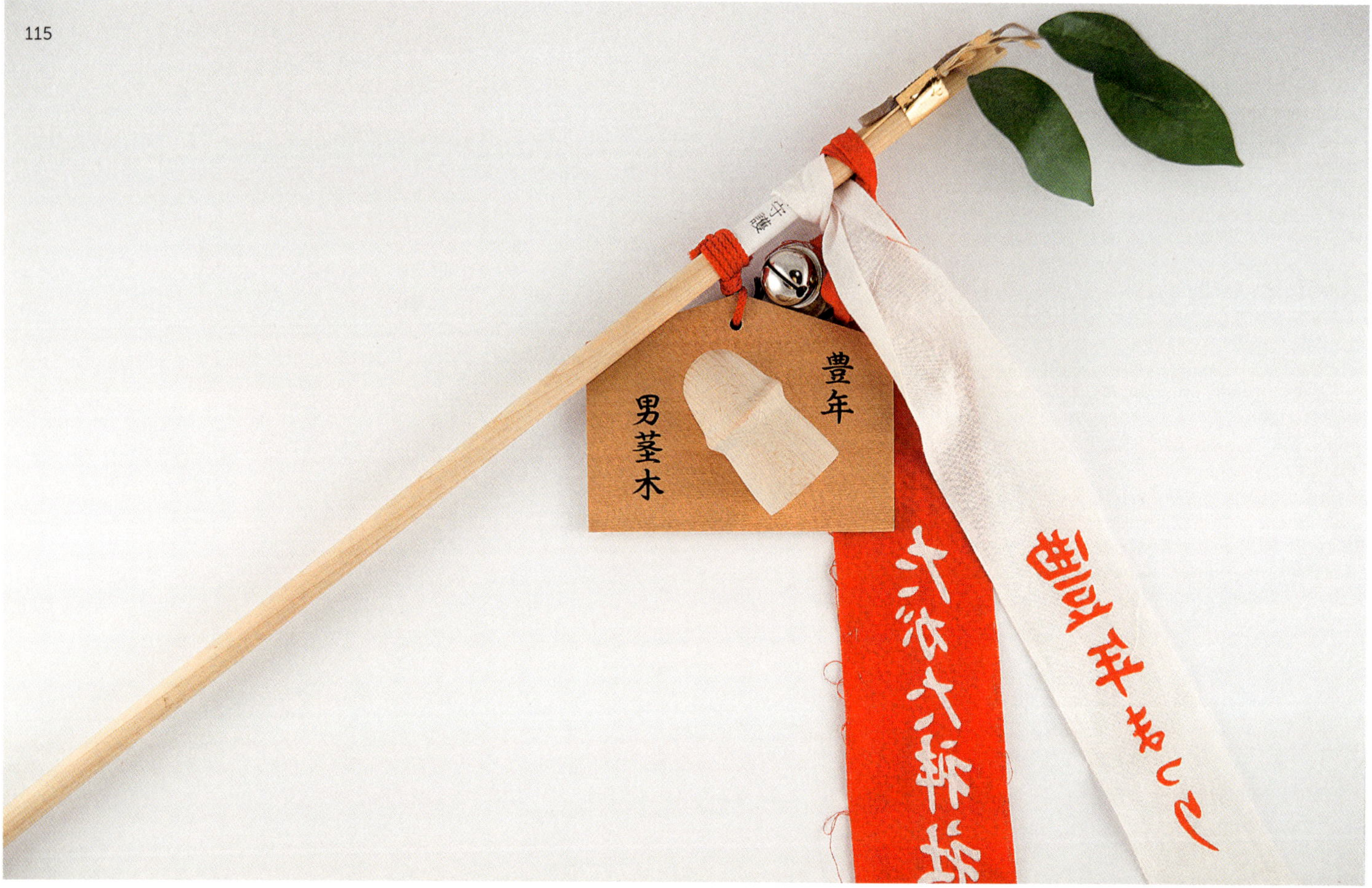

Rooster on top of barrel of sake 酒の樽の上に雄鶏 *(sake no taru no ue ni ondori)*

112
Umemiya Taisha 梅宮大社. Ukyo Ward, Kyoto. Early 21st century. W. 15.2 cm
The inscriptions read:
醸造祖神 = *Jōzō Sojin* (ancestral deity of sake brewing)
安産授子 = *anzan jushi* (easy childbirth; to be granted a child)

Sake brewers worship at the shrine and offer barrels of sake there every year, because it enshrines *Oyamazumi-no-kami* (the deity who first brewed sake).

Also enshrined is his daughter *Konohana-no-sakuyahime-no-mikoto*. As she gave birth to a child the day following her marriage, the shrine attracts women wishing for *kodakara* (the treasure that is children) or *anzan* (easy delivery). A woman can ask for *kodakara* by sitting on *matage ishi* (a large stone with two egg-shaped stones on top of it).

Rabbit 兎 *(usagi)*

113
Okazaki Jinja 岡崎神社. Sakyo Ward, Kyoto. Early 21st century. W. 13.5 cm
The inscriptions read:
東天王 = *Higashi Tennō* (location of shrine)
岡崎神社 = *Okazaki Jinja*

The *usagi* (rabbit) is one of the zodiac animals, but this particular *ema* is not meant to celebrate the Year of the Rabbit. Since early times the originating shrine has served as a place to pray for fertility, easy delivery and warding off evil. The rabbit is considered a helper spirit of the shrine (because of the many rabbits in the mountain behind the shrine).

Phallus 男根 *(dankon)*

Ema with a *dankon* (phallus) design are often associated with a desire for fertility or a wish to be cured from a venereal disorder [TS-10; IR; RT-194].

114
Tagata Jinja 田縣神社. Komaki, Aichi Prefecture. Late 20th century. W. 10.6 cm
The inscription reads: 祈 [り] = *inori* (prayer)

115
Tagata Jinja 田縣神社. Komaki, Aichi Prefecture. Late 20th century. W. 10.0 cm; stick L. 50 cm
The inscriptions read:
豊年 = *hōnen* (fruitful year)
男茎木 = *okō ki* (male stem tree)
たがた神社 [on red banner] = *Tagata Jinja*
豊年まつり [on white banner] = *Hōnen matsuri* (lit. fruitful year festival)

116
Kanayama Jinja 金山神社 (in precincts of *Wakamiya Hachimangū*). Kawasaki, Kanagawa Prefecture. Early 21st century. W. 14.3 cm
The inscriptions read:
金山神社 = *Kanayama Jinja*
奉納 = *hōnō* (dedication, offering)
川崎市大師駅前鎮座 = *Kawasakishi Daishi ekimae chinza* (enshrined near Kawasaki City Daishi station)

Kanayama Jinja houses the god of blacksmiths. Each spring, *Kanamara matsuri* (Festival of the steel phallus) is held. This festival owes its name to the legend of a sharp-toothed demon who resided in the vagina of a young woman and wielded his sharp teeth against her male companions. The woman sought help from a blacksmith, who forged an iron phallus to break the demon's teeth. The festival was originally popular among prostitutes, who prayed for prosperous business and protection from venereal diseases, but it is now celebrated to wish for children, marriage, marital harmony, and easy delivery. In recent years, it has also been used to raise funds for HIV/AIDS research.

117

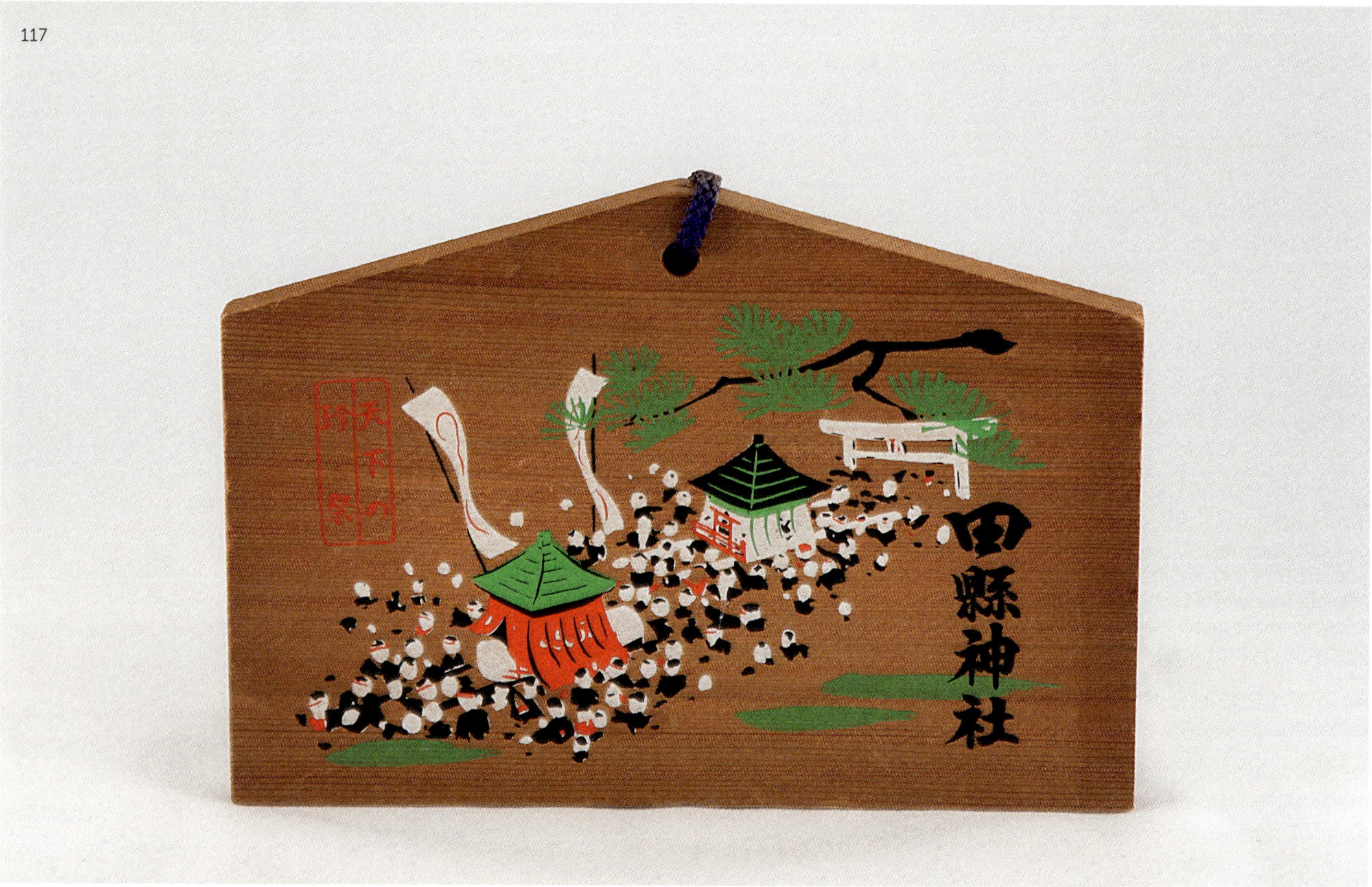

118

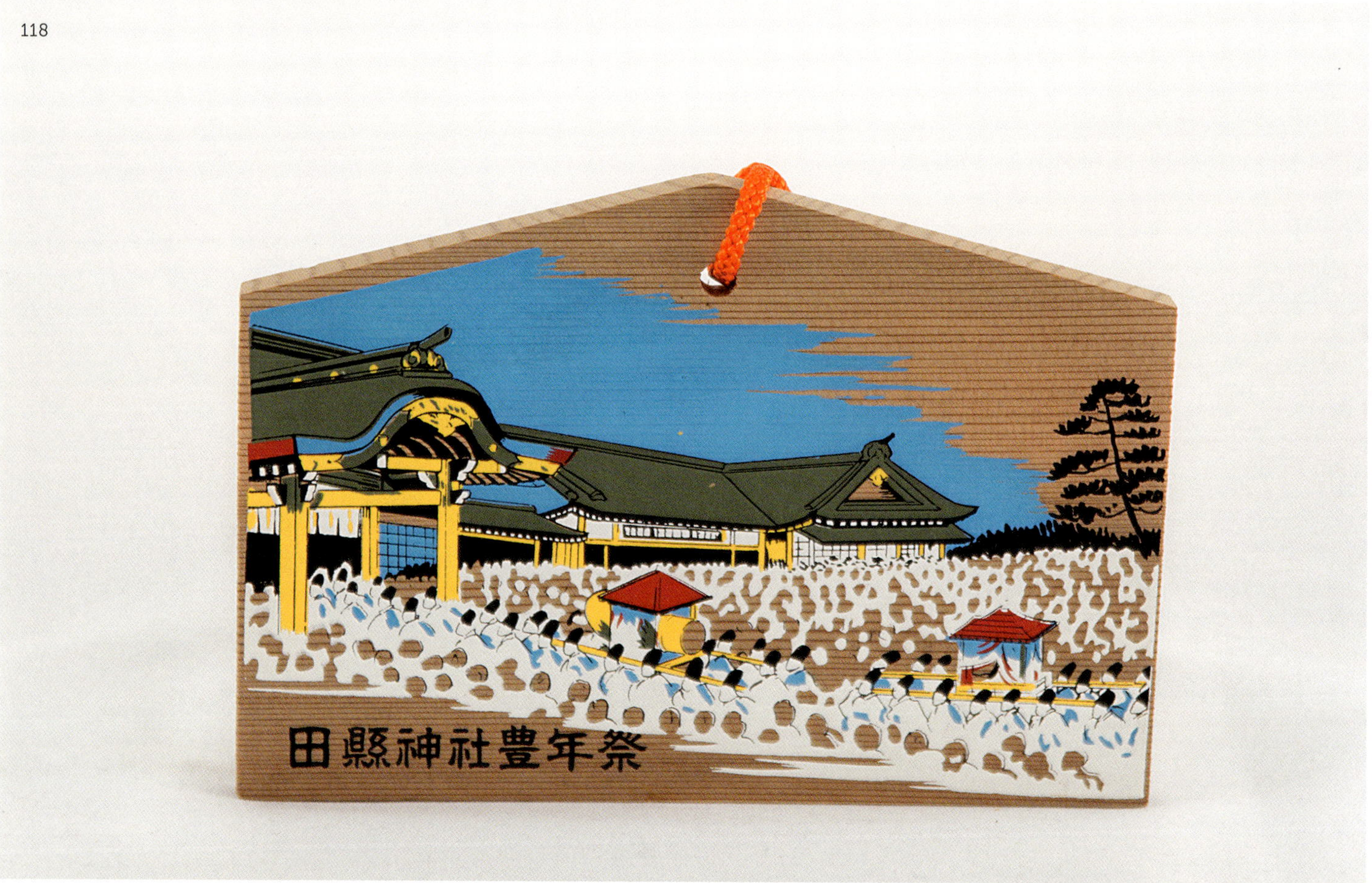

Giant stalk shape 大男茎形 *(ōotoko kukinari)*

During the year, *Tagata Jinja* (Aichi Prefecture) is mostly visited by couples who come to ask for *kodakara* (the treasure that is children) or to give thanks for *anzan* (easy delivery).

On 15 March of each year, the shrine becomes the stage for *Hōnen matsuri* (Fruitful year festival). This festival was organised in the past to ensure a bountiful harvest, but now also celebrates other kinds of prosperity and fertility [5]. The *ema* presented below portray the procession in which a giant "stalk shape" (wooden phallus) is carried in a *mikoshi* (portable shrine) to symbolise the visit of a male deity (*Takeinadane*) to its female counterpart (*Tamahime-no-mikoto*).

117

Tagata Jinja 田縣神社. Komaki, Aichi Prefecture.
Late 20th century. W. 16.6 cm.
The inscription on the right reads:
田縣神社 = *Tagata Jinja*

118

Tagata Jinja 田縣神社. Komaki, Aichi Prefecture.
Mid-20th century. W. 16.8 cm
The inscription reads:
田縣神社豊年祭 = *Tagata Jinja hōnen matsuri*
(*Tagata* shrine fruitful year festival)

119

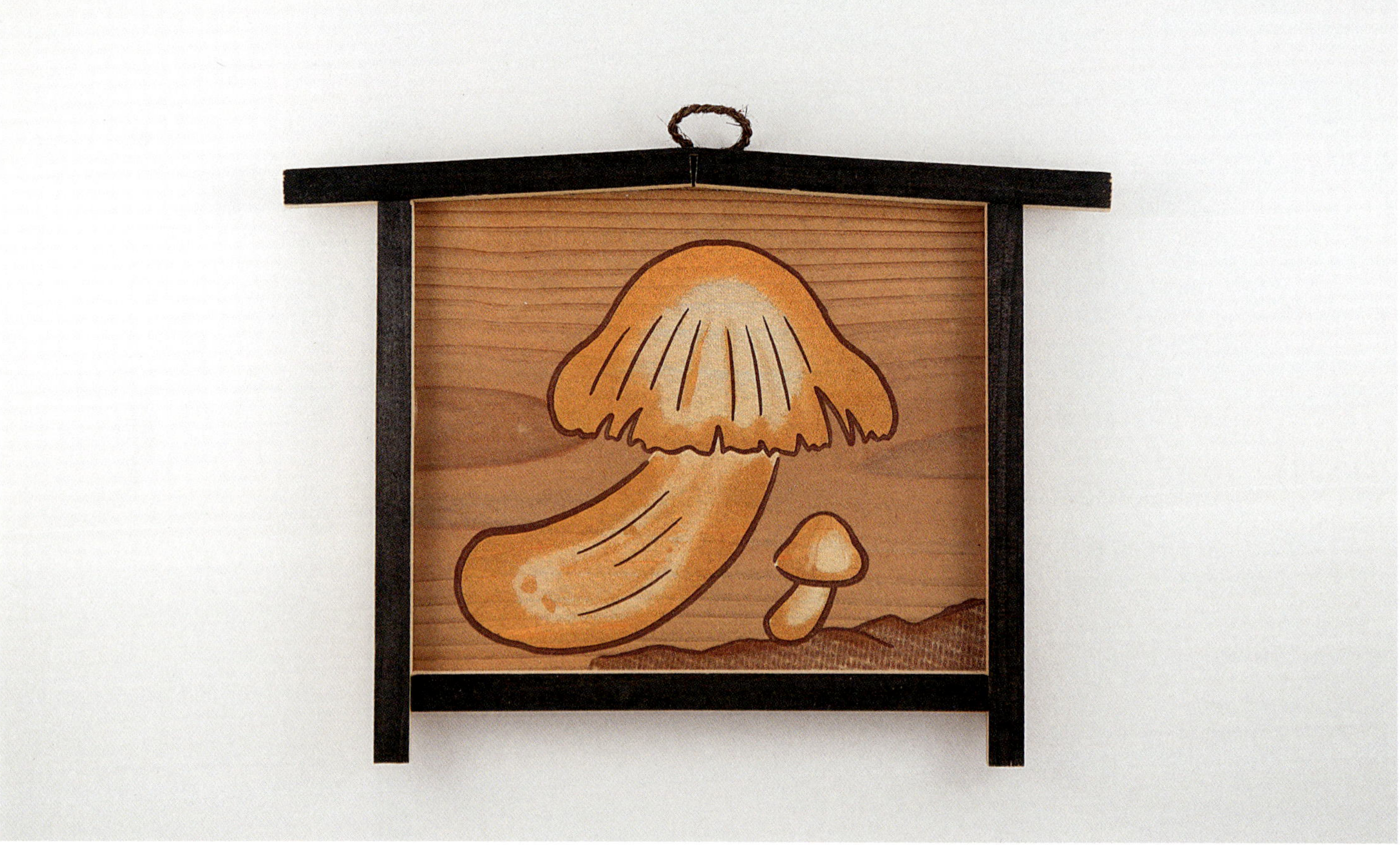

120

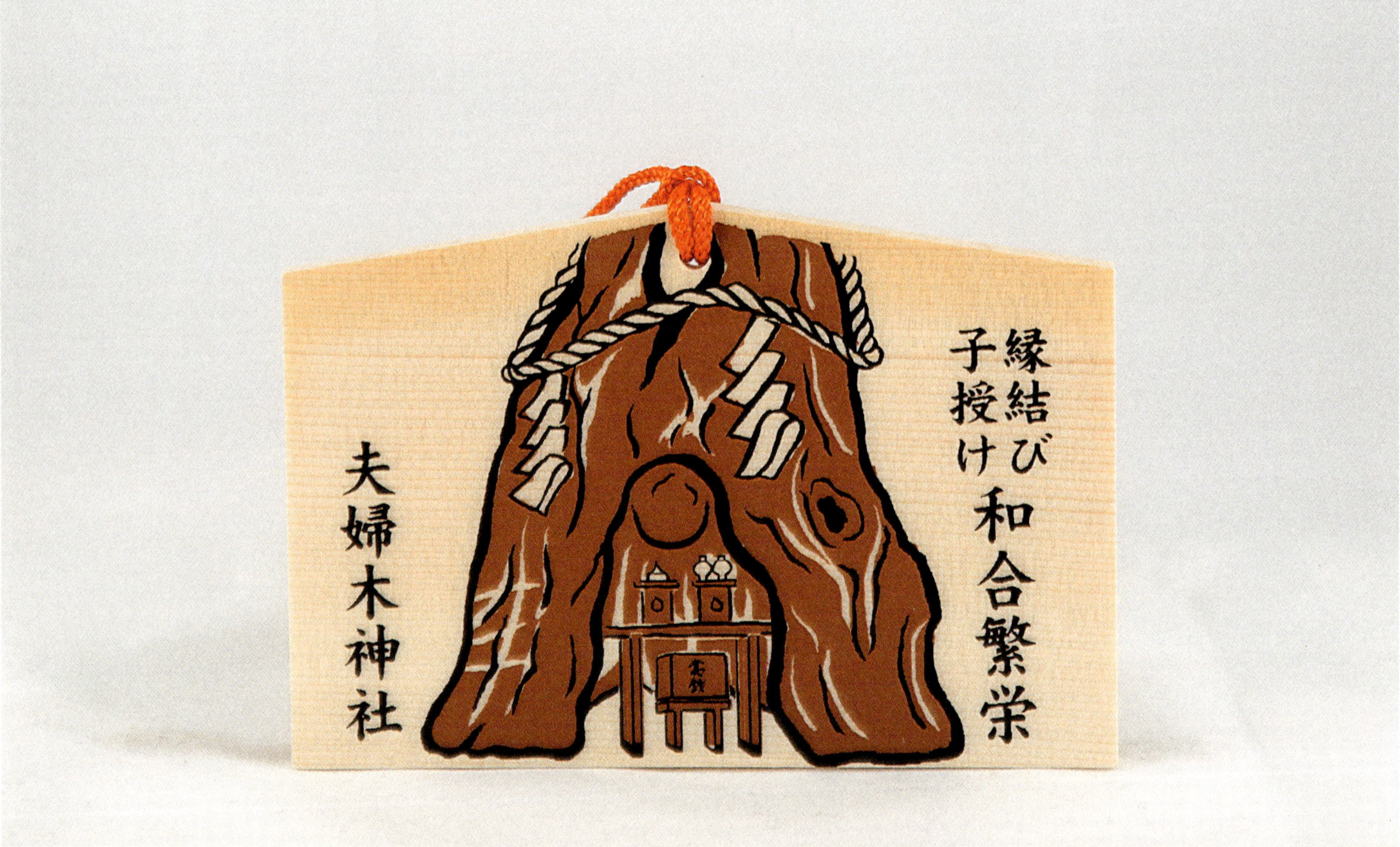

Mushroom 松茸 *(matsutake)*

Since the mushroom resembles a phallus, its display on *ema* can serve as a phallic symbol [TS-16].

119
Hand-painted reproduction for a Japanese club of *ema* collectors called *Nihon Ema Tomo no Kai* (Friends of Japanese Ema Society). No.222. Late 20th century. W. 17.9 cm

Sacred tree 霊木 *(reiboku)*

120
Meotogi Jinja 夫婦木神社. Kofu, Yamanashi Prefecture. Early 21st century. W. 13.5 cm
The inscriptions read:
縁結び = *enmusubi* (joining two people together in love/marriage)
子授け = *kosazuke* (to be blessed with a child)
和合繁栄= *wagō hanei* (harmonious prosperity)
夫婦木神社 = *Meteogi Jinja*

When the first three kanji of the shrine's name are read separately, they mean "husband wife tree". There is a sacred tree at the shrine in the shape of *joseiki* (female genitalia). It is worshipped for *kodakara* (the treasure that is children).

There was also a sanctuary in Japan which offered an *ema* design (not illustrated here) that explicitly portrayed the female genitalia [TS-10].

121

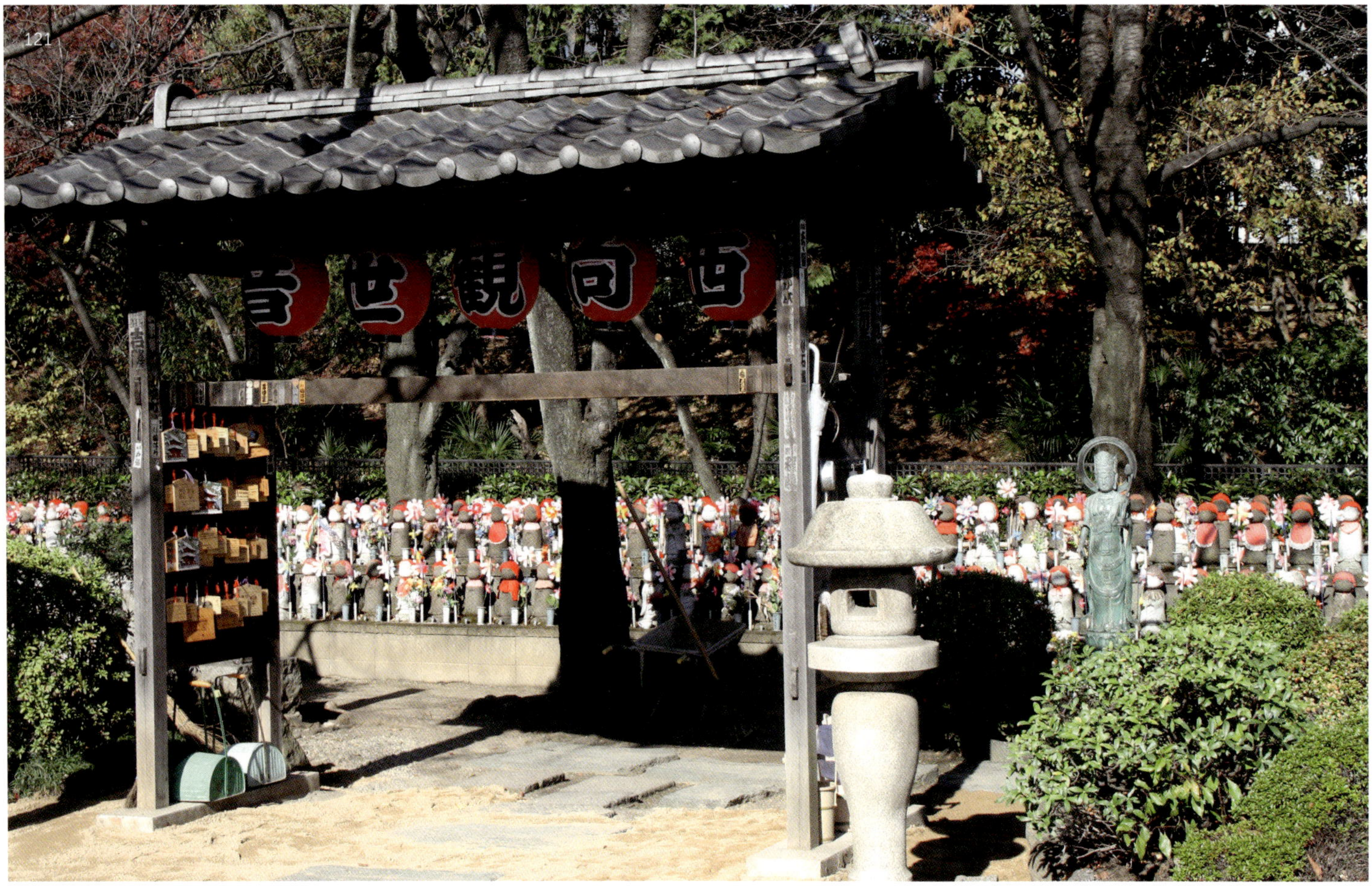

122

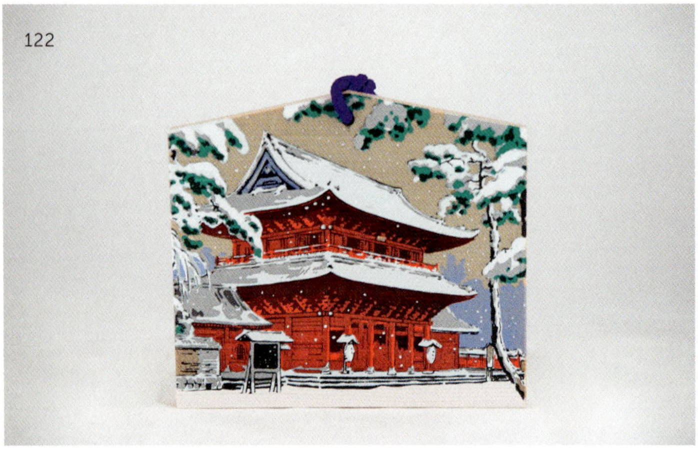

123

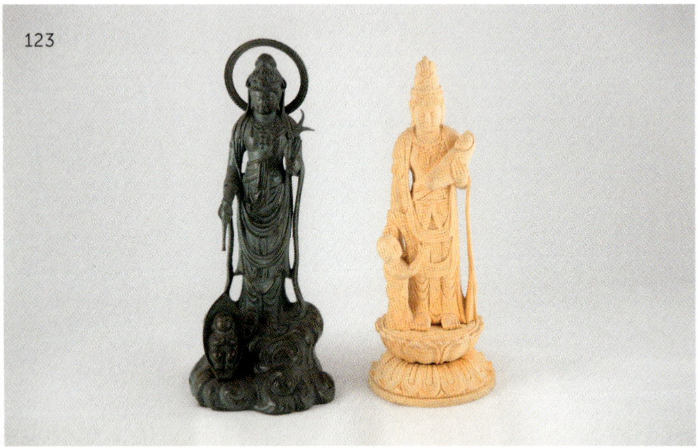

124

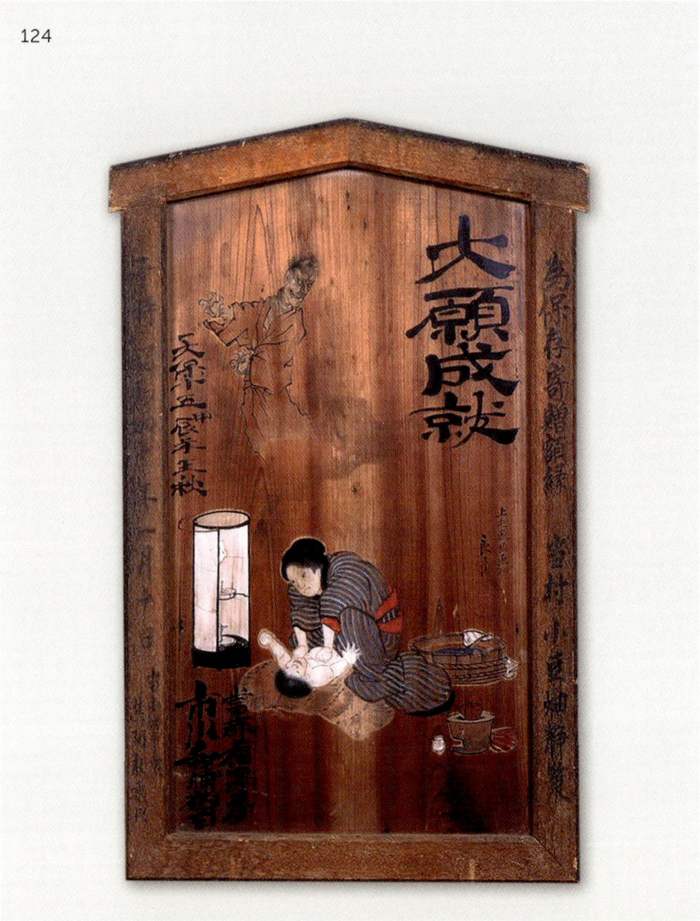

Abortion
流産
(*ryūzan*)

Background

An abortion can be either spontaneous (*shizenryūzan*) or induced (*jinkōryūzan*). Japan was one of the first countries in the world to legalise induced abortion. In the aftermath of World War II, many women with unwanted pregnancies died or suffered other serious consequences from unsafe illegal abortions. To protect women from such consequences, the Eugenic Protection Law came into force in 1948. Its enactment elicited a very large increase in the number of legally performed and officially reported abortions in Japan. The Law included a clause that allowed for abortion if having the child would cause severe economic problems, and most abortions were carried out under this clause. In addition, other reliable birth control methods were not available at the time (Japan would later refuse to allow the birth control pill). In 1957, more than 1.1 million abortions were recorded, leading to an abortion rate of 71.6 per 100 live births (the actual figures may have been even higher due to underreporting). In subsequent decades, there was a long period of decline until the figures stabilised in the early 1990s. In 2003, almost 320,000 abortions were reported, giving an abortion rate of 28 per 100 live births. Among the reasons why the induced abortion rate has remained substantial over the years may have been the relatively low use of oral contraceptives in Japan [1].

The Japanese term for an aborted, stillborn or miscarried foetus is *mizuko* 水子 (lit. water child). In the past, it was believed that a *mizuko* (who has never sinned) is easily reborn. As babies were not seen as full human beings, abortion was seen as relatively easy to do and no extensive funeral ritual was carried out afterwards. It has been suggested that thischanged in the 1970s, when commercially driven entrepreneurs started to campaign for *mizuko kuyō* (religious memorial services for *mizuko* at Buddhist temples) by means of frightening accounts of foetal wrath and spirit attacks in tabloids and other mass media. However, this suggestion is not correct. The media indeed paid much attention to the subject in the 1970s, but the first *mizuko* rituals had already been performed earlier. The instigators were women who had abortions under the economic clause but later (as Japan's economy recovered) found they could support a child. They felt bad about having had abortions and began performing rituals to apologise. The practice of *mizuko kuyō* developed from this. *Mizuko kuyō* is not a traditional Buddhist ritual. It is most often practised by women or families who have experienced an abortion in the recent or more distant past. People often have services done for the *mizuko*, purchase a stone *Jizō* (a well-known protector of children who has become the dominant deity in *mizuko* rituals) and/or offer *ema*. Such *ema* are commonly provided with a personal prayer (e.g., sleep peacefully), an apology (e.g., forgive me), or a request to the *mizuko* spirit to become a guardian spirit for the family. Sometimes when people have later had a child they will ask the *mizuko* spirit to become the protector of that child [EO-78; MS; 2].

121
Garden entrance at *Zōjōji* 増上寺 (Minato Ward, Tokyo)

Zōjōji offers *mizuko* services to commemorate aborted, stillborn or miscarried foetuses. This picture shows the entrance to its special garden for stone *Jizō* statues. The statues are wearing red caps and red bibs, and represent either *Mizuko Jizō* or *Kosodate Jizō* (Child rearing *Jizō*). *Ema* picturing the temple itself are hanging on the *ema* rack on the left.

122
Ema portraying *Zōjōji* in the snow. Early 21st century. W. 17.5 cm

123
Statues of *Mizuko Kannon* 水子観音
Wood (right) and metal (left). Late 20th century or early 21st century. H. 19 cm and 20 cm

Although *Mizuko Jizō* is undeniably the most prominent deity in *mizuko* rituals, a number of temples have given a specific *mizuko* role to *Kannon*, because *Kannon* is considered female and is often associated with childbirth and child rearing [MS].

124
Infanticide 間引き (*mabiki*) scene on large *ema Shōrenji* 青蓮寺. Ota, Gunma Prefecture. Mid 19th century. Cultural Properties Division, Ota City Hall (Ota, Gunma Prefecture)
The large inscription in the top right corner reads: 大願成就 = *taiganjōju* (realisation of a great ambition).

Abortion and infanticide (*mabiki*) were already practised in the Edo period, particularly in times of famine. They were not accompanied by apologising *ema*, because children under the age of seven were not yet seen as fully human beings. In the 18th century, a counter-movement emerged which rejected and condemned infanticide. Throughout the 19th century, this movement produced scrolls, large *ema*, pamphlets and posters that associated infant-killing mothers with evil demons. The large *ema* illustrated here fits in this tradition. In the foreground, a mother is smothering her infant. Disapproval of this act is expressed by the portrayal of a demonic figure hovering over her [3].

125

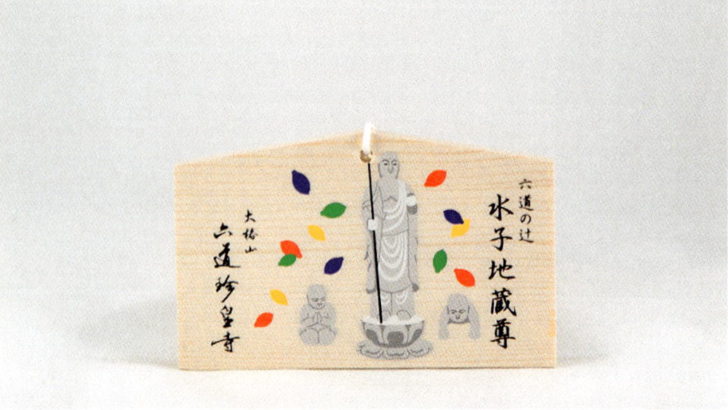

126

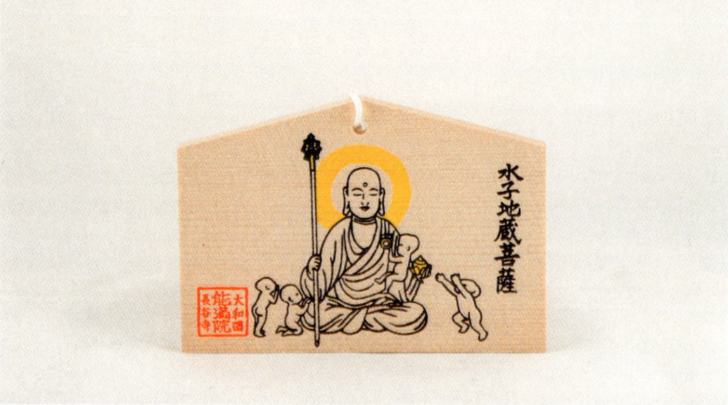

127

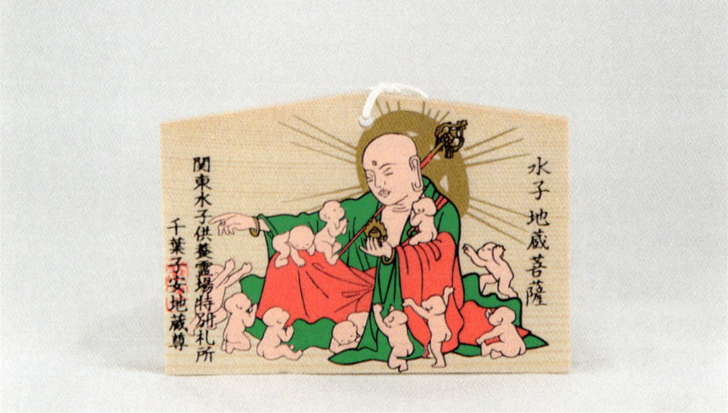

128

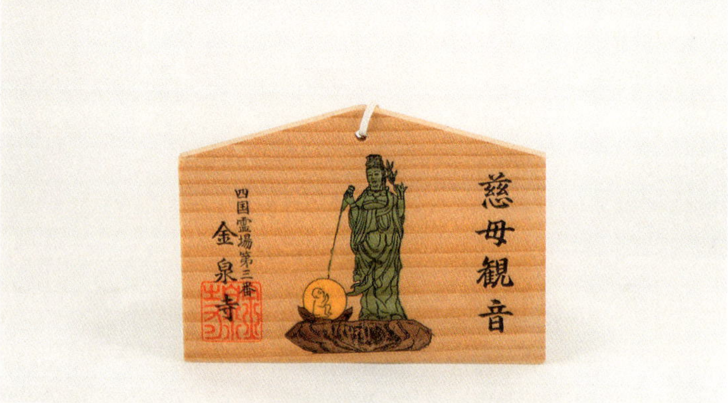

129

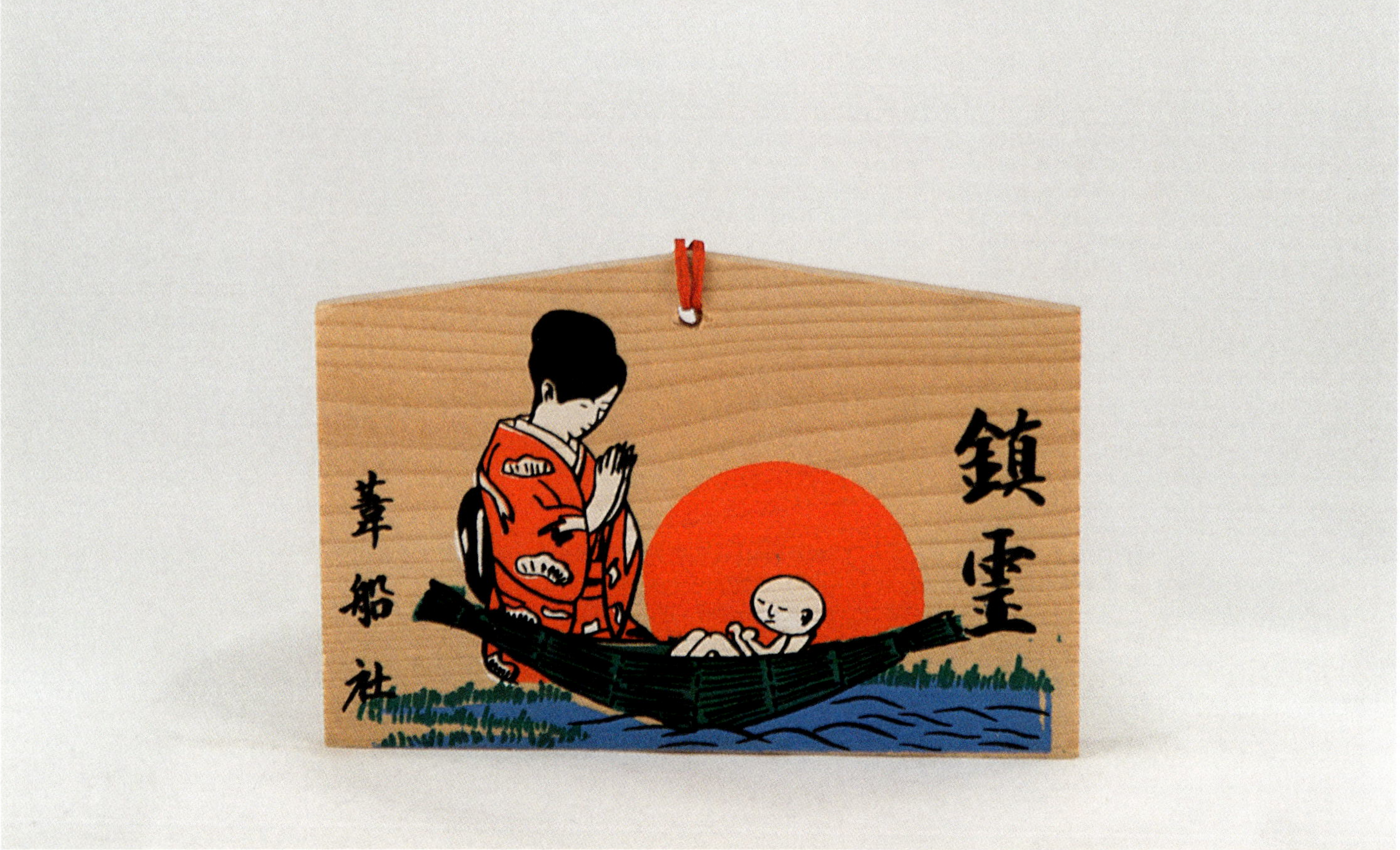

Ema designs

Mizuko Jizō 水子地蔵

Mizuko Jizō is the most prominent figure of worship in *mizuko kuyō* (religious memorial services for *mizuko* at Buddhist temples). Temples that sell or have sold *ema* with an image of *Mizuko Jizō* include *Nakayamadera* (Takarazuka, Hyogo Prefecture) [EO-140], *Rokudōchinnōji* (Kyoto), and *Nōmanin* near *Hasedera* (Sakurai, Nara Prefecture).

125
Rokudōchinnōji 六道珍皇寺. Higashiyama Ward, Kyoto. Early 21st century. W. 13.1 cm
The inscriptions read:
六道の辻 = *rokudō no tsuji* (at the crossroad of the six realms)
水子地蔵尊 = *Mizuko Jizōson*
六道珍皇寺 = *Rokudōchinnōji*

126
Nōmanin 能満院 near *Hasedera* 長谷寺 Sakurai, Nara Prefecture. Early 21st century. W. 12.6 cm
The inscriptions read:
水子地蔵菩薩 = *Mizuko Jizō Bosatsu*
大和国 = *Yamato no kuni* (former Yamato Province which is now located in Nara Prefecture)
能満院 = *Nōmanin*
長谷寺 = *Hasedera*

Koyasu Jizō 子安地蔵

127
Chiba Koyasu Jizōson 千葉子安地蔵尊 Togane, Chiba Prefecture. Early 21st century. W. 14.0 cm.
The inscription on the left reads:
千葉子安地蔵尊 = *Chiba Koyasu Jizōson*

Although the name of the temple refers to *Koyasu Jizō* (Safe Childbirth *Jizō*), the temple's website specifies this votive tablet as a *mizuko kuyō ema*.

Jibo Kannon 慈母観音 (Affectionate Mother Kannon)

In the Edo Period, outlawed Christians would secretly venerate the Virgin Mary by praying to a statue of *Jibo Kannon*. In recent times, *Jibo Kannon* has become a *Mizuko Kannon* who can take the place of the parents and affectionately provide for their *mizuko* in the other world [MS].

128
Konsenji 金泉寺. Itano town, Tokushima Prefecture. Late 20th century. W. 12.5 cm
The inscriptions read:
慈母観音 = *Jibo Kannon*
四国霊場第三番 = *Shikoku reijō daisanban* (third temple on the Shikoku pilgrimage)
金泉寺 = *Konsenji*

This *ema* depicts how *Jibo Kannon* offers a salvation lifeline to a *mizuko* in a bubble (which may refer to the womb). At the temple, there is a *Kannon* statue that also depicts this scene.

Mizuko in reed boat 葦船 *(ashibune)*

129
Ashifunesha 葦船社 on the grounds of *Kotohira Jinja* 金刀比羅神社 (commonly known as *Koyasu Jinja*). Hachioji, Tokyo Metropolis. Early 21st century. W. 13.7 cm.
The inscriptions read:
鎮霊 = *chin rei* (pacifying the spirits [of the dead])
葦船社 = *Ashifunesha*

Koyasu Jinja refers to *koyasu* (safe childbirth) but *Ashifunesha* offers *mizuko* services. The *ema* shown here depicts a *mizuko* (water child) aboard a reed boat and is meant to apologise to or pray for an aborted foetus. The mythological background is that *Hiruko* (child of *Izanagi* and *Izanami*) was deformed as a result of *Izanami*'s mistake in speaking first to *Izanagi* during their courtship. Because of his deformity, *Hiruko* was set adrift in a reed boat. In later times, he was identified with *Ebisu*, one of the *Shichifukujin* (Seven Gods of Good Fortune) [KU; MS].

130

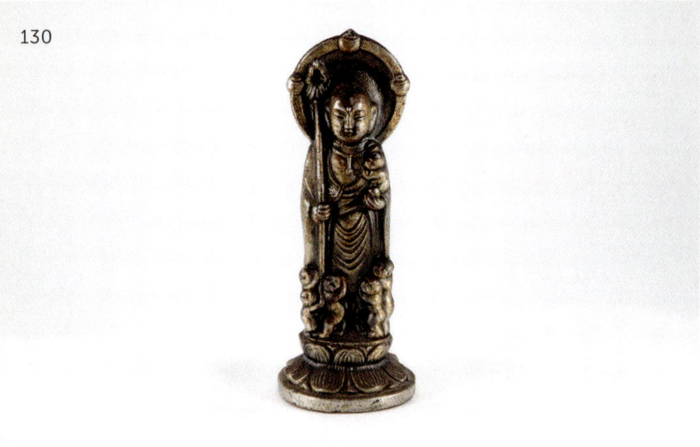

131

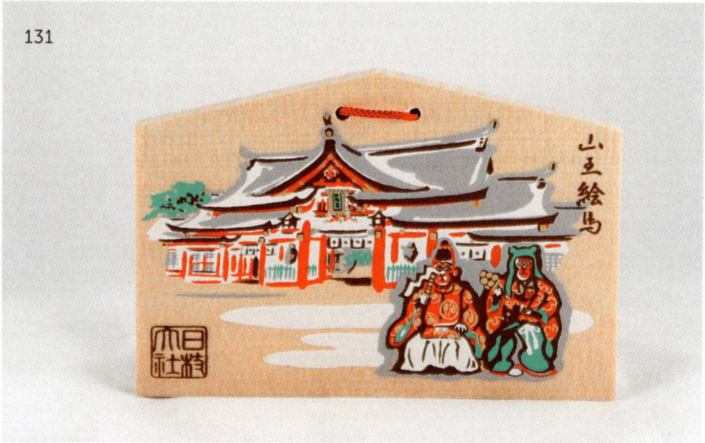

132

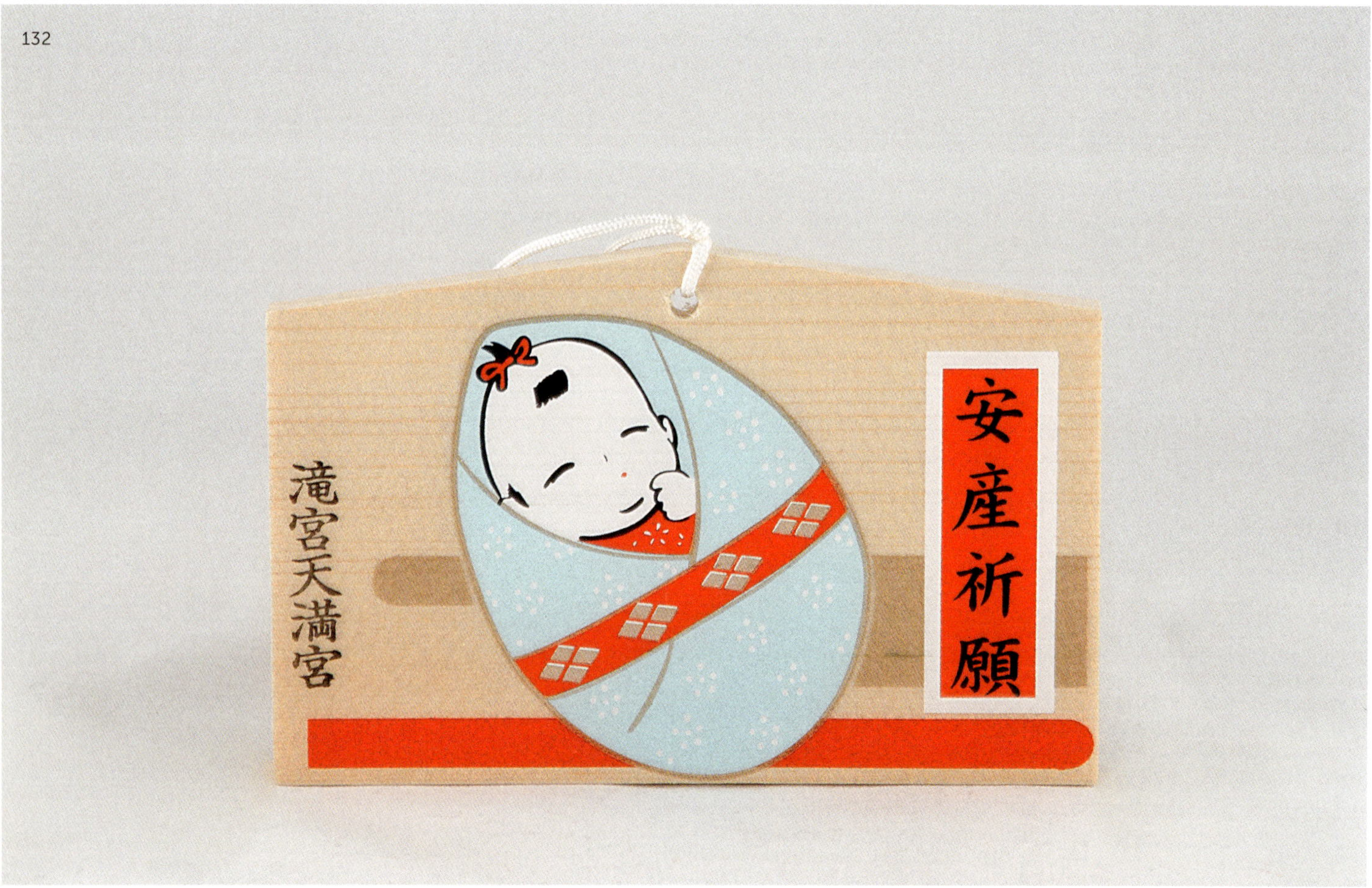

133

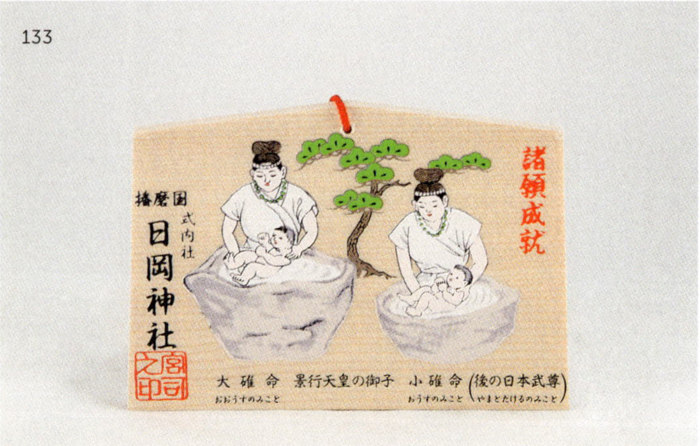

134

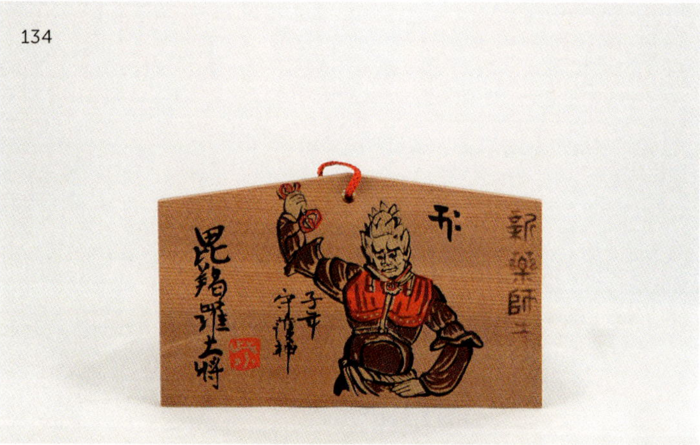

Easy childbirth 安産 (*anzan*)

Background

The most common modern cause of maternal death in Japan is haemorrhage and this was probably also the case in the past. Around 1900, the maternal death rate in Japan was one hundred times higher than today (410 versus 4.1 per 100,000 births). In the same period, the neonatal death rate decreased more than fifty times (from 79.0 to 1.5 per 1000 live births) [HSJ; 1]. In view of these figures it is unsurprising that *anzan* (easy childbirth) and *koyasu* (safe childbirth) were prominent among the benefits sought at shrines and temples, especially in earlier times.

Even though healthcare has improved significantly, these benefits remain popular today. On websites reviewing the benefits of Japanese shrines and temples, *anzan* (easy childbirth) and *kodakara* (the treasure that is children) are often grouped together and constitute an important main category. Such websites list almost as many or even more entries for *kodakara/anzan* as they do for recovery from illness in general (i.e., not counting entries concerning specific illnesses) [GK; 2].

Numerous figures of worship have been developed to cater for these needs in both the Shinto and Buddhist traditions. One prominent Shinto deity for fertility and easy delivery is the water goddess *Suijin*. Another Shinto divinity for easy childbirth is the mythical princess *Konohana Sakuya Hime*, also known as *Koyasu-sama*, who is worshipped at various *Asama* shrines. Buddhist counterparts are various forms of the figures *Kannon* and *Jizō* such as *Koyasu Kannon*, *Koyasu Jizō*, and *Anzan Jizō*. Another Buddhist figure of worship for fertility, easy childbirth and the guarding of children is *Kishibojin*, also called *Kariteimo*. A figure who can appear in Shinto or Buddhist guises in connection with fertility, safe childbirth and harmonious marriage is *Sarugami* (Monkey God) or *Sannō Gongen* (Mountain King Avatar), to whom numerous *Hie* shrines are dedicated. *Sarugami* is commonly considered to be the *tsukai* (Shinto messenger) or *gongen* (Buddhist avatar) of *Sannō*, the central figure of worship for the Buddhist Tendai sect founded on Mount Hiei [MS].

130
Statue of *Koyasu Jizō* 子安地蔵 (Easy Childbirth *Jizō*). Metal. Mid to late 20th century. H. 16 cm

This form of *Jizō* grants easy and safe delivery and is often depicted holding a child, or with children in his lap or at his feet [MS].

131
Sannō Gongen 山王権現. *Hie Jinja* 日枝神社 Chiyoda Ward, Tokyo. Early 21st century. W. 17.5 cm
The inscription reads: 山王絵馬 = *Sannō ema*

Hie Jinja is dedicated to *Sannō Gongen*, which means avatar of *Sannō* (literally Mountain King). He dwells on Mt. Hiei (the home mountain of the Buddhist Tendai Sect) and *Masaru* (monkey) is his *gongen* (avatar) or *tsukai* (messenger). *Masaru* is also known as Demon Queller, based on the word play that *saru* in Japanese can mean monkey as well as expel, depending on how it is written.

The *ema* displays the *shinmon* (shrine gate) and the two statues of *Sannō Gongen* guarding it. The male statue on the left is holding a *gohei* (wand with paper streamers) while the female counterpart on the right has a *suzuki* (ritual purification wand adorned with bells). She cradles a baby in her arms and is considered the patron of safe childbirth and harmonious marriage [MS].

Ema designs

Infant 幼児 *(yōji)*

132
Takinomiya Tenmangū 滝宮天満宮. Ayagawa, Kagawa prefecture. Early 21st century. W. 13.8 cm
The inscriptions read:
滝宮天満宮 = *Takinomiya Tenmangū*
安産祈願 = *anzan kigan* (prayer for easy childbirth)

133
Hioka Jinja 日岡神社. Kakogawa, Hyogo Prefecture. Early 21st century. W. 16.0 cm
The red inscription reads:
諸願成就 = *shogan jōju* (fulfilment of all vows/wishes)

The black kanji give日岡神社 = *Hioka Jinja* and the names of the two princes and of their legendary father Emperor *Keikō*.

This *ema* shows the first bath of two legendary twins, the elder Prince *Ōusu* and the younger Prince *Ousu* (who would become known as Prince *Yamato Takeru*). After growing up, the former killed the latter. The shrine can be visited to pray for *anzan* (easy delivery) and *shoganjōju* (fulfillment of various prayers).

General Bikara 毘羯羅大将 *(Bikara Taishō)*

Bikara (Vikarāla in Sanskrit) is one of the *Jūni Shinshō* (Twelve Divine Generals) serving and protecting *Yakushi Nyorai* (Medicine Buddha). His images are commonly holding up a ritual *vajra* weapon that symbolises the properties of a diamond (indestructibility) and a thunderbolt (irresistible force) [MS].

134
Shin-Yakushiji (New *Yakushiji*) 新薬師寺. Nara, Nara Prefecture. Late 20th century or early 21st century. W. 13.6 cm
The inscriptions read:
新薬師寺 = *Shin-Yakushiji*
子安守護神 = *koyasu shugojin* (safe childbirth guardian deity)
毘羯羅尊 = *Bikarason*

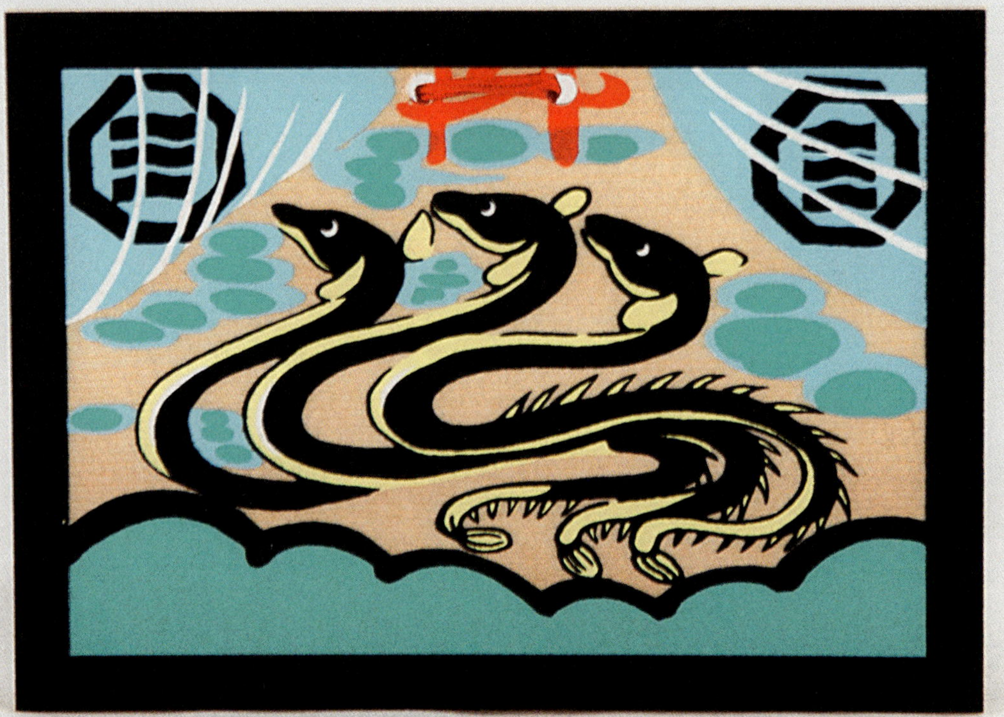

Eels 鰻 *(unagi)*

The *ema* design of three *unagi* (eels) can be used for *anzan kigan* (prayer for easy childbirth) and for *hōjō* (abundant offspring). The underlying analogies are that the eel is slippery (allowing for easy delivery) and lays an enormous number of eggs [AE; TS-6; IH2-46].

135
Mishima Jinja 三嶋神社. Higashiyama Ward, Kyoto. Early 21st century. W. 15.4 cm

Mishima Jinja also offers an *ema* with two eels for child wishes and for marital harmony (see p.69).

136

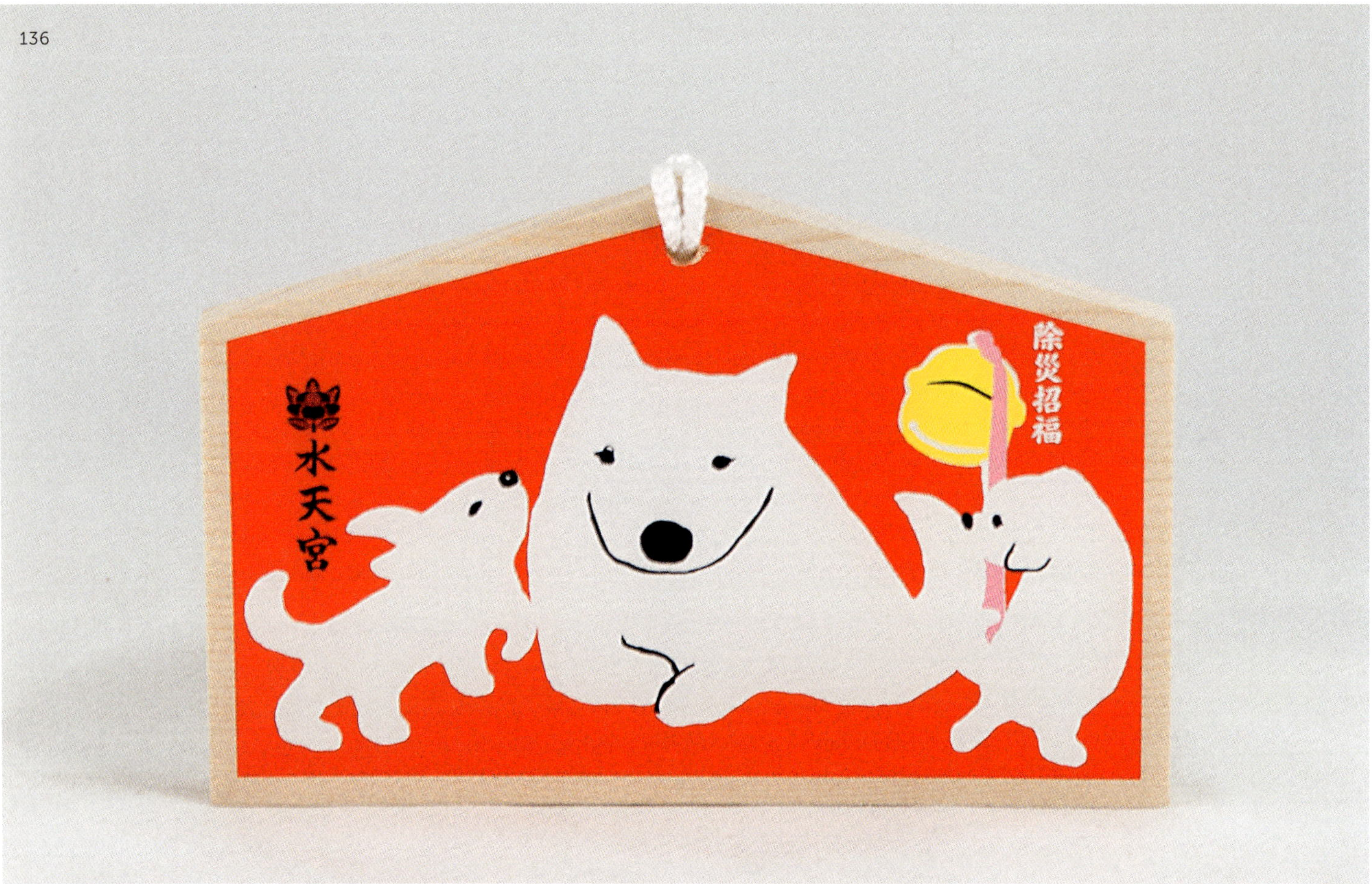

137

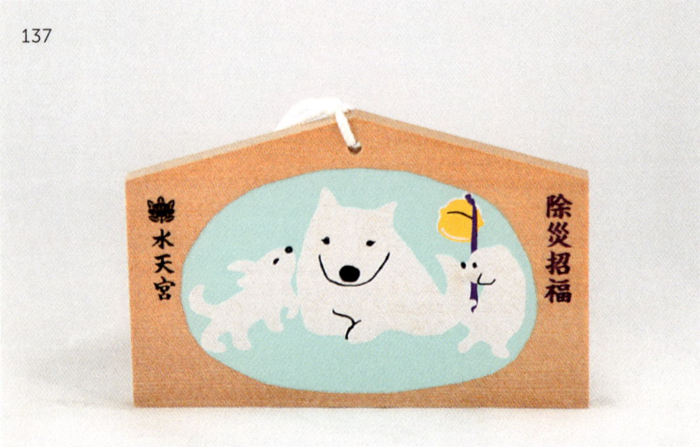

138

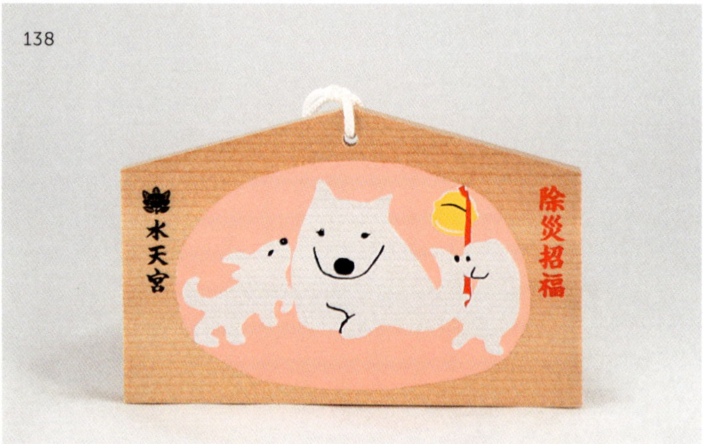

139

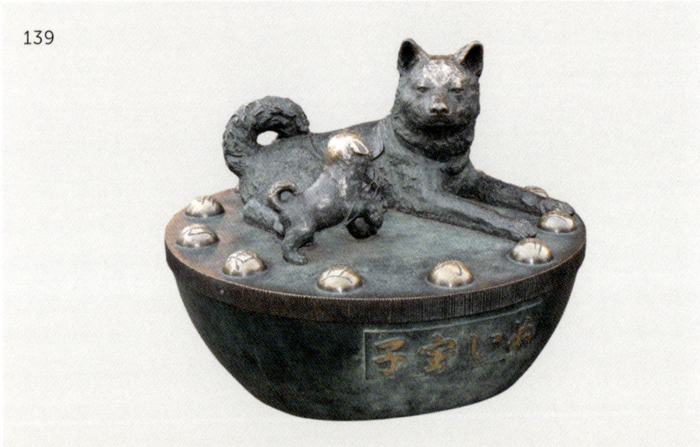

140

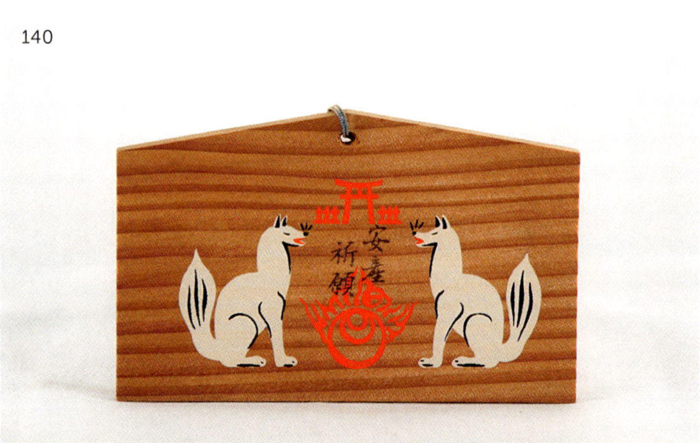

Dog 犬 *(inu)*

Ema portraying an *inu* (dog) often represent this animal as a zodiac sign. However, they can relate to *kodakara* (the treasure that is children) and/or *anzan kigan* (prayer for easy childbirth), when they are inscribed as such or portray a mother dog with puppies. The traditional association is that dogs give birth easily [EO-183 ; GG2-2013/04].

136-138

Dog with puppies 子犬と犬 (*koinu to inu*). *Suitengū* 水天宮. Chuo Ward, Tokyo. Early 21st century. W. 14.5 cm
The inscriptions read:
除災招福 = *josai shōfuku* (removing disaster inviting good luck)
水天宮 = *Suitengū*

The shrine has more than local significance and is well-attended by parents expecting a baby (to pray for safe childbirth). Often people who have prayed for safe delivery return to the shrine to give thanks for this, and to ask the deity to keep their baby safe. Pregnant women preferably visit the shrine on *inu-no-hi* (the day of the dog which returns every 12th day). The *ema* with the red background is sold only on this day. The former website of the shrine described this *ema* as *kodakara fuku* while the other two were only referred to as *fuku* (blessing) *ema*. The former website of the shrine described this *ema* as kodakara fuku while the other two were only referred to as fuku (blessing) *ema* [IR-31; 3].

139

Famous statue called *kodakara inu* (dog for the treasure that is children) at *Suitengū*. It represents a mother dog with a puppy surrounded by the twelve zodiac signs. It is believed that touching the statue (or one's zodiac sign) will bring safety to mother and child. The statue also featured on an *ema* of *Suitengū* (not illustrated here).

Facing foxes 向い狐 *(mukai kitsune)*

Ema with foxes facing each other are generally intended to pray for *gokokuhōjō* (abundant harvest) and *shōbai hanjō* (prosperous business), but this design has occasionally been used for *kosazuke* (being blessed with a child) or *anzan* (easy delivery). Cf. the entry on foxes on p.27.

140

Origin unclear. Late 20th century. W. 14.6 cm
The inscription reads: 安産祈願 = *anzan kigan* (prayer for easy delivery)

141

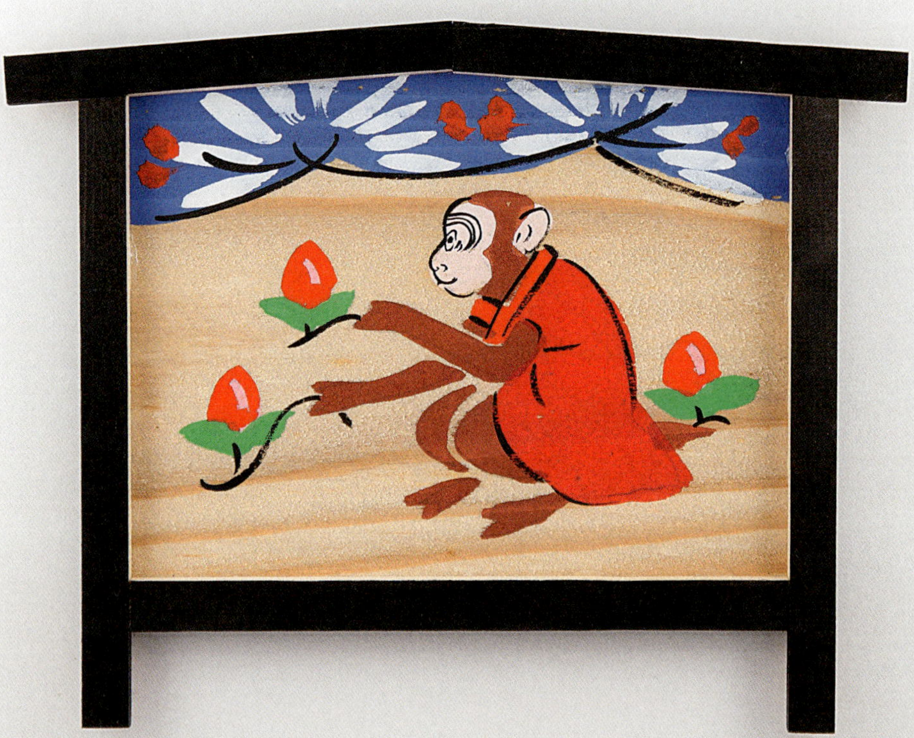

142

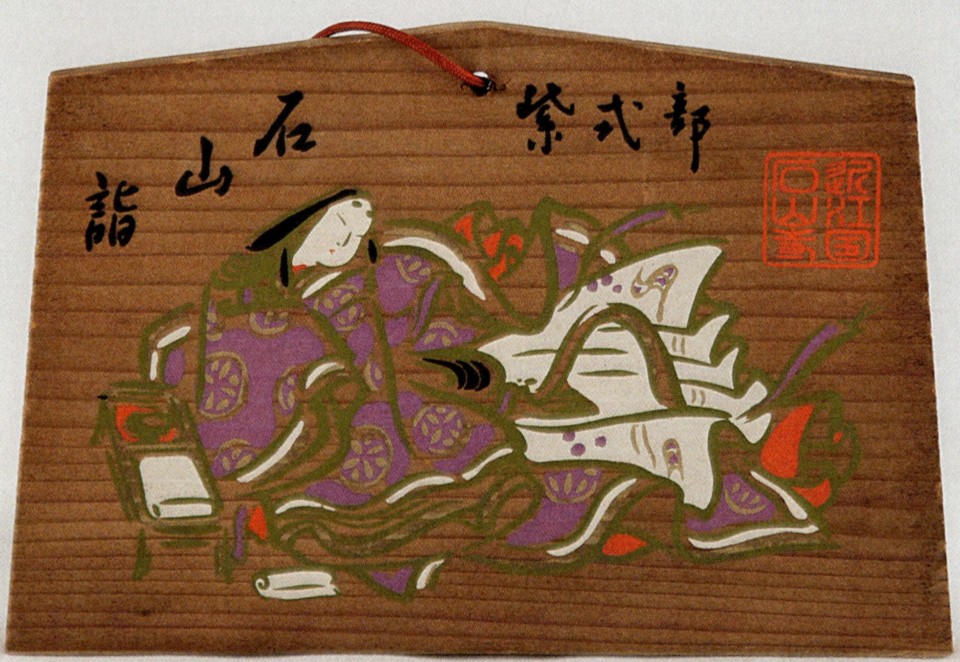

Monkey with peach(es) 桃持猿 *(momo ji saru)*

The monkey is not only a zodiac animal but is also connected to *Kōshin* worship (see the entry on *Shōmen-Kongō* on p.51). The peach can be a symbol of vitality and longevity.

Ema designs of a monkey holding one or two peaches are primarily presented for *anzan* (easy delivery), but they have also been used at times for *kosazuke* (to be blessed with a child) or *fujinbyō heiyu* (recovery from women's illnesses) [TS-23; IH2-42].

141
Hand-painted reproduction for a Japanese club of *ema* collectors called *Nihon Ema Tomo no Kai* (Friends of Japanese Ema Society). No.289. Late 20th century. W. 17.9 cm. Original design probably from *Shōsenji,* Ome, Tokyo Metropolis. Used for *anzan* (easy delivery).

Murasaki Shikibu 紫式部

142
Ishiyamadera 石山寺. Otsu, Shiga Prefecture. Late 20th century. W. 15.3 cm
The inscriptions read:
紫式部 = *Murasaki Shikibu*
石山詣 = *Ishiyama mōde* (visit to *Ishiyama*)

This *ema* design is used for easy childbirth and for a good marriage. The figure depicted is *Murasaki Shikibu*, a female writer from the Heian Period. It is believed that she began writing her famous *Tale of Genji* (a classic work of Japanese literature) at *Ishiyamadera*.

143

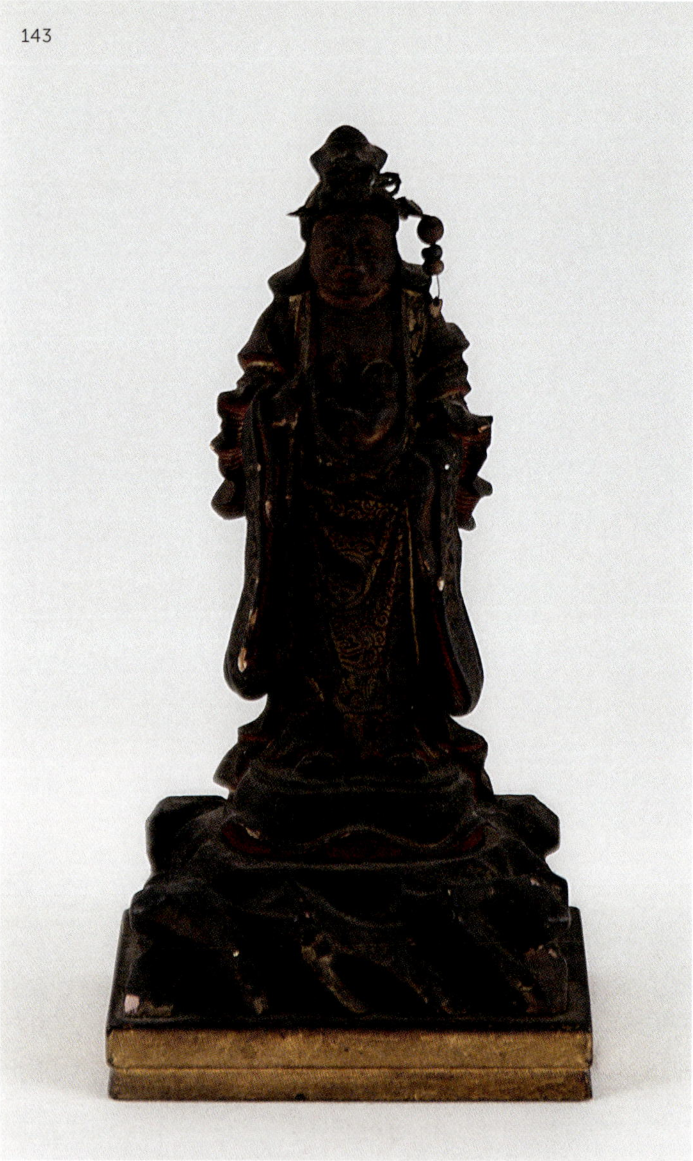

144

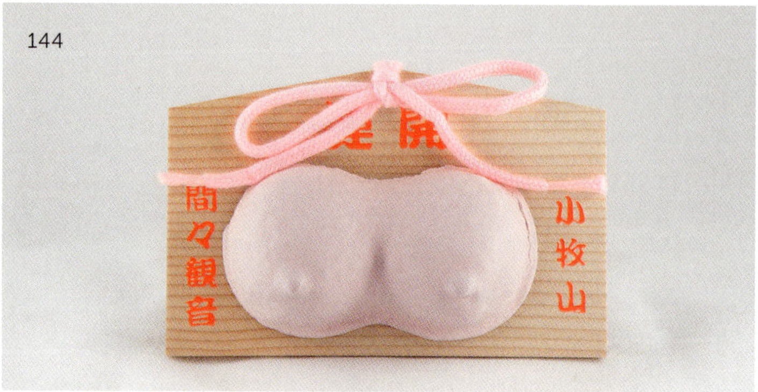

145

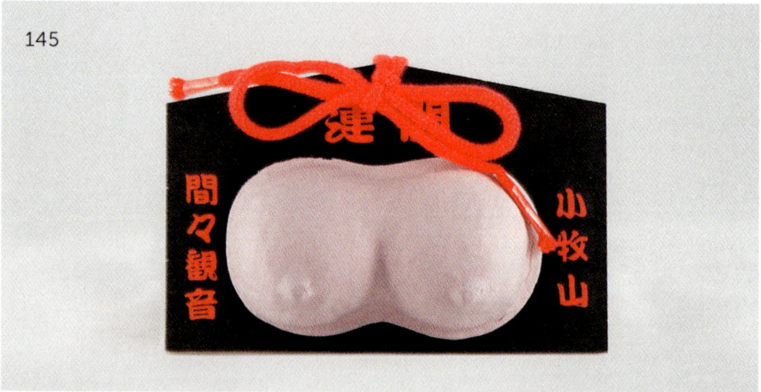

146

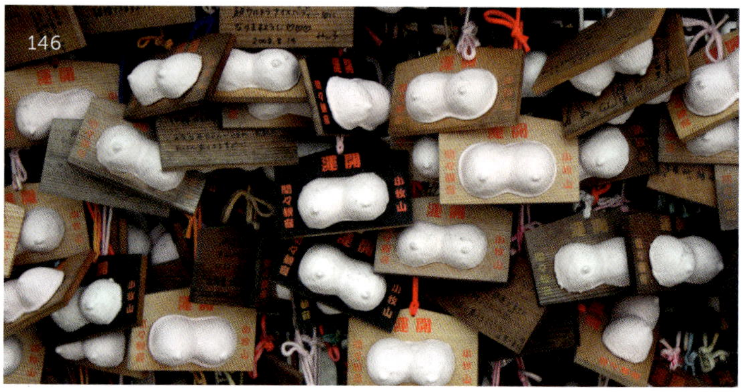

147

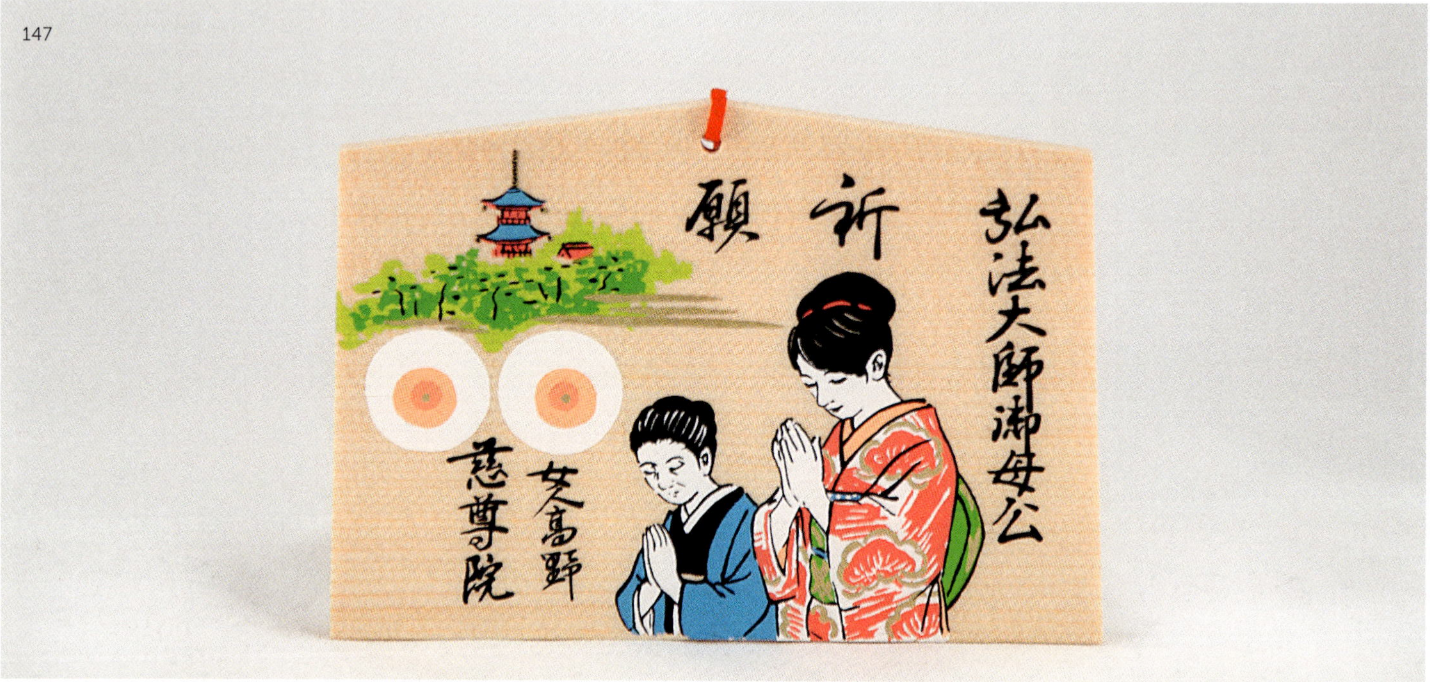

Breastfeeding 授乳 (*junyū*)

Background

In the Edo period, breastfeeding was the only way of feeding infants in Japan. Cow's milk was not much used as a substitute until the end of the 19th century. One of the reasons may have been connected with the inhibition of cattle breeding due to the Buddhist rule that the eating of red meat was forbidden. Breastfeeding was continued until the child was 2 to 3 years old. However, it was not unusual for rich parents to hire a wet nurse to breastfeed the child until the age of 7 years to further the child's health and to reduce the risk of dying. In the mid-20th century, the use of bottle feeding increased rapidly and since then, less than half of mothers rely exclusively on breastfeeding at one month after birth. Instead, breastfeeding is often combined with bottle feeding [1].

Buddhist figures of worship who can be invoked for abundant breast milk include *Yakushi*, *Jizō*, *Kannon* and *Kishibojin* [2]. For example, there is a statue of *Chichi Yakushi* (Healing Buddha of Breasts) at *Sōhonzan Zentsūji* (Zentsuji, Kagawa Prefecture). Women who do not have enough breast milk for their baby come here to pray. If their prayer is answered they return to offer a small replica of a breast in gratitude.

143
Polychrome wooden statue of *Kishibojin* 鬼子母神. 18th century. H.14.5 cm

Kishibojin (also known as *Kishimojin* or *Kariteimo*) is a Buddhist goddess for *kosazuke* (to be blessed with a child), *anzan* (easy delivery), *junyū* (breastfeeding) and *kosodate* (child rearing). She is often shown with a baby on her left arm and/or a pomegranate (symbol of fertility due to its many seeds) in her right hand [MS].

Ema designs

Breasts 乳 *(chichi)*

Ema with *chichi* (breasts) are used to petition for abundant breast milk or for enlargement of the bust line. Sometimes they are also used for breast cancer (see the entry on breasts in the section of women's illnesses on p.191) [TS-4,15; RT-243].

144-145
Ryūonji 龍音寺 (commonly called *Mama Kannon* or *Mama Chichi Kannon*). Komaki, Aichi Prefecture. Early 21st century. W. 15.4 cm
The inscriptions read:
小牧山 = *Komakiyama* (Mount Komaki)
開運 = *kaiun* (opening up good luck)
間々観音 = *Mama Kannon*

Mount Komaki was the original location of the temple. Its *ema* were at first intended for the sufficient production and easy flow of breast milk, but are now also offered to pray for beautiful breasts. According to legend, a woman who could not provide breast milk to her newborn baby was suddenly able to do so, after praying to *Kannon* at the temple. This miracle took place more than 170 years after the temple's foundation. The temple also provides related benefits, from conceiving children and safe childbirth to memorial services for aborted children [RT-243].

146
Ema rack at *Ryūonji* (Komaki, Aichi Prefecture).

147
Jisonin 慈尊院. Kudoyama, Wakayama Prefecture. Early 21st century. W. 15.8 cm
The inscriptions read:
弘法大師御母公 = *Kōbō Daishi go bo kō* (Kobo Daishi's honourable mother)
祈願 = *kigan (prayer)*
女人高野 = *nyonin Kōya* (women's Koya)
慈尊院 = *Jisonin*

Besides a pair of breasts, this *ema* depicts the pagoda of the temple and two praying females (one older and one younger). The same praying females also occur in an *ema* design sold by another shrine [IY-65].

Jisonin is dedicated to the mother of *Kōbō Daishi*. *Kōbō Daishi* introduced Shingon Buddhism to Japan in the early 9th century and turned *Kōyasan* (Mount Koya) into the centre of this important Buddhist sect. Until 1973 women were not allowed in the sacred area of *Kōyasan*. Instead, they would go to the temple dedicated to *Kōbō*'s mother (who had lived just outside Koya's sacred boundaries to be near her son).

148

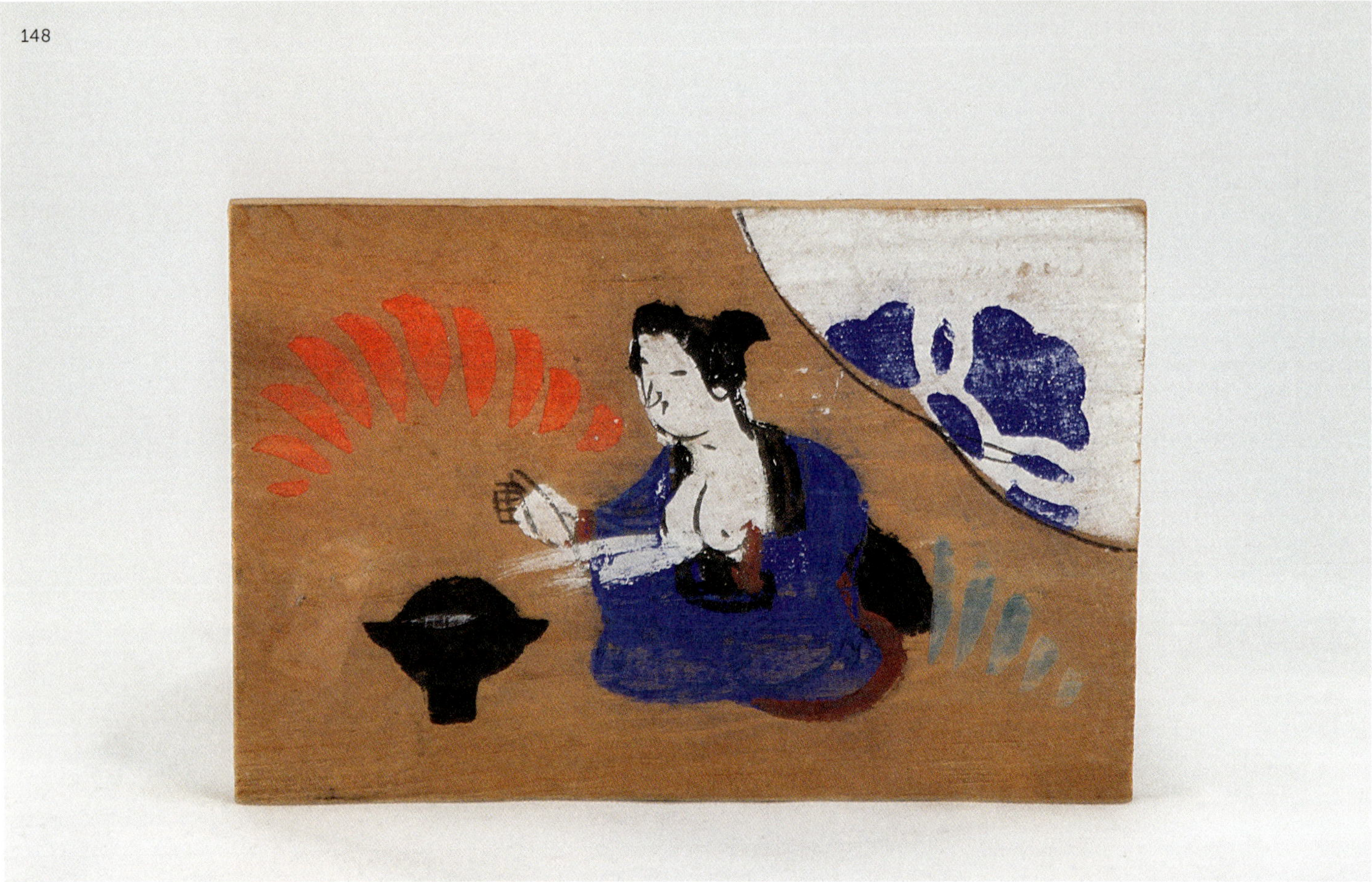

149

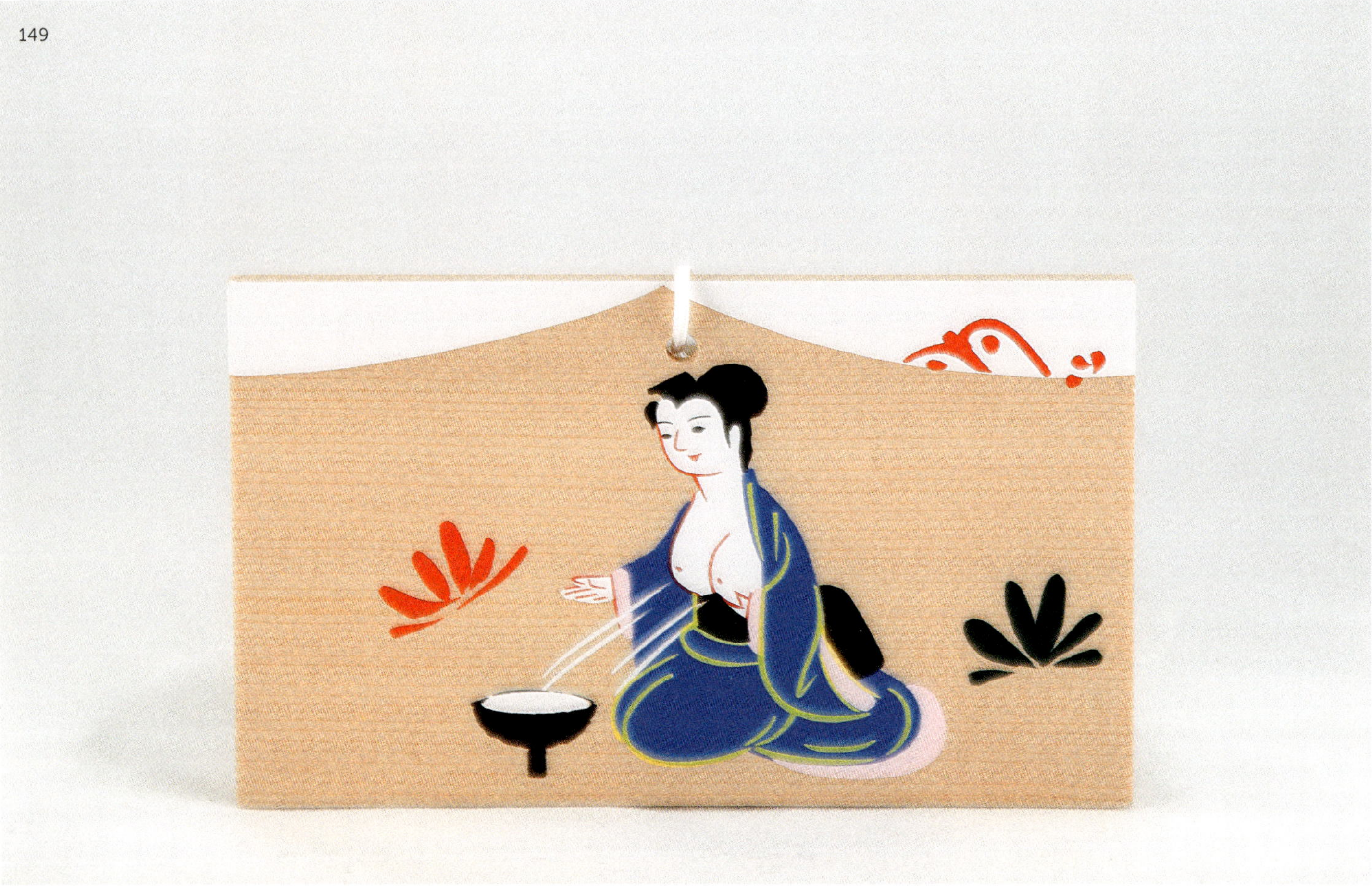

Breasts spurting milk* 乳しぼり *(chichishibori)

Ema with this design were used to ask for *chichi sazuke* (milk bestowed). They are reminiscent of an Edo woodblock print of an *uba* (wet nurse) who is squeezing milk out of her breasts to show her suitability for the job [3].

148
Shitennōji 四天王寺. Tennoji Ward, Osaka. Hand-painted *ema*. Mid-20th century. W. 15.1 cm

Over the years, different versions of this *ema* design have served at *Hoteidō* (*Hotei* Hall) of *Shitennōji* as a prayer for the abundant production and easy flow of breast milk. The same sanctuary also had an *ema* that showed actual breastfeeding [FS-19; IJ-80; TS-15; IH2-54].

149
Shitennōji 四天王寺. Tennoji Ward, Osaka. Printed *ema*. Early 21st century. W. 15.0 cm

Today, the temple is still associated with lactation, nursing, praying for large amounts of breast milk, and the safe delivery of babies.

150

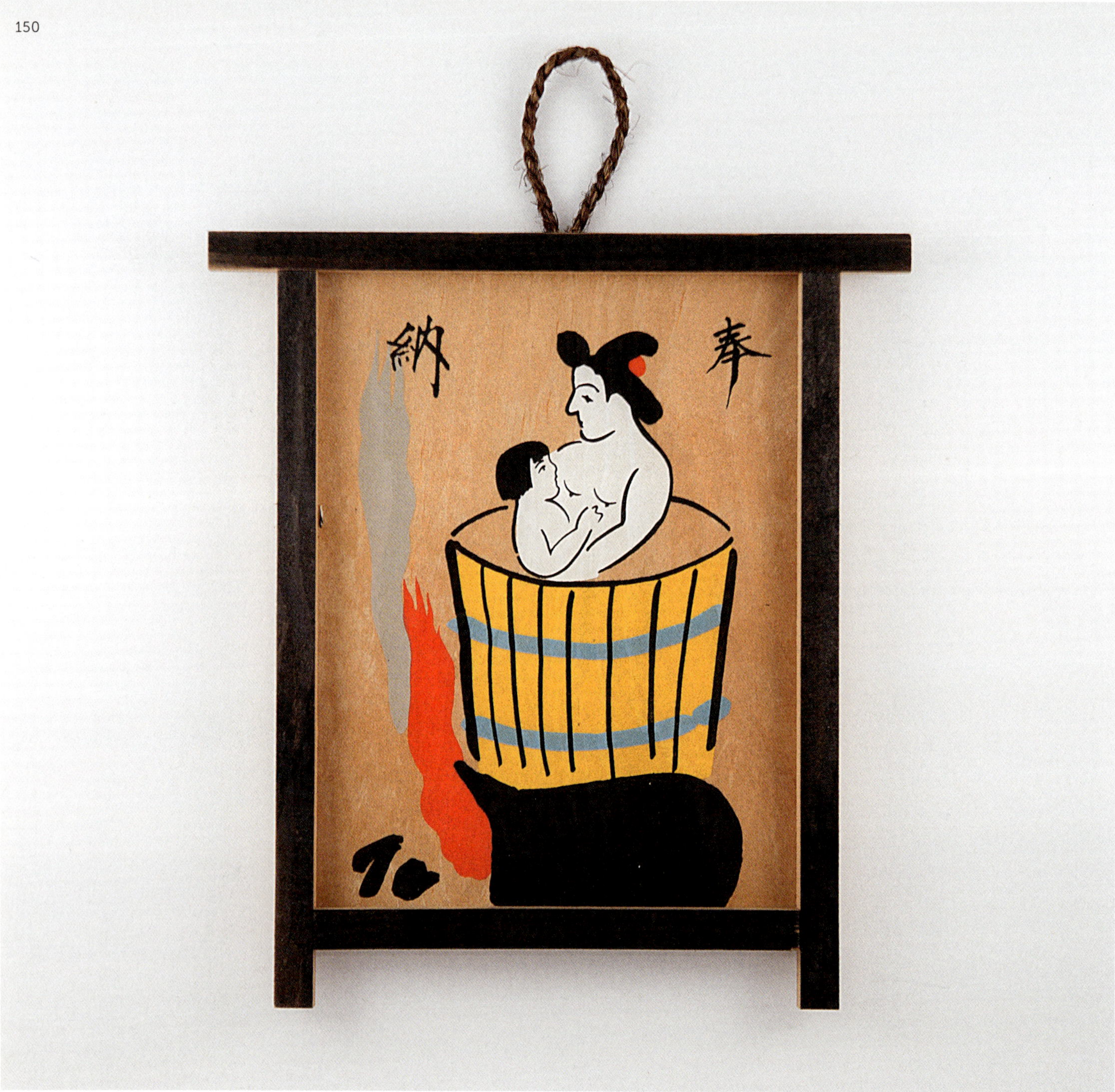

151

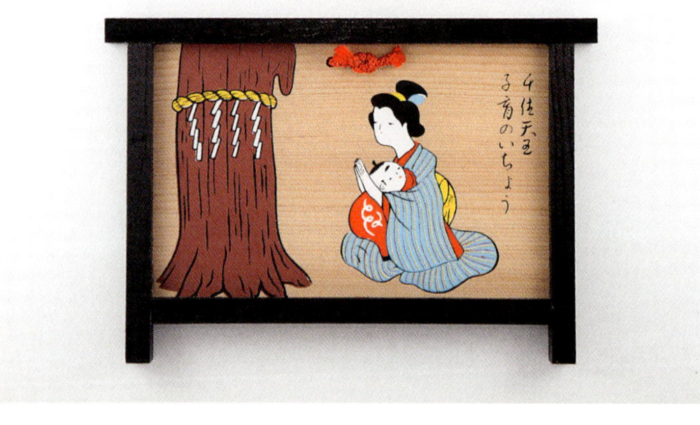

152

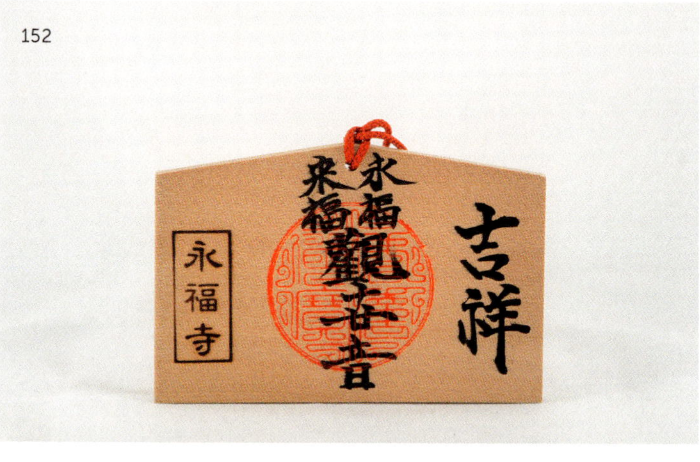

Child rearing 子育て (*kosodate*)

Background

Raising children in good health was a major concern of the Japanese population in the past. Judging from historical figures of infant mortality, newborns had a substantial risk of dying before they reached the age of one (about 1 in 6.5 live births in 1900 compared to 1 in 357 in 2004) [GG1-2011/07; HSJ].

Some shrines and temples offer *kosodate* (child rearing) in addition to *junyū* (breast-feeding) or *anzan* (easy childbirth).

150
Bathing mother and child 母子入浴 (*boshi nyūyoku*). Hand-painted reproduction for a Japanese club of *ema* collectors called *Nihon Ema Tomo no Kai* (Friends of Japanese Ema Society). No.106. Late 20th century. W. 14.5 cm. Original design from the Kansai region.

The *ema* designs of *shōni nyūyoku* (bathing young child) and *boshi nyūyoku* (bathing mother and child) show the bathing of an infant or young child in a short, steep-sided wooden bathtub known as *furo*. They were used to take away *nyūyokukirai* (dislike of bathing) in young children [TS-15; IH2-56].

Ema designs

Ginkgo tree of child rearing 子育て銀杏 *(kosodate ichō)*

151
Susanoo Jinja 素盞雄神社. Minami-Senju, Arakawa Ward, Tokyo. Early 21st century. W. 19.0 cm
The inscriptions read:
千住天王 = *senju tennō* (may refer to the *Senju Tennōsai* festival held at the shrine)
子育てのいちょう = *kosodate no ichō* (ginkgo tree of child rearing)

This *ema* shows a mother with child, who is praying to a ginkgo tree with a *shimenawa* rope ornamented with *shide* (zigzag-shaped paper streamers). The ginkgo tree grows in the grounds of the shrine and is worshipped for abundant milk production and *kosodate* (child rearing). For the former purpose, the *ema* is a substitute for drinking a decoction of the ginkgo tree bark. For the latter purpose, the *ema* gives safe child growth for seven years.

Another *ichō* (ginkgo tree) that is worshipped for the production of breast milk is the *chichi ichō* near *Miyagino Hachiman Jinja* in Sendai, Miyagi Prefecture. It grows many aerial roots resembling *chichi* (breasts). According to legend, it was planted in the 8th century A.D. on the grave mound of an imperial wet nurse, who had expressed that to be her dying wish [1].

Kosodate Jizō 子育て地蔵 *(Child-Raising Jizō)*

152
Eifukuji 永福寺. Kakegawa, Shizuoka Prefecture. Early 21st century (2015). W. 14.1 cm
The inscriptions read:
吉祥 = *kisshō* (lucky omen)
永福 = *Eifuku*
来福 = *raifuku* (future good fortune)
観世音 = *Kanzeon* (formal name of *Kannon*)
永福寺 = *Eifukuji*

This *ema* is associated with *Kosodate Jizō* on the website of the temple.

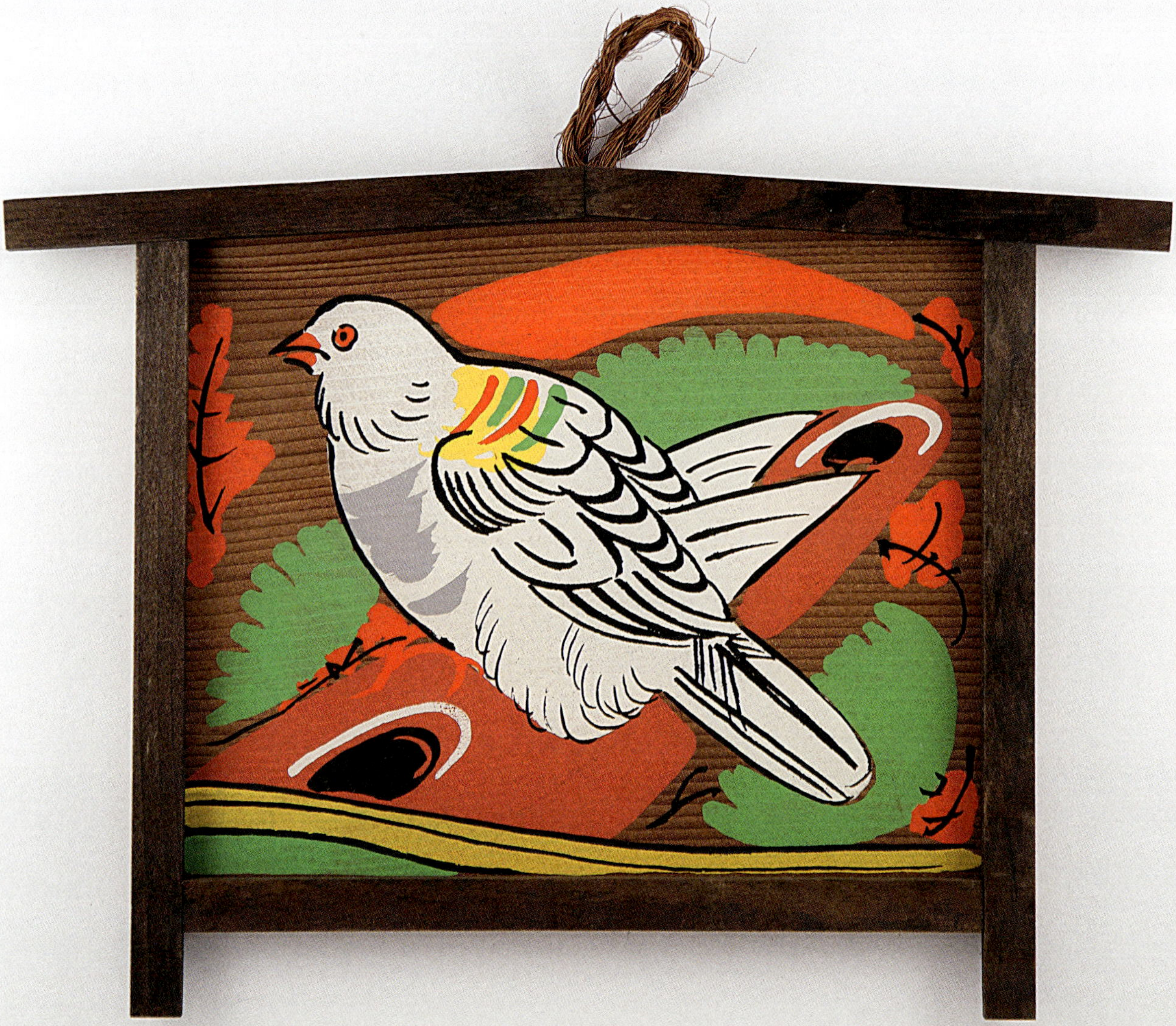

Pigeon 鳩 *hato*

The pigeon is a messenger of *Hachiman* (God of War). The *ema* design of a single pigeon could be used for different purposes, including *kosodate* (raising children) and the removal of *mame* (blisters, corns) [TS-22]. Cf. the entries on pigeons on p.161 and p.185

153
Hand-painted reproduction for a Japanese club of *ema* collectors called *Nihon Ema Tomo no Kai* (Friends of Japanese Ema Society). No.87. Late 20th century. W. 18.0 cm. Original design from a *Hachiman Jinja* in Tokyo

154

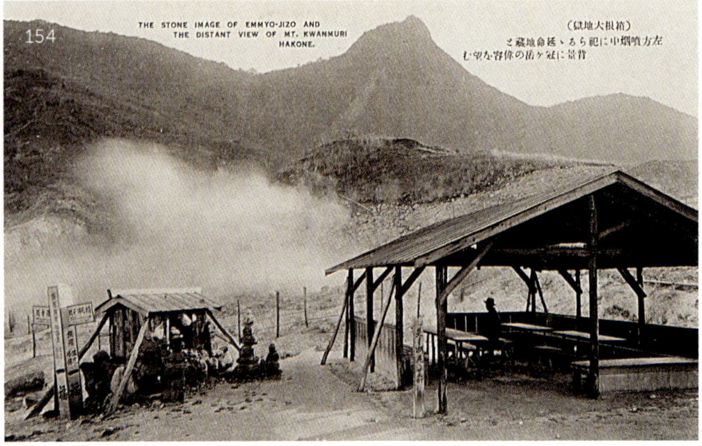

155

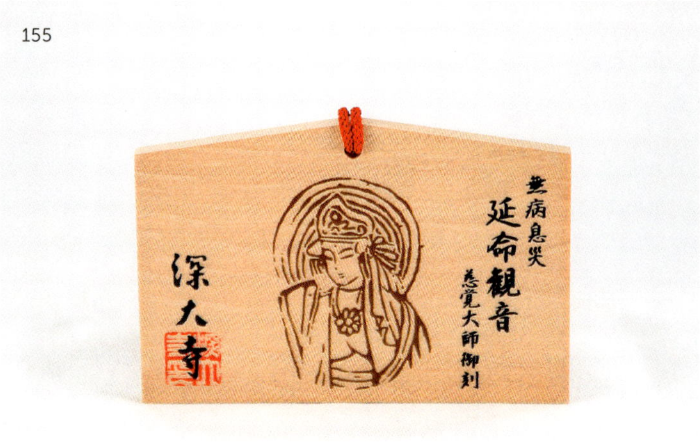

156

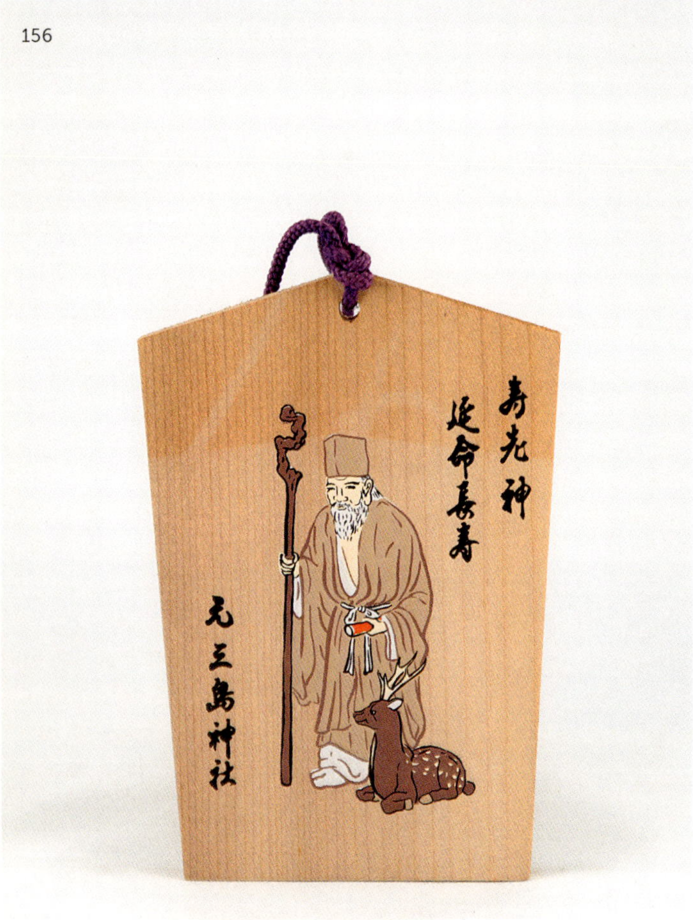

157

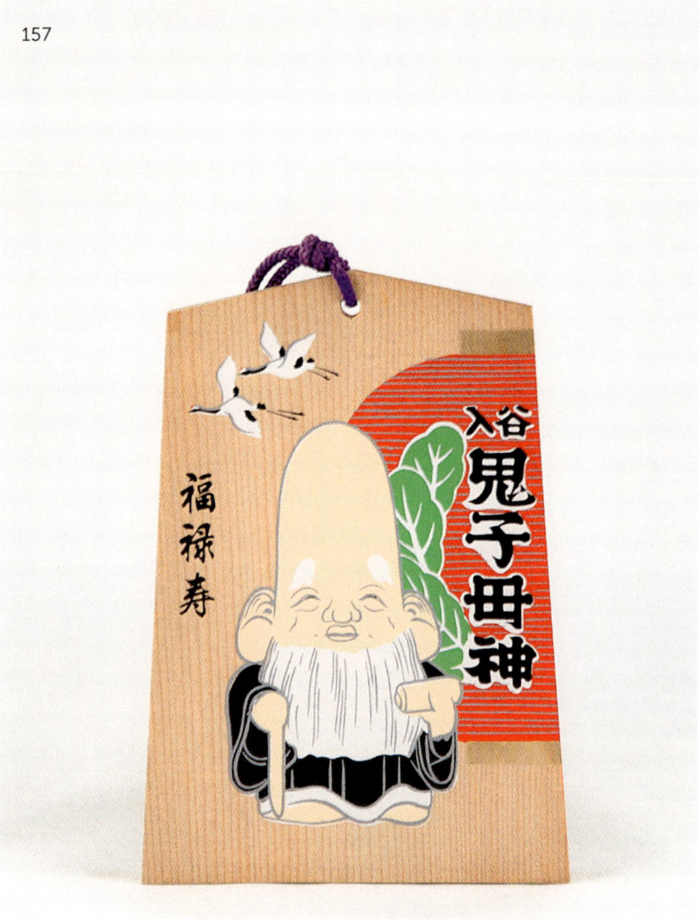

158

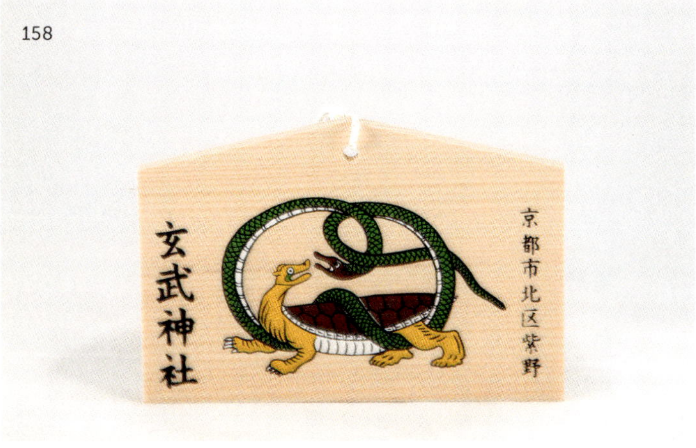

159

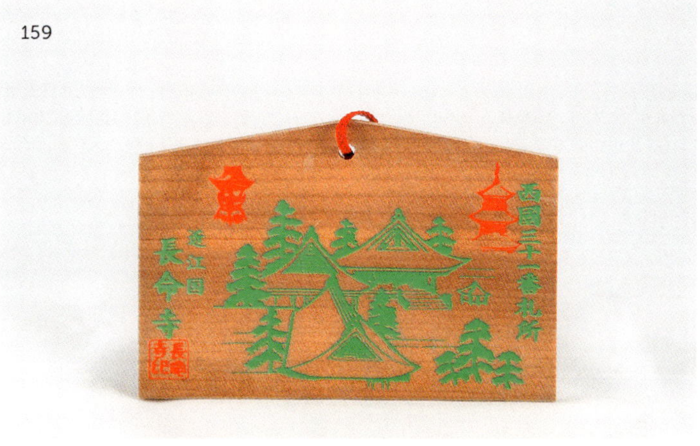

Longevity/long life 長寿／長命 (*chōju/chōmei*)

Background

Japan is among the countries with the highest life expectancy in the world. Depending on the methodology used, it may even rank as number one with an overall life expectancy of about 83 to 84 years.

Important Buddhist figures of longevity are *Enmei Jizō* and *Enmei Kannon* (*enmei* means life-prolonging). Two Taoist deities of longevity (both belonging to the Seven Deities of Good Fortune) are *Jurōjin* and *Fukurokuju* [MS].

If the numerous Japanese words for longevity and the number of symbols for longevity in Japanese art (Table 7) are indicative, there can be little doubt that the Japanese attach great value to longevity. They have a special verb (*jumyōwonobasu*) that means "to prolong one's life" and a whole series of longevity celebrations for reaching specific old ages (e.g., *yonenoiwai* for the celebration of one's 88th year) [KU].

154
Early Japanese postcard showing roadside sanctuary of *Emmyō Jizō* near Mount Kanmuri in the Hakone Mountains, Kanagawa Prefecture.
Emmyō Jizō is a different spelling of *Enmei Jizō* and translates as Life-prolonging *Jizō*.

Ema designs

Longevity is more of a *hito no isshō* (human life) issue than a medical theme, and no attempt has been made here to offer an extensive review of *ema* designs for longevity. Instead, some representative examples of *ema* with figures of worship, temples, symbols and inscriptions are presented that are all associated with longevity (*chōju*) or long life (*chōmei*).

Enmei Kannon 延命観音 (*Life-prolonging Kannon*)

155
Jindaiji 深大寺. Chofu, Tokyo Metropolis.
Early 21st century. W. 13.5 cm
The inscriptions read:
無病息災 = *mubyōsokusai* (sound health)
延命観音 = *Enmei Kannon*
慈覚大師御刻 = *Jikaku Daishi gokoku* (honorable carving by *Jikaku Daishi*, an ascetic living in the 9th century)
深大寺 = *Jindaiji*

Table 7 Derived from Temple CR. Traditional themes in Japanese art. Berkeley: Regent Press, 2008

Japanese symbols of *chōju* (longevity)

Bamboo	Gourd	Mannetake	Salmon
Bream	Heron	Nanten	*Shoki*
Cicada	*Ho-o*	Orange	Stork
Chrysanthemum	*Jo* and *Uba*	Pine	Tortoise/turtle
Crane	Lobster	Sacred fungus	*Yuzuri*
Deer			

Jurōjin 寿老人

Jurōjin is a Taoist deity of longevity who belongs to the *Shichifukujin* (Seven Gods of Good Fortune). He is commonly represented with a staff and a scroll (on which the lifespan of all living things is written). He is often accompanied by a deer (which itself is a symbol of longevity).

156
Motomishima Jinja 元三島神社. Taito Ward, Tokyo. Late 20th century. W. 11.0 cm
The inscriptions read:
寿老人 = *Jurōjin*
延命長寿 = *enmei chōju* (life-prolonging and longevity)
元三島神社 = *Motomishima Jinja*

Fukurokuju 福禄寿

Fukurokuju is a Taoist deity of longevity who belongs to the *Shichifukujin* (Seven Gods of Good Fortune). He is usually portrayed as a bald dwarf with a high forehead. He has a cane and a scroll which contains either a magical scripture or the lifespan of every person on earth.

157
Shingenji 真源寺. Taito Ward, Tokyo.
Late 20th century. W. 11.2 cm
The inscriptions read:
入谷鬼子母神 = *Iriya Kishiboin*
福禄寿 = *Fukurokuju*
The temple houses not only the *Shichifukujin* (Seven Gods of Good Fortune) but also a famous statue of *Kishiboin* (goddess of childbirth and children).

Genbu 玄武

Genbu (Black Tortoise) is a god of Chinese origin who rules over the northern heavens. He is a constellation representing the north and the winter season. He is one of the guardian spirits that protect Kyoto, more specifically the northern part where *Genbu Jinja* is located. He is usually depicted as a snake coiling around a tortoise, both of which symbolise longevity.

158
Genbu Jinja 玄武神社. Kita Ward, Kyoto.
Early 21st century. W. 13.6 cm
The inscriptions read:
京都市北区紫野 = *Kyōtoshi Kitaku Murasakino*
玄武神社 = *Genbu Jinja*

Long life temple 長命寺 (*Chōmeiji*)

As indicated by the name of the temple (*chōmei* = long life), it can be visited to pray for longevity.

159
Chōmeiji 長命寺. Omihachiman, Shiga Prefecture. Late 20th century. W. 13.5 cm
The inscriptions read:
西国三十一番札所 = *Saikoku sanjū-ichi ban fudasho* (amulet-issuing temple no.31 of the Saikoku [Pilgrimage])
近江国 = *Ōmi kuni* (old province which today comprises Shiga Prefecture)
長命寺 = *Chōmeiji*

160

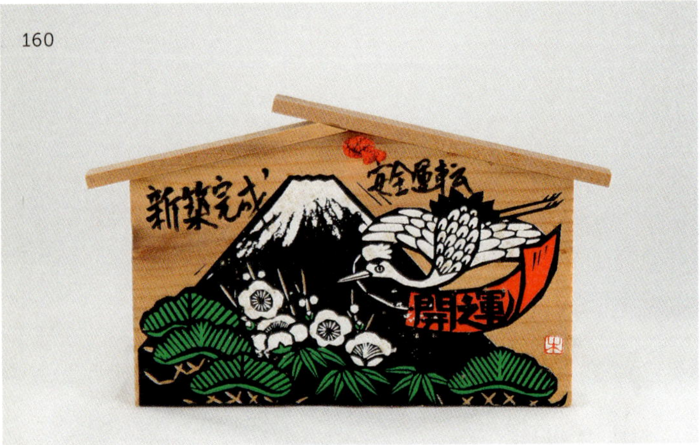

161

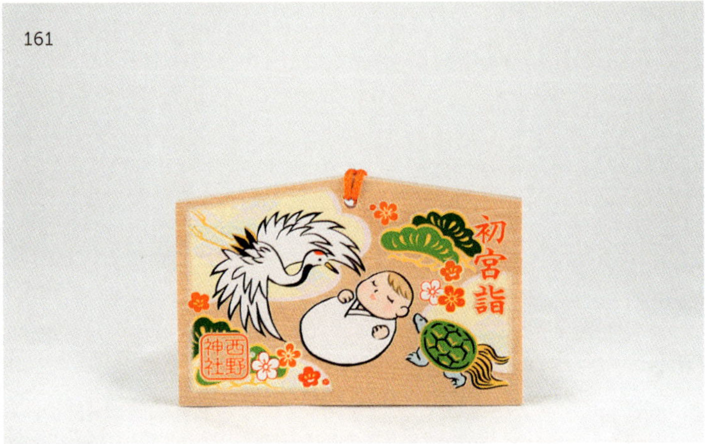

162

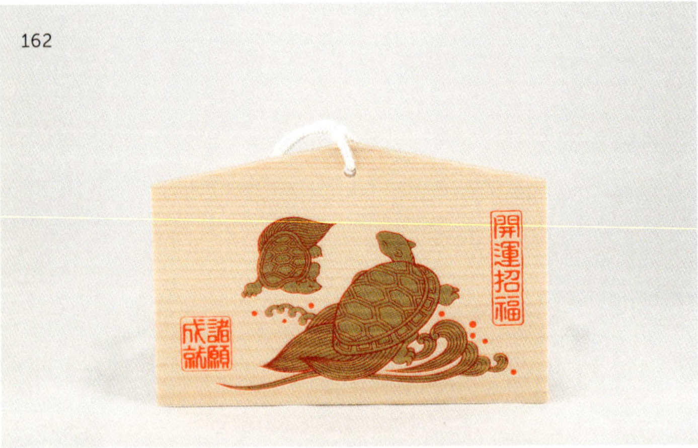

164

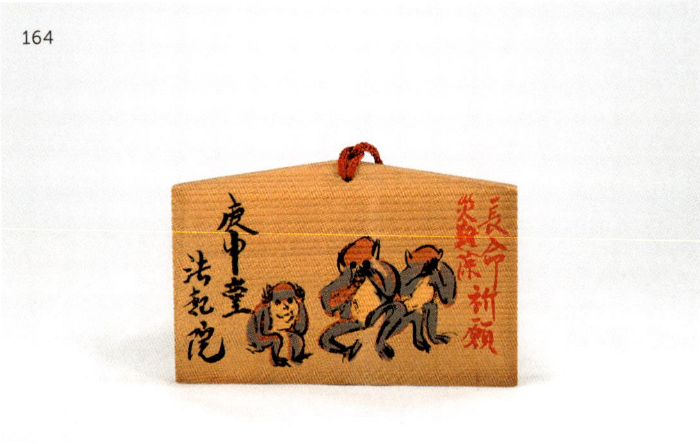

163

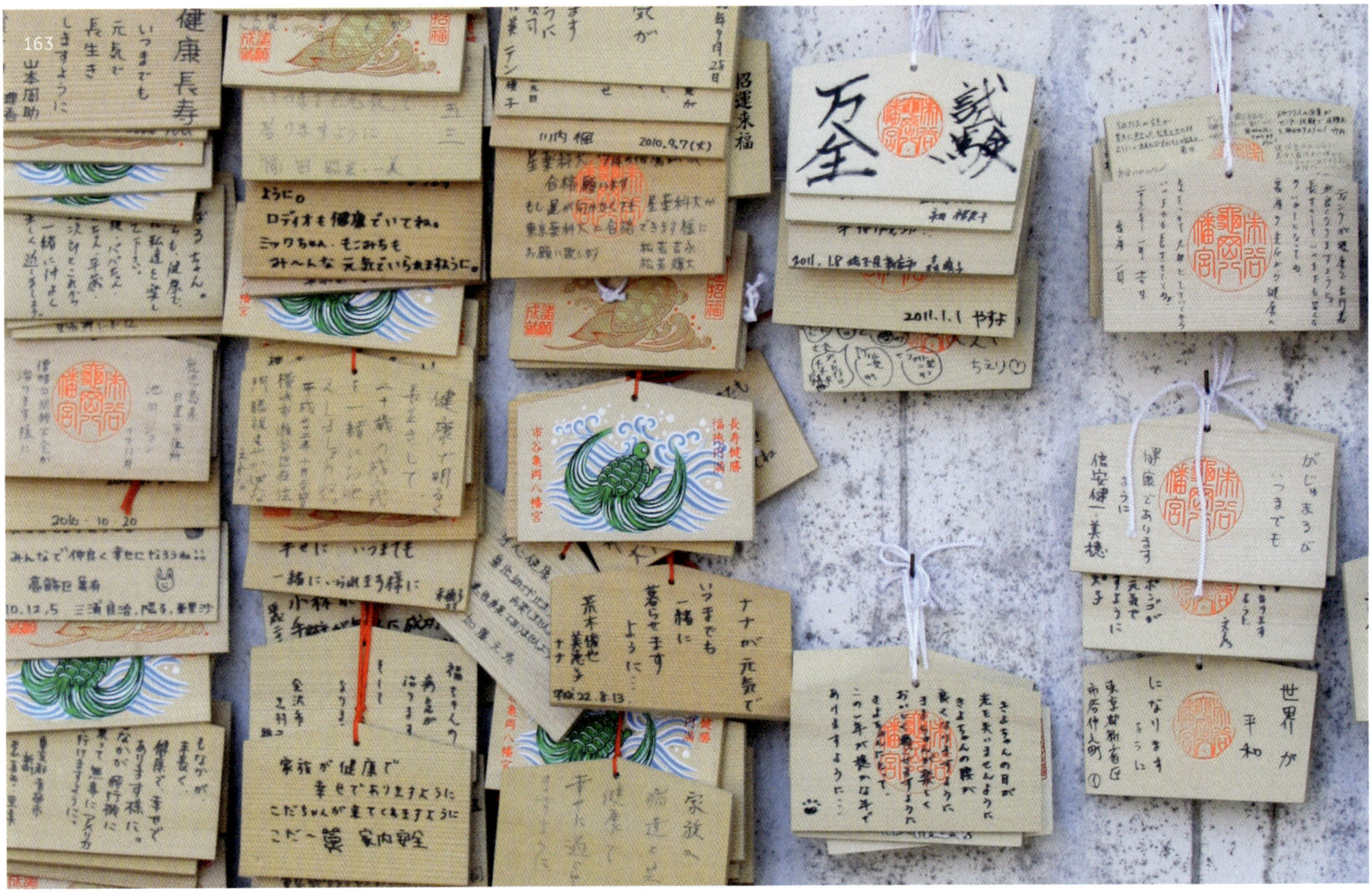

Crane 鶴 *(tsuru) and Three Friends of Winter* 松竹梅 *(shōchikubai)*

The long-living *tsuru* (crane) is regarded as a symbol of longevity. *Shōchikubai* is composed of three different plants (pine, bamboo and plum). It symbolises steadfastness, perseverance, and resilience, because unlike many other plants its components do not wither in wintertime.

160
Origin unclear. Late 20th century. W. 17.5 cm
The inscriptions read:
安全運転 = *anzen unten* (safe driving)
開之運 = *kainoun* (opening up good luck)
新築完成 = *shinchiku kansei* (completion of new building)

The *ema* shows Mount Fuji at the background.

Crane and tortoise/turtle 鶴亀 *(tsurukame)*

161
Nishino Jinja 西野神社. Sapporo, Hokkaido Prefecture. Early 21st century. W. 13.7 cm
The inscriptions read:
初宮詣 = *hatsumiyamairi*
西野神社 = *Nishino Jinja*

Hatsumiyamairi is the first visit of a newborn child to the shrine (usually a month after birth).

Tortoise/turtle 亀 *(kame)*

162
Ichigaya Kamegaoka Hachimangū 市谷亀岡八幡宮. Shinjuku Ward, Tokyo. Early 21st century. W. 15.5 cm
The inscriptions read:
開運招福 = *kaiun shōfuku* (good luck charm for opening up good luck)
諸願成就 = *shoganjōju* (fulfilment of all wishes)

The name of the shrine contains the character for *kame* (tortoise/turtle). In Japanese art, the *kame* is a symbol of longevity. It is often depicted together with aged people or deities of longevity (such as *Jurōjin* and *Fukurokuju*).

163
Ema rack at *Ichigaya Kamegaoka Hachimangū* 市谷亀岡八幡宮 in Tokyo.

The gold-coloured *kame* is a recent replacement for a green-coloured *kame*.

Three Monkeys 三猿 *(sanzaru)*

See the entry on the *Kōshin* deity *Shōmen-Kongō* on p.51 for the *ema* design of the three monkeys (who see no evil, hear no evil, and speak no evil).

164
Kōshindō 庚申堂 at *Hokkiin* 法吉院
Hokkiin is just outside *Hasedera* 長谷寺, Sakurai, Nara prefecture. Late 20th century. W. 13.6 cm
The inscriptions read:
長命 = *chōmei* (long life)
災難除 = *sainanyoke* (eradication of disasters)
祈願 = *kigan*
庚申堂 = *Kōshindō*
法吉院 = *Hokkiin*

165
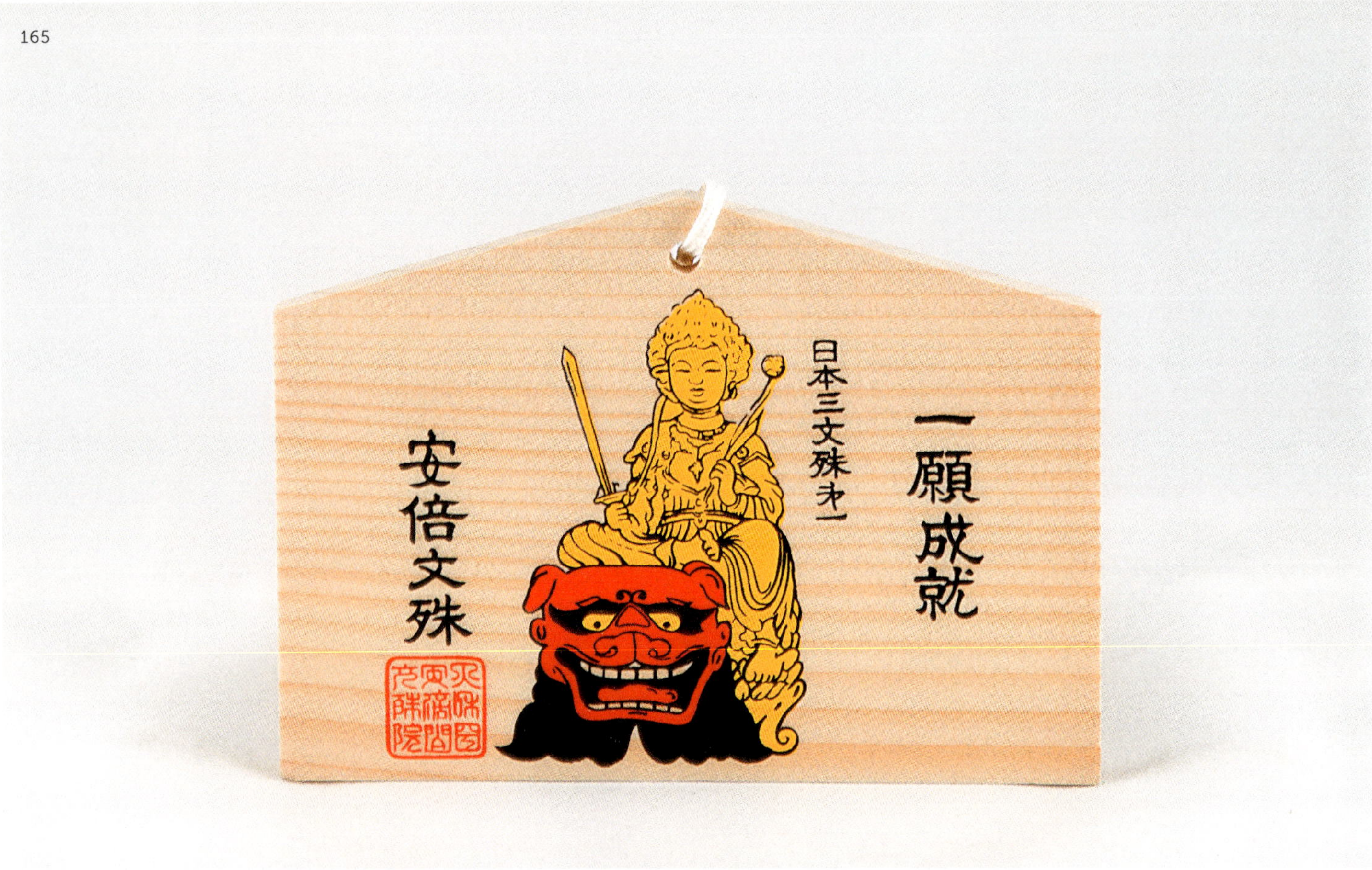

166
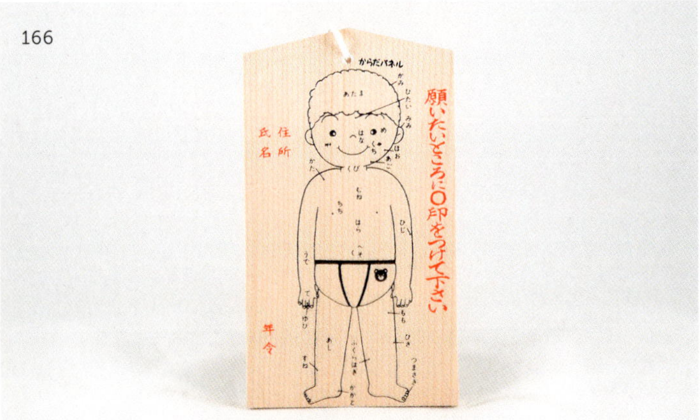

167
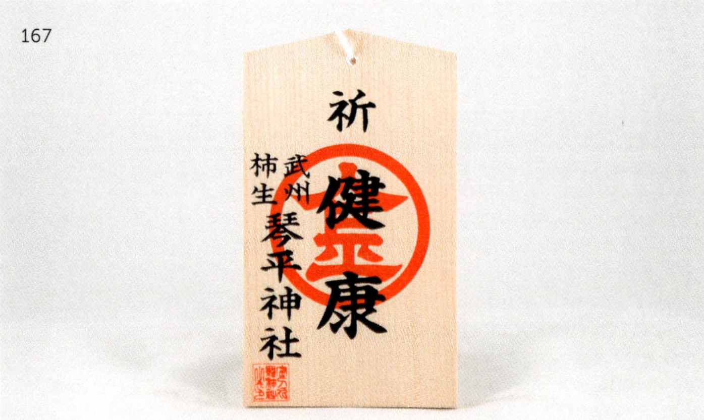

168
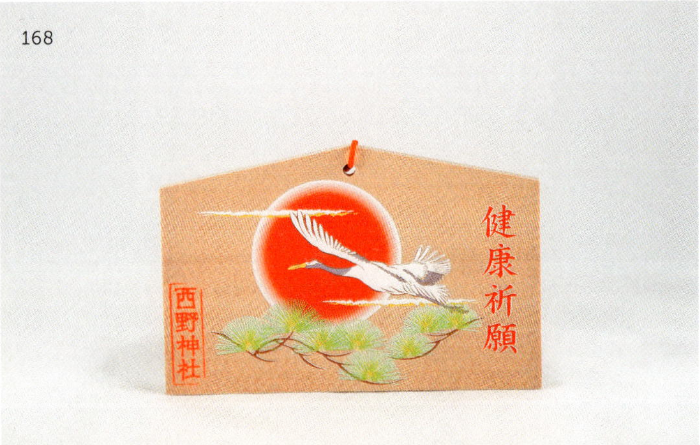

169
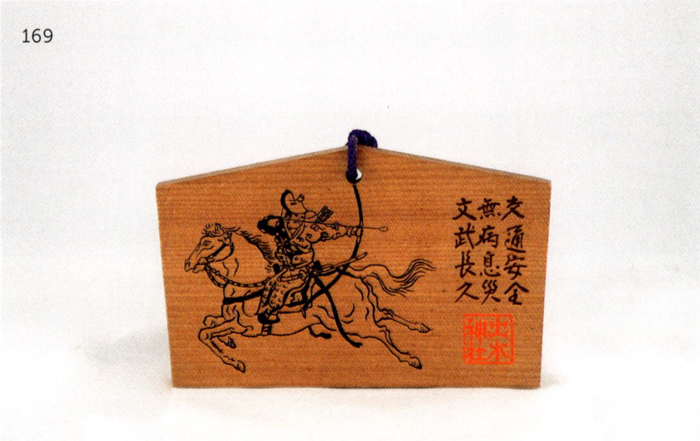

Health
健康 (*kenkō*)

165
Ema depicting statue of *Monju Bosatsu* 文殊菩薩 from *Abe Monjuin* 安倍文殊院. Sakurai, Nara Prefecture. Late 20th century or early 21st century. W. 12.6 cm
The inscriptions read:
一願成就 = *ichi gan jōju* (fulfilment of one prayer/wish)
日本三文珠第一霊場 = *Nihon san Monju dai ichi reijō* (first site on the Japan Three Monju Pilgrimage)
大和国 = *Yamato kuni* (Yamato kingdom; Yamato is an old name for Japan)
安倍文殊 = *Abe Monju*

The temple sells *boke sake* (wine made from quinces) that is said to maintain health. Its *ema* shows part of a seven-metre-high statue of the temple that represents *Monju Bosatsu* seated on a *sishi* (lion) and flanked by four attendants.

Ema designs

This section presents a few *ema* designs that are used for health in general. *Ema* for other human life issues have been reviewed in other sections of part three and *ema* designs for the healing or prevention of illnesses will be discussed in part four.

Human body 人体 *(jintai)*

166-167
Bushū Kakio Kotohira Jinja 武州柿生琴平神社 Kawasaki, Kanagawa Prefecture. Early 21st century. W. 9.0 cm
The inscription on the front reads:
願いたいところに○印をつけてください = *negaitai tokoro ni O in wo tsukete kudasai* (please place an O mark on the place which is the focus of your request)

An inscription on the reverse reads:
祈健康 = *ki kenkō* (wish for health)

A published *ema* with a similar design is attributed to a temple in Sendai (Miyagi Prefecture) [VO-197].

Crane and pine tree 鶴と松 *(tsuru to matsu)*

The crane and the pine tree are both symbols of longevity.

168
Nishino Jinja 西野神社. Sapporo, Hokkaido Prefecture. Early 21st century. W. 15.1 cm
The inscriptions read:
健康祈願 = *kenkō kigan* (prayer for health)

Horseback archery 流鏑馬 *(yabusame)*

Yabusame (horseback archery) is performed at sanctuaries to please and entertain the gods watching over Japan. An archer on a galloping horse has to shoot three special arrows at three wooden targets. He must control his horse with his knees, since he needs both hands to shoot his bow.

169
Izumi Jinja 出水神社. Kumamoto, Kumamoto Prefecture. Late 20th century. W. 15.6 cm
The inscriptions read:
交通安全 = *kōtsū anzen* (travel safety)
無病息災 = *mubyōsokusai* (sound health)
文武長久 = *bunbu chōkyū* (perpetuity of the pen and the sword; this refers to the samurai notion that military prowess should be aligned with scholarship and lead to long life).
西野神社 = *Nishino Jinja*

170

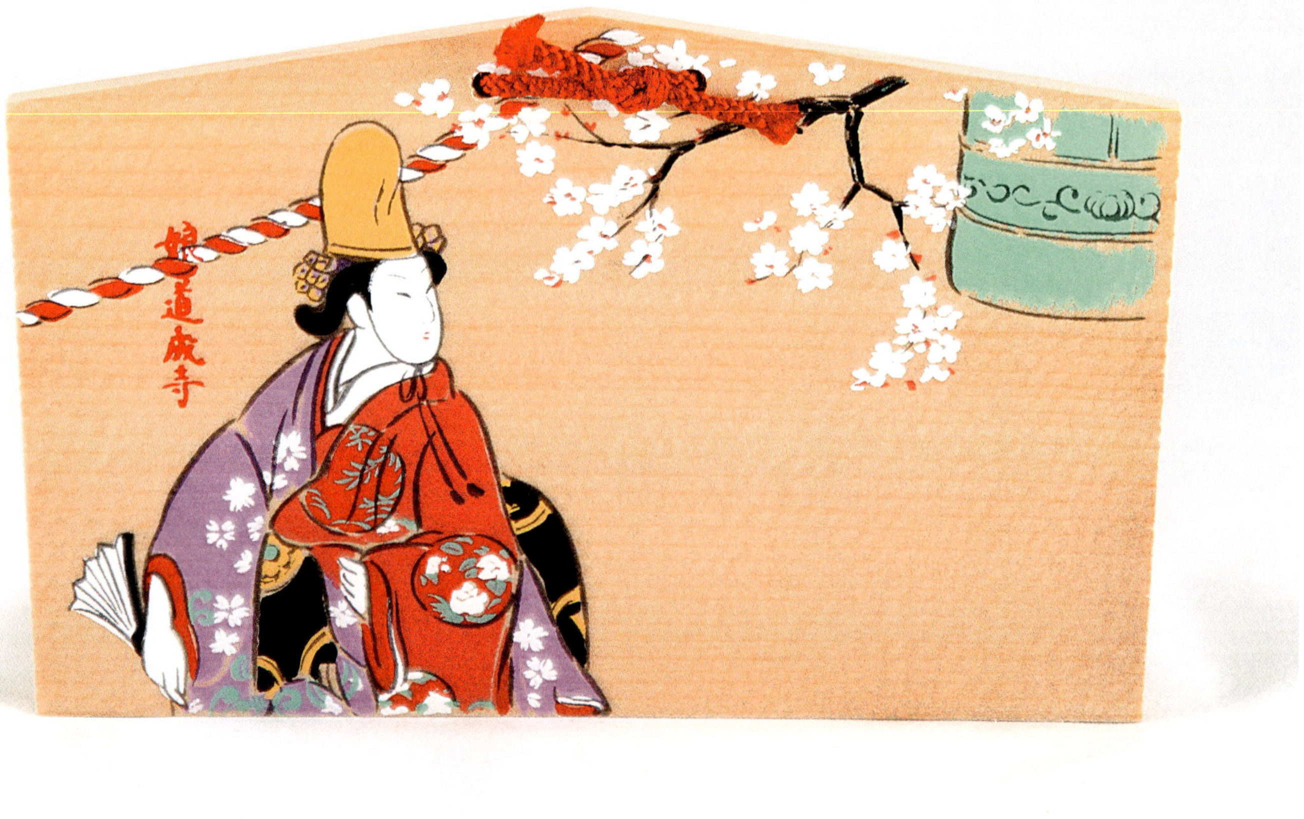

171

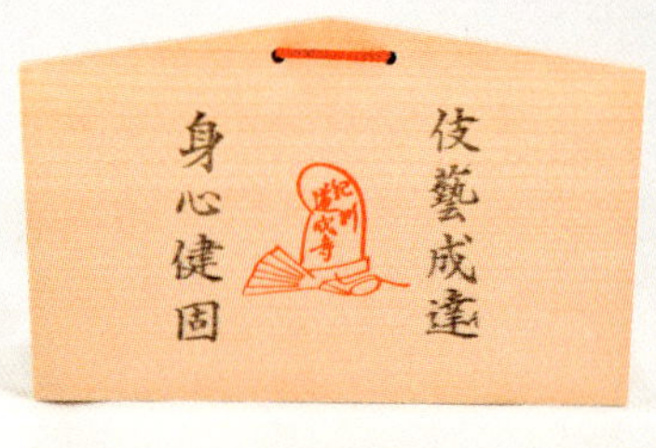

172

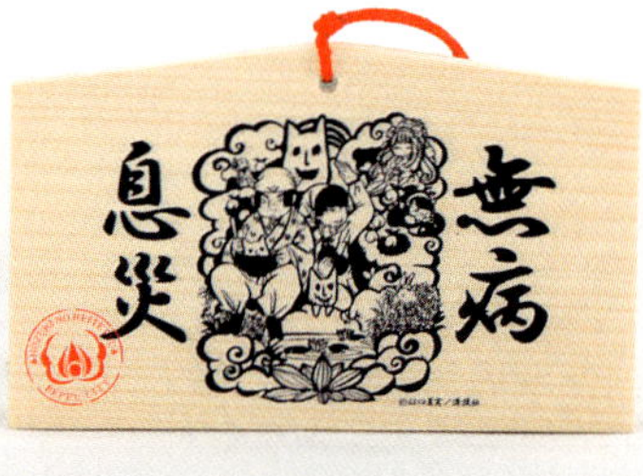

Musume Dōjōji 娘道成寺

Musume Dōjōji is a famous *kabuki* play (classical drama) that tells the story of the traveling priest *Anchin*. He falls in love with the beautiful *Kiyohime*, but manages to overcome his desire and refrains from further meetings. When she starts to pursue him in a furious rage, he flees and hides under the temple bell of *Dōjōji*. In the meantime, *Kiyohime* transforms into a large serpent and coils around the bell, making it white-hot and thereby burning the priest inside to death.

170–171

Dōjōji 道成寺. Hidakagawa, Wakayama Prefecture. Early 21st century. W. 17.1 cm
The kanji on the reverse read:
伎藝成達 = *gigei jōtatsu* (progress/skilful development in the arts)
紀州道成寺 = *Kishū Dōjōji* (Kishu is the traditional name for the Wakayama region where the temple is)
身心健固 = *shinshin kengo* (strengthening of mind and body)

This *ema* is reproduced here because its reverse is inscribed with *shinshin kengo*. The front of the *ema* shows *Kiyohime* in a gorgeous kimono and part of the temple bell in the upper right corner.

Manga characters 漫画 キャラ *(manga kyara)*

172

Beppu, Oita Prefecture. Early 21st century
The inscription reads:
無病息災 = *mubyō sokusai* (sound health)

The *ema* design portrays characters from a Japanese manga series called *Hōzuki no Reitetsu* 鬼灯の冷徹.

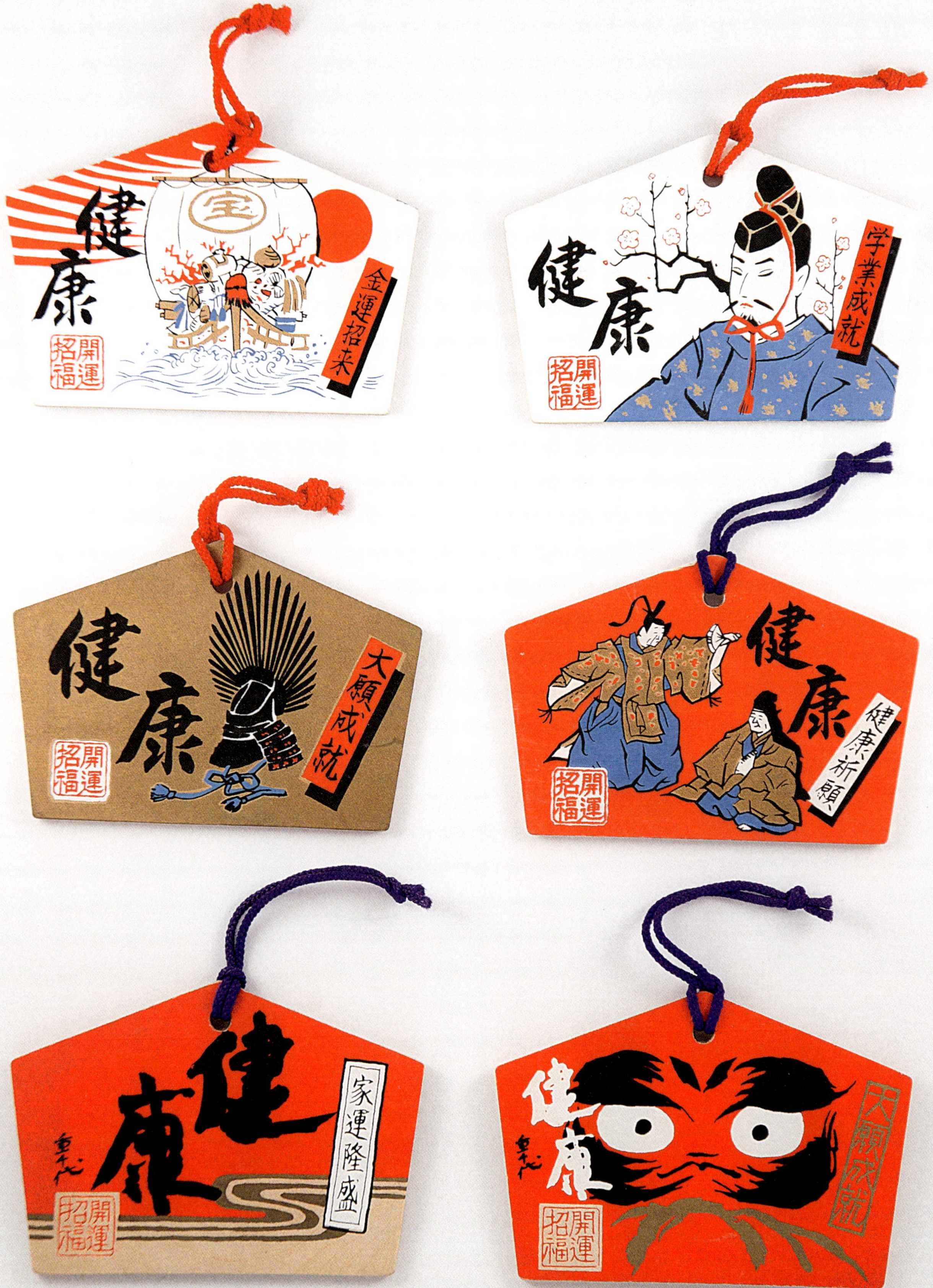
健康
金運招来
開運招福
健康
学業成就
開運招福
健康
大願成就
開運招福
健康
健康祈願
開運招福
健康
家運隆盛
開運招福
健康
大願成就
開運招福

Inscription with 健康 = kenkō (health)

173
Six small *ema* of unclear origin that have different designs but all share 健康 = *kenkō* (health) as inscription. The seals also read the same: 開運招福 = *kaiun shōfuku* (good luck charm for opening up good luck).

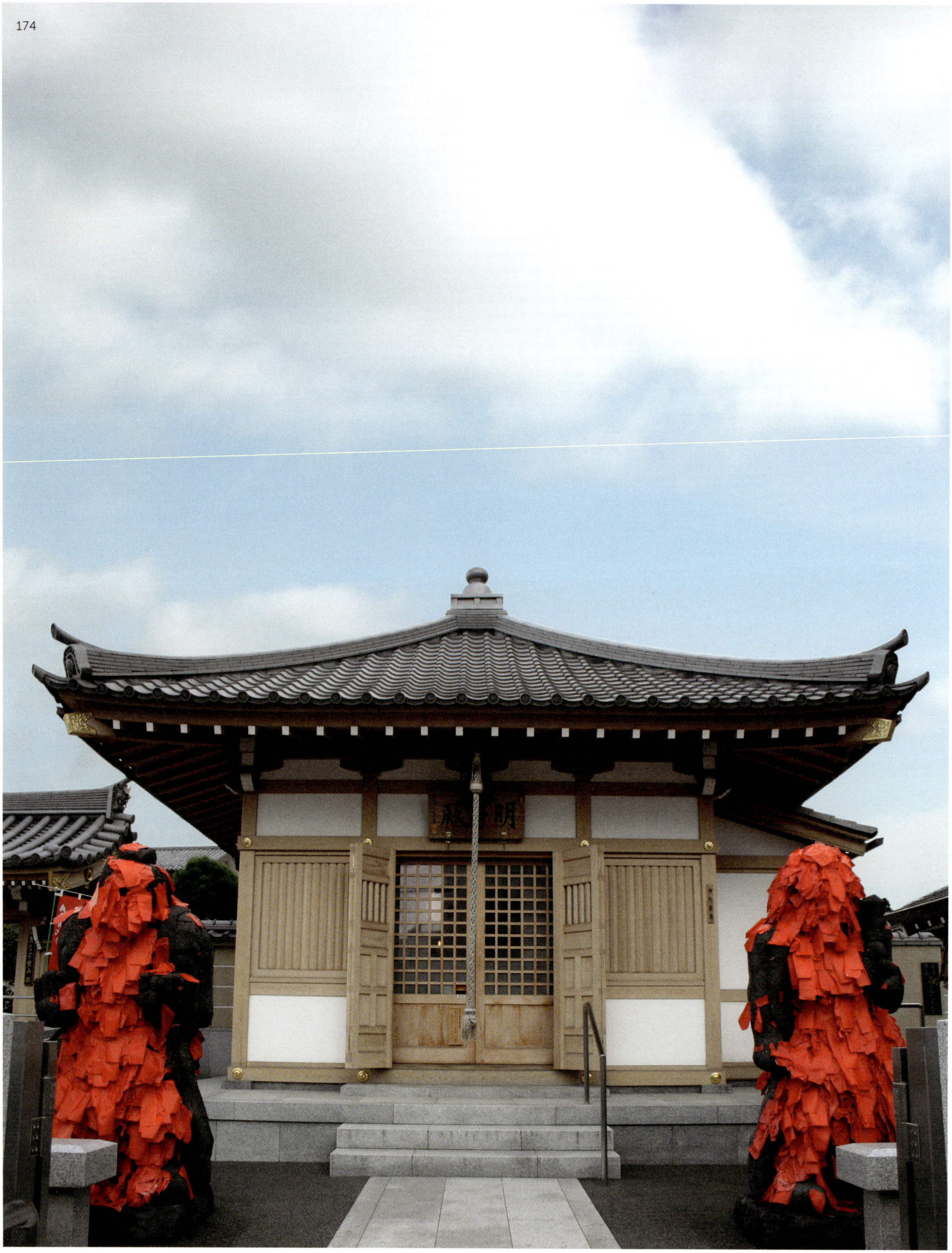

4 Illnesses 病気 (*Byōki*)

174
Two guardian Deva kings 仁王 (*Niō*) standing in front of *Akagami Niō Togakuji* (Kita Ward, Tokyo). People who want to be cured of an illness affecting a specific body part purchase two red papers in the temple shop. They paste the first red paper on the corresponding part of the right-hand *Niō* statue and then paste the other red paper on the left-hand statue in the hope that they will be cured.

Similar practices occur elsewhere. For instance, there is a *Yakushi* statue at *Kegonji* (Ibi District, Gifu Prefecture) that is completely covered with prayer slips. People put a prayer slip on the statue in the place where they feel pain or problems in their own bodies, then throw water over the statue and the prayer slip while praying. In such ways their pains/problems are symbolically removed from the sufferer and healed or absorbed by *Yakushi*.

This part presents different categories of *ema* designs for recovery from illness. *Ema* for maintaining good health and other human life issues are discussed in part three (p.67).

175

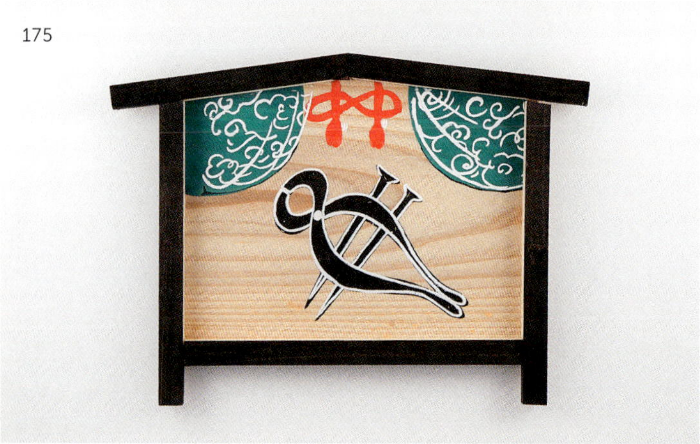

176

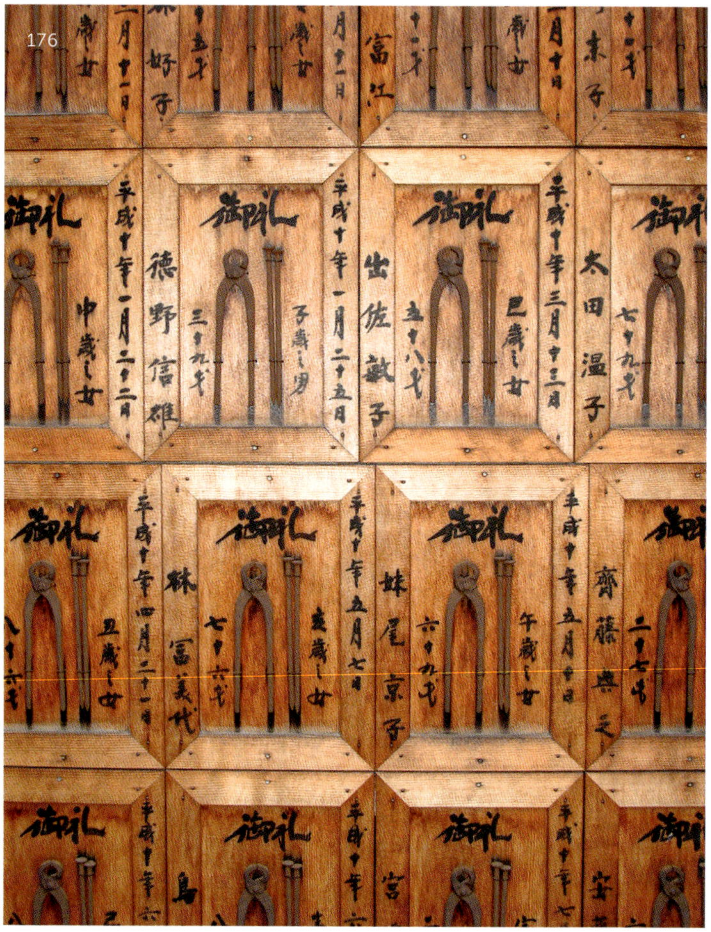

177

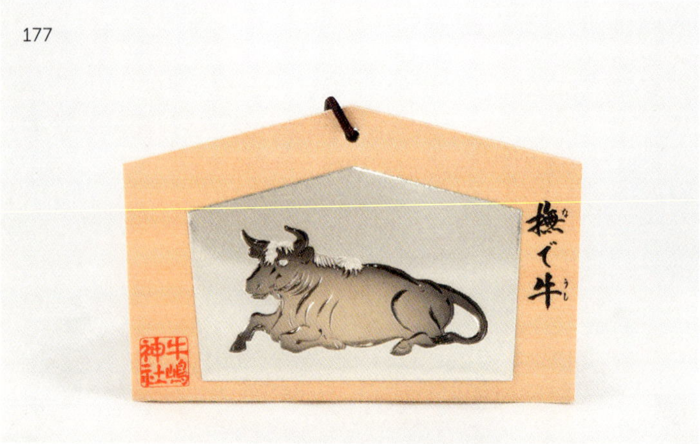

178

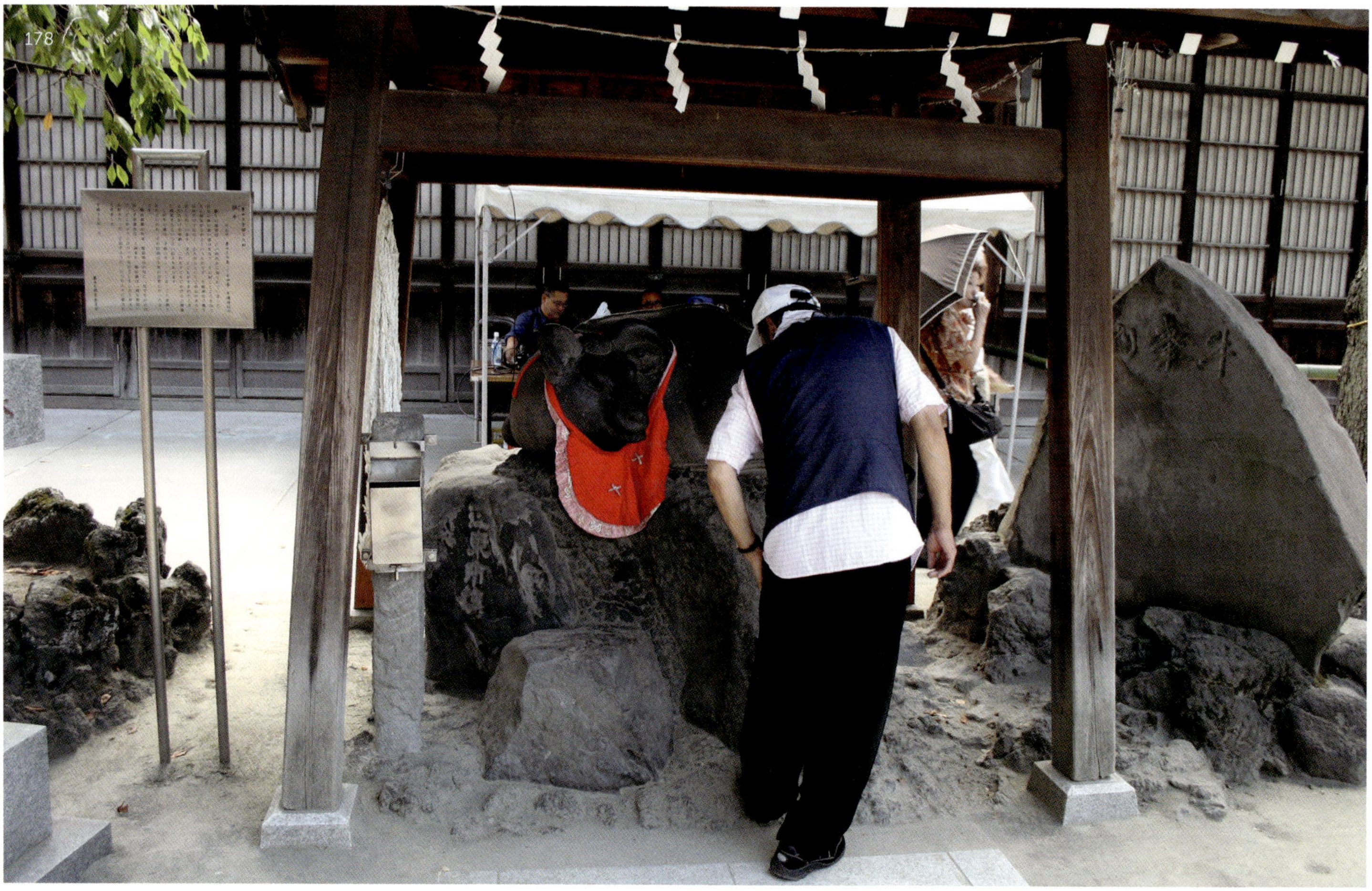

Recovery from illness 病気平癒 (*byōki heiyu*)

This section presents examples of *ema* designs for recovery from illness in general. *Ema* for specific categories of illnesses are reviewed in later sections of part four.

Ema designs

Pincers and nail(s) 釘と釘抜 (*kugi to kuginuki*)

Ema designs with pincers and one or two nails were used for pulling out pains and illnesses from the body [TS-4].

175
Hand-painted reproduction for a Japanese club of *ema* collectors called *Nihon Ema Tomo no Kai* (Friends of Japanese Ema Society). Late 20th century. W. 18.3 cm. Original design possibly from the Omi region (now Shiga Prefecture) [1].

176
Ema with *kuginuki* (pincers, nail puller) and *kugi* (nail). *Shakuzōji* 石像寺. Kamigyo Ward, Kyoto
The inscription on top reads: 御礼 = *orei* (thanking, expression of gratitude).

The temple enshrines *Kuginuki Jizō* (Nail-Pulling *Jizō*) who is addressed for good health and recovery from illness. This is based on the legend of a merchant who suffered from severe pain in his hands and came to pray to *Jizō* in *Shakuzōji* for seven days so that his pain would go away. During the night of the 7th day, *Jizō* showed him two nails in a dream and told him that he was suffering because in a former life he had been sticking nails into a straw doll to curse people. When the man woke up his pain was gone and when he hurried to the temple he saw two bloody nails in front of the statue of *Jizō*. The man gratefully promised to pay the temple one hundred other visits. From that time on, *Jizō* has been called *Kuginuki Jizō* and people have come to him to get rid of all kinds of pain and physical or mental hardships. *Kuginuki* (Nail-Pulling) is also a pun with *ku* = pain and *nuki* = without [GG3-2013/01].

Cow/ox to be rubbed 撫で牛 (*nadeushi*)

177–178
Ushijima Jinja 牛島神社. Sumida ward, Tokyo. Early 21st century. W. 15.0 cm
The inscription reads:
撫で牛 (*nadeushi*)

There is a *nadeushi* statue at *Ushijima Jinja* to which healing effects are attributed. To benefit, one has alternately to touch one's own sick body part and the corresponding part of the *nadeushi* statue. The older man in the lower picture repeatedly first rubbed the *nadeushi* statue with his hand and then his left knee.

Various sanctuaries in Japan have statues that are used in this way. These are not limited to cows/oxen and other animals (such as *nadeusagi* = rabbit to be rubbed), but also include Buddhist figures of worship such as *Yakushi*, *Binzuru*, and *Jizō* [MS].

179

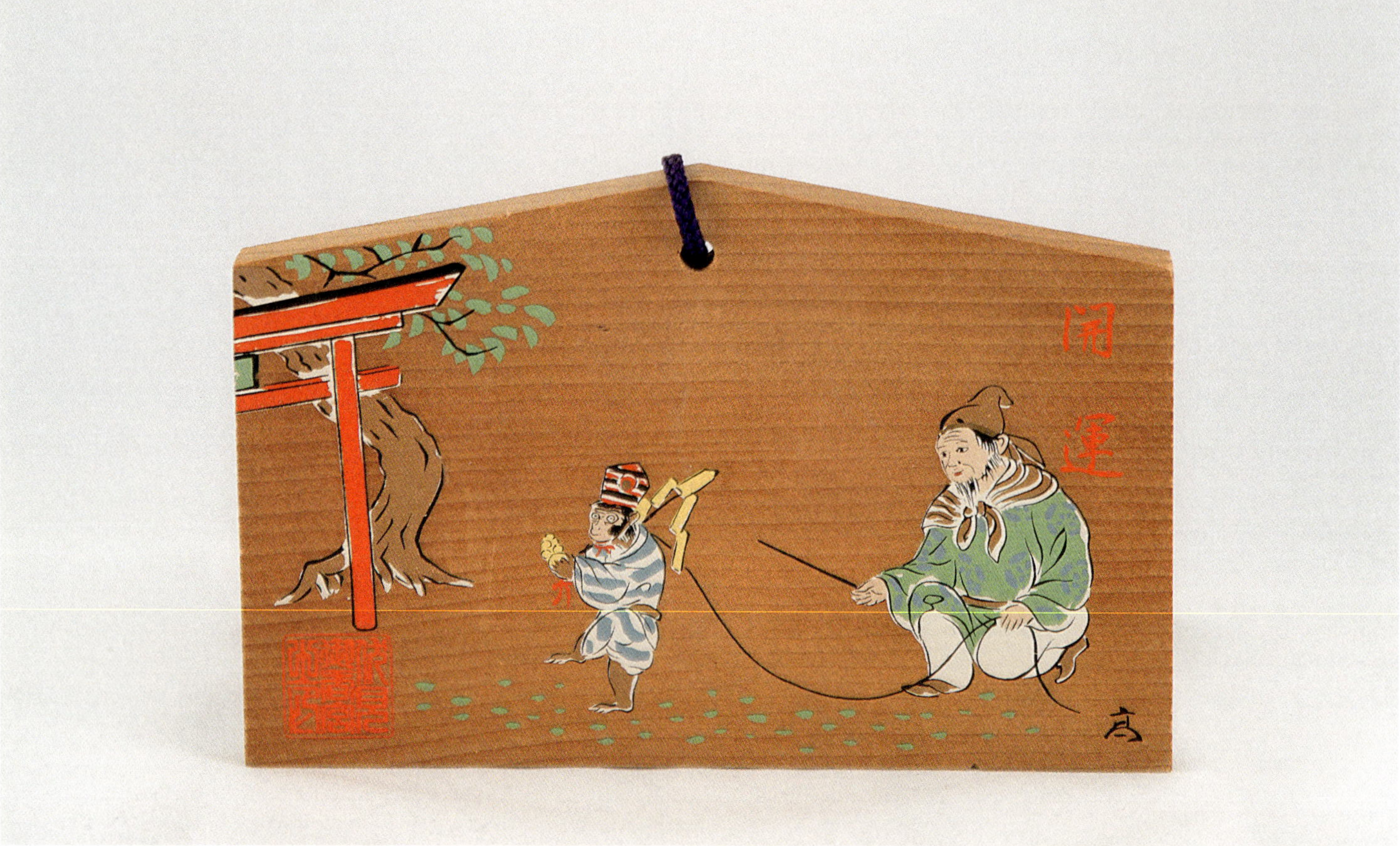

180

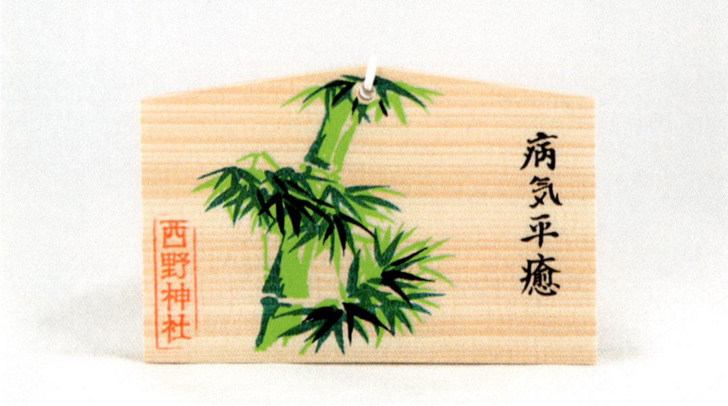

181

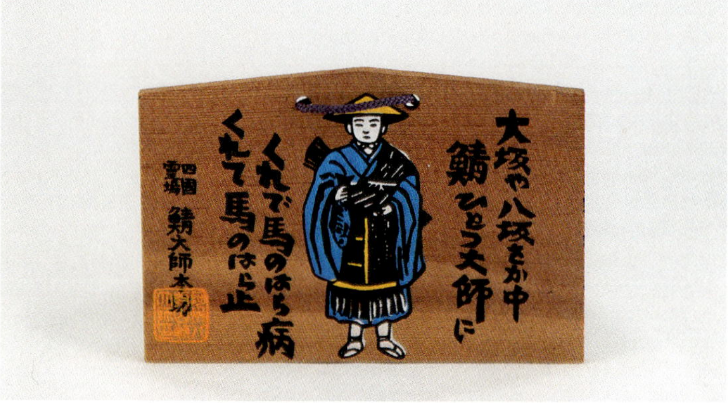

182

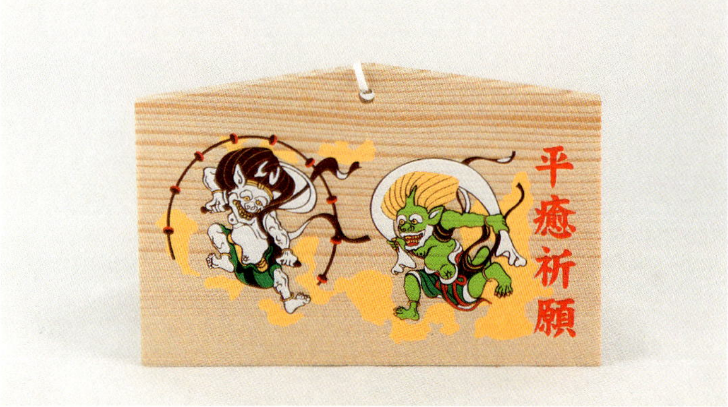

183

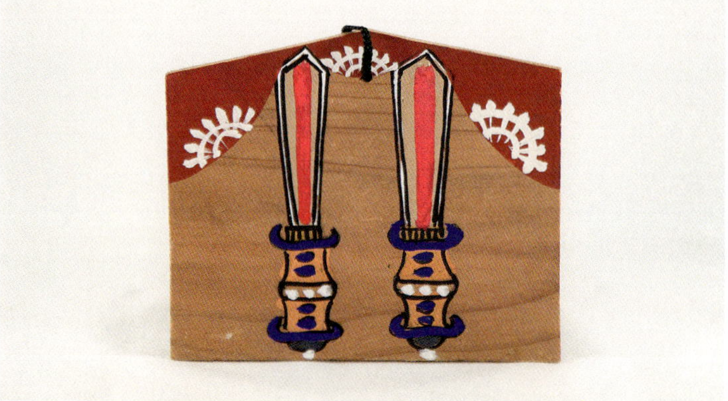

Monkey trainer 猿回し *(sarumawashi)*

179
Gokōnomiya Jinja 御香宮神社. Fushimi Ward, Kyoto. Late 20th century. W. 17.6 cm
The inscription on the right reads:
開運 = *kaiun* (opening up good luck)

This *ema* design is based on the legend of a *sarumawashi* (showman who trains performing monkeys) who had fallen ill. He was cured by drinking *gokōsui* water brought to him by his monkey. *Gokōnomiya* means shrine of aromatic water (from a spring yielding very pure water).

Green bamboo 青竹 *(aodake)*

Aodake symbolises health and youthfulness. There is an *ema* design of bamboo shoots on a wooden stand in the literature that was meant for healthy growth [TS-9].

180
Nishino Jinja 西野神社. Sapporo, Hokkaido Prefecture. Early 21st century. W. 13.8 cm
The inscriptions read:
病気平癒 = *byōki heiyu* (recovery from illness)
西野神社 = *Nishino Jinja*

Saba Daishi 鯖大師

Saba Daishi Honbō (Kaifu District, Tokushima Prefecture) can be visited for *byōki heiyu* (recovery from illness) and *kodakara* (the treasure that is children). The principal object of worship is a statue of *Kōbō Daishi* (founder of Shugon Buddhism) with a *saba* (mackerel) in his hand. According to the temple's foundation legend, he once met a merchant with a pack horse loaded with dried mackerel. When he asked the merchant for a mackerel, the latter refused and walked away. After a while, the horse stumbled and fell ill, and the merchant realised his mistake. He rushed back to *Kōbō Daishi* to ask for forgiveness and for a cure for his horse. *Kōbō Daishi* uttered a spell over a pot of sea water and, when this water was given to the horse, it quickly recovered. The merchant gave a mackerel to *Kōbō Daishi*, who placed it in the sea and said a prayer, whereafter the fish came to life again and swam away. The merchant built a sanctuary on the spot that would become known as *Saba* (Mackerel) *Daishi* [2].

181
Saba Daishi Honbō 鯖大師本坊, Kaifu District, Tokushima Prefecture. Late 20th century. W. 13.4 cm
The inscriptions read:
大坂や八坂さか中鯖ひとつ大師にくれで馬のはら病くれて馬のはら止 = *Ōsaka ya Yasaka-sa ka chū saba hitotsu daishi ni kure de uma no hara-byō kurete uma no hara tome* (poem referring to the foundation legend)
四国霊場 = *Shikoku reijō* (Shikoku Pilgrimage site)

According to an inscription on the reverse of the *ema*, one must promise not to eat mackerel for three years to make wishes come true.

Fūjin 風神 *and Raijin* 雷神

Fūjin is the Shinto God of the Wind who can be recognized by the large bag of winds around his shoulders. *Raijin* is the Shinto God of the Thunder and is usually surrounded by a ring of drums [MS].

182
Mikuriya Jinja 御厨神社. Akashi, Hyogo Prefecture. Early 21st century. W. 14.0 cm
The inscription reads:
平癒祈願 = *heiyu kigan* (prayer for recovery)

This *ema* design is available not only at *Mikuriya Jinja*, but also at *Haruna Jinja* (Numata, Gunma Prefecture). It is based on a famous painting by the Edo painter *Tawaraya Sotatsu* and depicts *Fūjin* on the right and *Raijin* on the left.

Swords 剣 *(ken)*

183
Origin unknown. Late 20th century. W. 14.7 cm

A published example of this *ema* design is described as swords of *Fudō* and was used against evil spirits and illness [TS-18]. It is unclear whether the specimen shown here served the same purposes.

An additional *ema* design (not illustrated here) that was probably used for recovery from illness consisted of flowers made of wheat straw at *Kinosaki Jinja* 城崎神社 (Nantan, Kyoto Prefecture) [TS-4].

184

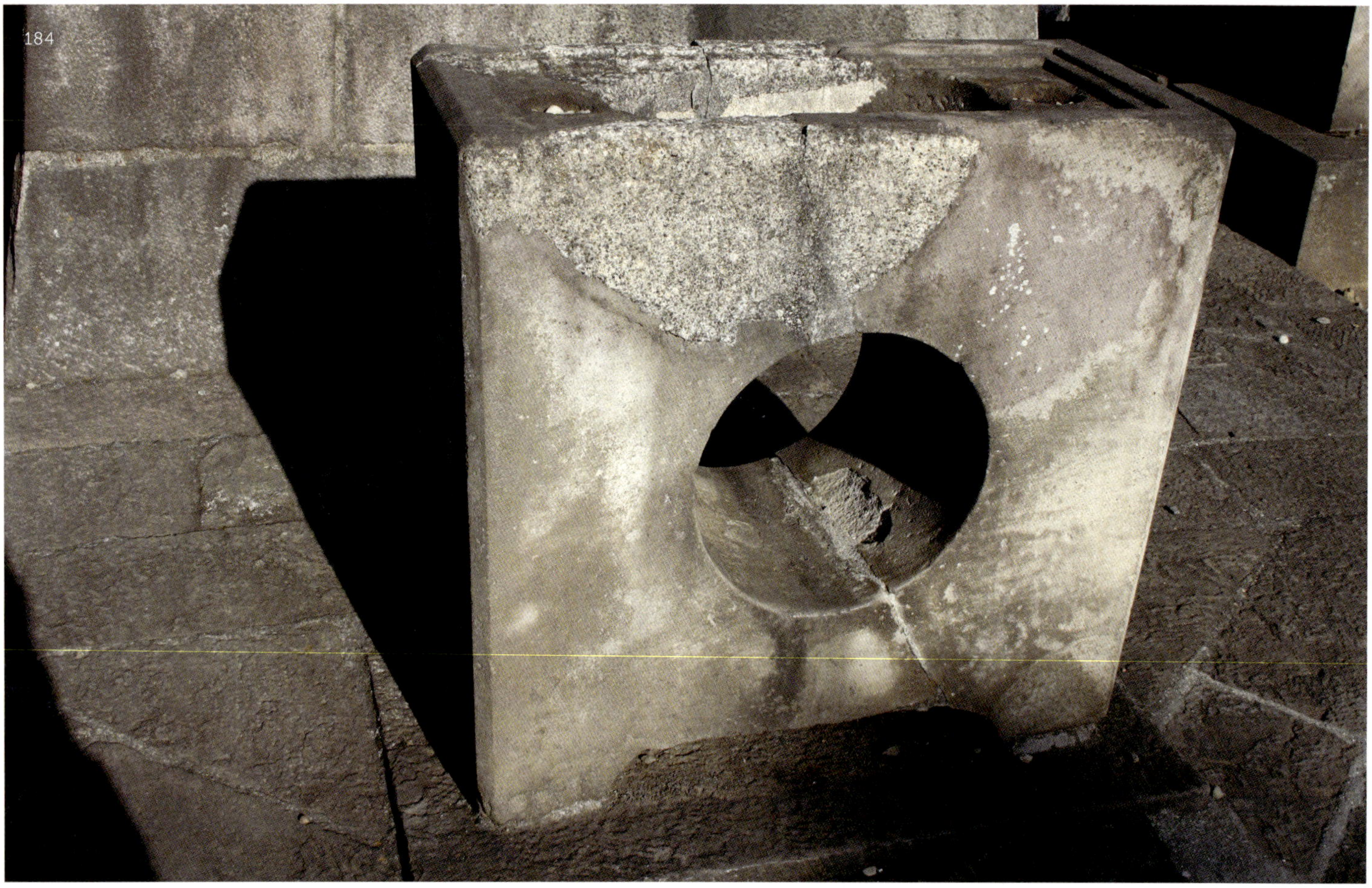

185

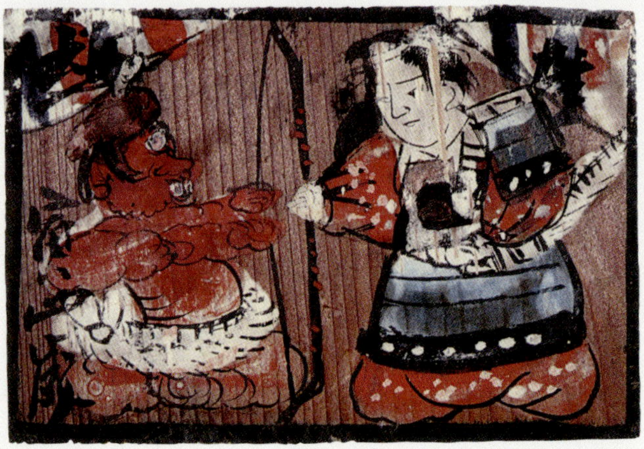

186

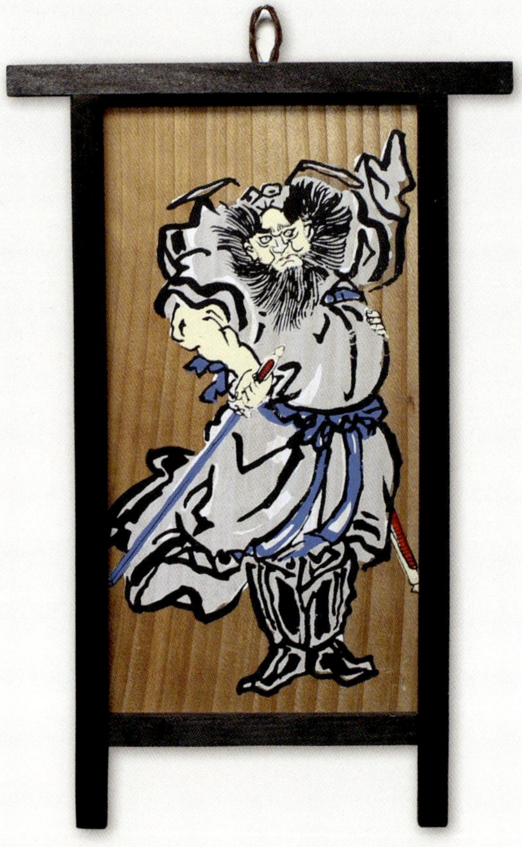

Epidemics
疫癘 (*ekirei*)

Background

The period from 700 to 1050 has become known as the age of plagues, because in those days the Japanese population suffered from repeated outbreaks of epidemic diseases such as smallpox, measles, influenza and diarrhoeal diseases (e.g., dysentery). Such diseases had a profound influence on religious activities. When Buddhism was introduced to Japan, early believers reached out to this new religion because it promised protection from sickness. Figures of worship it brought with it, such as *Yakushi* (Medicine Buddha), proved especially popular in this context. After the spread of a smallpox epidemic around 735-737, the spread of Buddhism was furthered by an imperial decision to erect the great temple *Tōdaiji* in Nara with branch temples throughout the country [WF].

Epidemic diseases such as smallpox, measles, influenza and diarrhoeal diseases caused problems and took their toll throughout much of Japanese history, and well into the Edo period (1600-1868). It is estimated, for example, that at least 10% of the population succumbed to smallpox around 1849 (when the first smallpox vaccine was introduced). It was a particularly common cause of death among children under 5 years old. Measles claimed far fewer victims over time than smallpox, because its epidemics were rarer. Yet it remained a dreaded affliction, because (unlike smallpox) it seemed to come out of nowhere and infected adults as well as young children. Since measles occurred only infrequently the population would be very susceptible to new outbreaks and when these occurred people would largely fall ill at once. Concerns about such issues were probably a factor also in the severe restrictions that the Japanese imposed on their foreign contacts, allowing trade only through their port of Nagasaki. Measles epidemics usually spread from this south-eastern gateway to the major cities of Kyoto, Osaka and Edo, and from there to the more remote parts of central and northern Japan [AJ].

The recurrent epidemics in the Edo period led to the donation of *ema* in the hope that one's family would be spared these disasters. An impressive example is a votive panel now in the British Museum, which dates from 1860 when Edo (now Tokyo) was plagued by measles and influenza. The panel depicts the Shinto deity *Susanoo no Mikoto* making a pact with thirteen spirits of illnesses (see p.19).

Towards the end of the Edo period, it was still common to ward off smallpox by magical means, such as certain potions and spells, pilgrimages and red-coloured folk toys or woodblock prints. According to folk belief, the colour *aka* (red) could avert smallpox and the Shinto deity *Hōsōgami* who caused smallpox. It was thought that a patient was dangerously ill if his skin turned purple, whereas he was more likely to recover if his skin turned red. Folk toys representing a red cow (*akabeko*) were valued as charms against smallpox and other serious infections. They could expel the demons responsible or keep them away. These toys were considered as omens of good luck and prosperity and served as gifts on auspicious occasions such as New Year (see p.63) [MS].

Hōsō-e (woodblock prints against smallpox) were printed entirely or predominantly in red and were therefore known as *aka-e* (red pictures). These prints were believed to be particularly powerful, if they portrayed *Shōki*, a demon queller. *Hashika-e* (measles pictures) were used in similar ways for protection against or recovery from measles. These woodblock prints depicted how the gods of measles were defeated or provided instructions on what to do or eat and what should be avoided [1].

184
Measles stone. Cemetery adjacent to *Yūtenji* 祐天寺. Meguro Ward, Tokyo

This stone served as a magical treatment for preventing or curing measles. When measles were prevalent, long lines of parents with their children would wait before the stone in the belief that their child would recover or be spared from measles if they were to put the child three times back and forth through the hole, while murmuring "I hope it will not be serious". The background story is that once the Jodo priest *Yūten* succeeded in conquering the devil in a long argument about religion. The belief gradually spread that a priest so powerful as to subdue the devil could also prevail against serious childhood ailments. After *Yūten*'s death, his residence was rebuilt by his disciples into a temple which was named *Yūtenji* after him [GS-173]. In the past, the temple offered an *ema* depicting the legendary priest *Yūten*, but late 2015 this *ema* was no longer available.

Ema designs

When an *ema* design shows a festival or charm with roots in the epidemic past, it does not automatically follow that that particular *ema* is currently in use for protection against epidemic diseases. For instance, the annual *Yasurai* Festival in Kyoto once started in response to epidemics, but present-day *ema* depicting this festival are not recommended for this specific purpose. Likewise, an *ema* portraying an *akabeko* charm (folk toy in the form of a red cow) is not used today as a protector against smallpox. Such *ema* have not been included in this section but in part two which deals with health-related images of festivals and charms (p.53 and p.63)

Ema for infections that primarily affect a specific body part or function are not discussed here either, but in the relevant section about that issue (e.g., lung tuberculosis in the section on respiratory symptoms/complaints).

Minamoto no Tametomo 源為朝

Ema for protection against smallpox often depicted heroic figures, such as the 12th century samurai *Minamoto no Tametomo*, in combat with a smallpox *oni* (demon). This motif is also seen in *hōsō-e* (woodblock prints for smallpox). According to legend, *Tametomo* was banished to the small island of *Hachijyo Jima*, which is believed to be the reason smallpox never occurred there [TS-33; IH2-92].

185
Image reproduced with permission of the publisher from Iwai H. *Ema ni negai o*. Tokyo: Nigensha, 2007:92

Shōki 鍾馗

Shōki is a Japanese Demon Queller, who protects against evil spirits and illness, expels the demons of plague, and guards the safety of hearth and home. His Chinese counterpart is the Taoist deity *Zhōng Kui*, whose ghost came to the 8th century emperor *Xuanzong* in a dream and saved him by vanquishing the demon that was making him ill. In the 17th century, the Japanese began using amulets depicting *Shōki* at the annual Boys' Festival to ward off smallpox and other illnesses [MS]. *Shōki* also features prominently in the *hōsō-e* (smallpox prints) of the 19th century.

186
Ema hand-painted by *Norihito Yasuda* (Nagoya) on commission from the Naito Museum of Pharmaceutical Sciences and Industry (Kakamigahara, Gifu Prefecture). Museum inv.no. Z22657. Late 20th century.

Used for the prevention of smallpox and *byōma taisan* (dispersal of the demons of illness). Inhabitants of the Kanto District tacked up an *ema* with *Shōki* at the entrances of their homes as a protection against evil spirits and smallpox [TS-18; NM-Z22657].

187

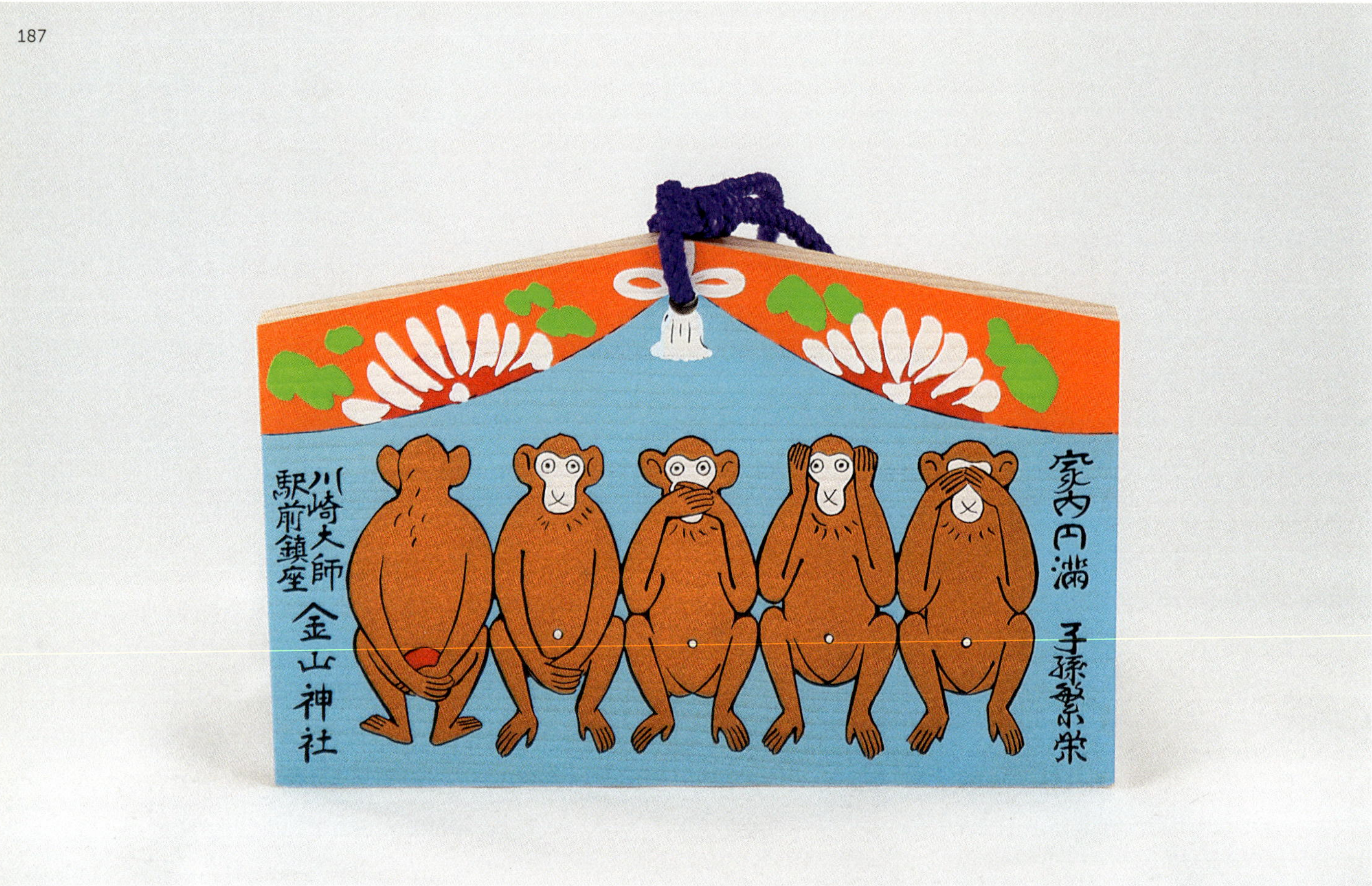

188

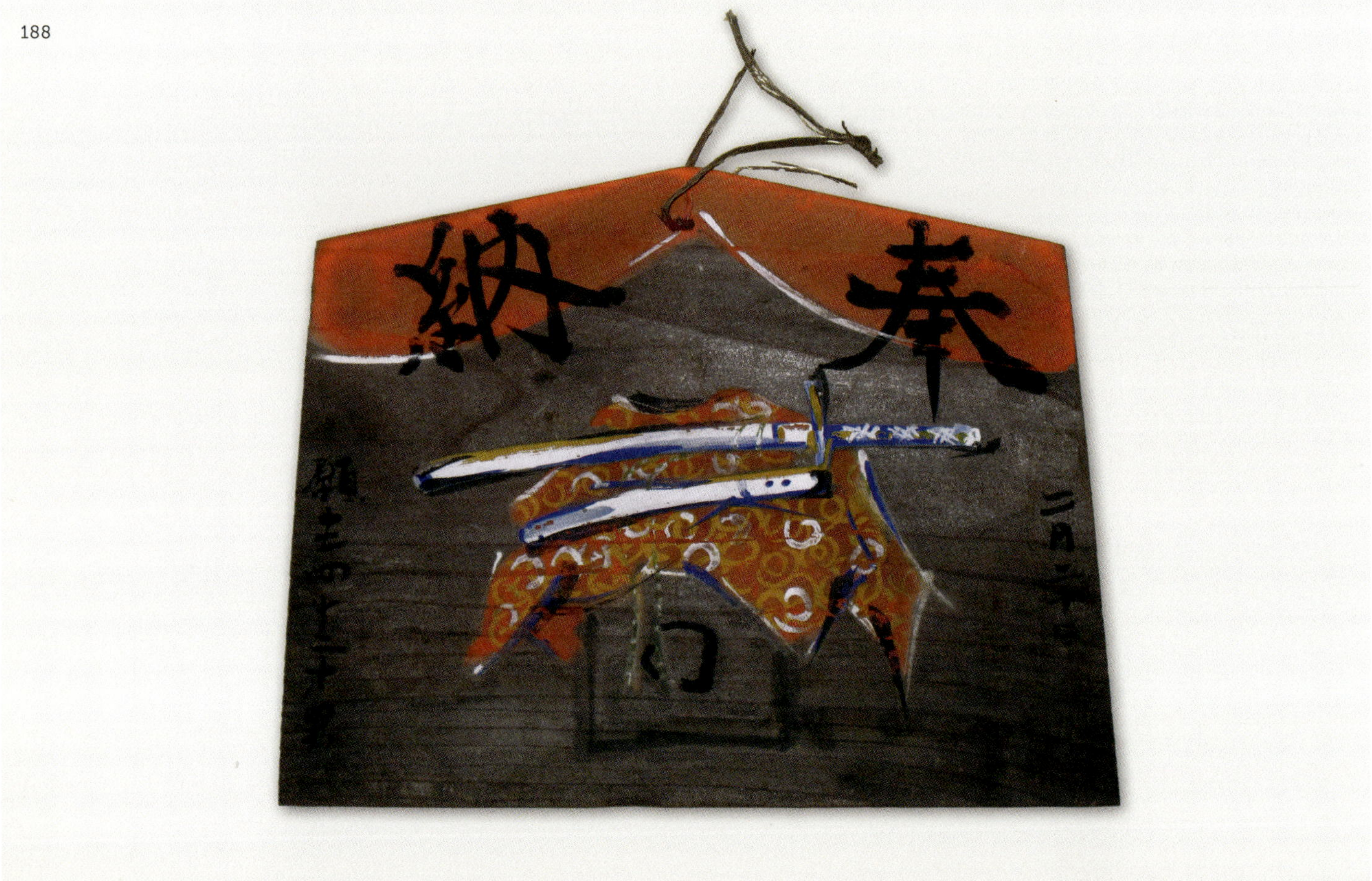

Protective monkeys 護猿 *(gosaru)*

The term *gosaru* (protective monkeys) is composed of *go* (which can mean five as well as protect) and *saru* (monkey). *Ema* with this design are sold by *Kanayama Jinja* to express commitment to safe sex (especially in the form of abstinence) and as protection against AIDS. The design reinforces the shrine's long association with benefits related to fertility and sexually transmitted diseases. The *ema* was created in the 1980s in rapid response to the AIDS epidemic. It gives educational advice on the prevention of AIDS by adding two monkeys that transmit no evil (*sesaru*) and receive no evil (*sasesaru*) to the popular three monkeys that see no evil, hear no evil, speak no evil (*misaru, kikasaru, iwasaru*) [RT-57].

187
Kanayama Jinja 金山神社. Kawasaki, Kanagawa Prefecture. Early 21st century. W. 17.5 cm
The inscriptions read:
家内円満 = *kanai enman* (harmony in one's home)
子孫繁栄 = *shison han'ei* (prosperity for one's offspring)
川崎大師 = *Kawasaki Daishi*
金山神社 = *Kanayama Jinja*
駅前鎮座 = *ekimae chinza* (shrine in front of the station)

Swords 剣 *(ken)*

The *ema* design of swords on a square wooden stand was used for the protection of children against measles, and in some districts for severing relationships [TS-11].

188
Ōsaki Hachimangū 国宝 大崎八幡宮. Sendai, Miyagi Prefecture. Early to mid-20th century. W. 23.9 cm
The inscription reads:
奉納 = *hōnō* (dedication, offering)
Tenri University Sankokan Museum (Tenri, Nara Prefecture). Museum inv.no. 74.248E1780 [acquired in 1975].

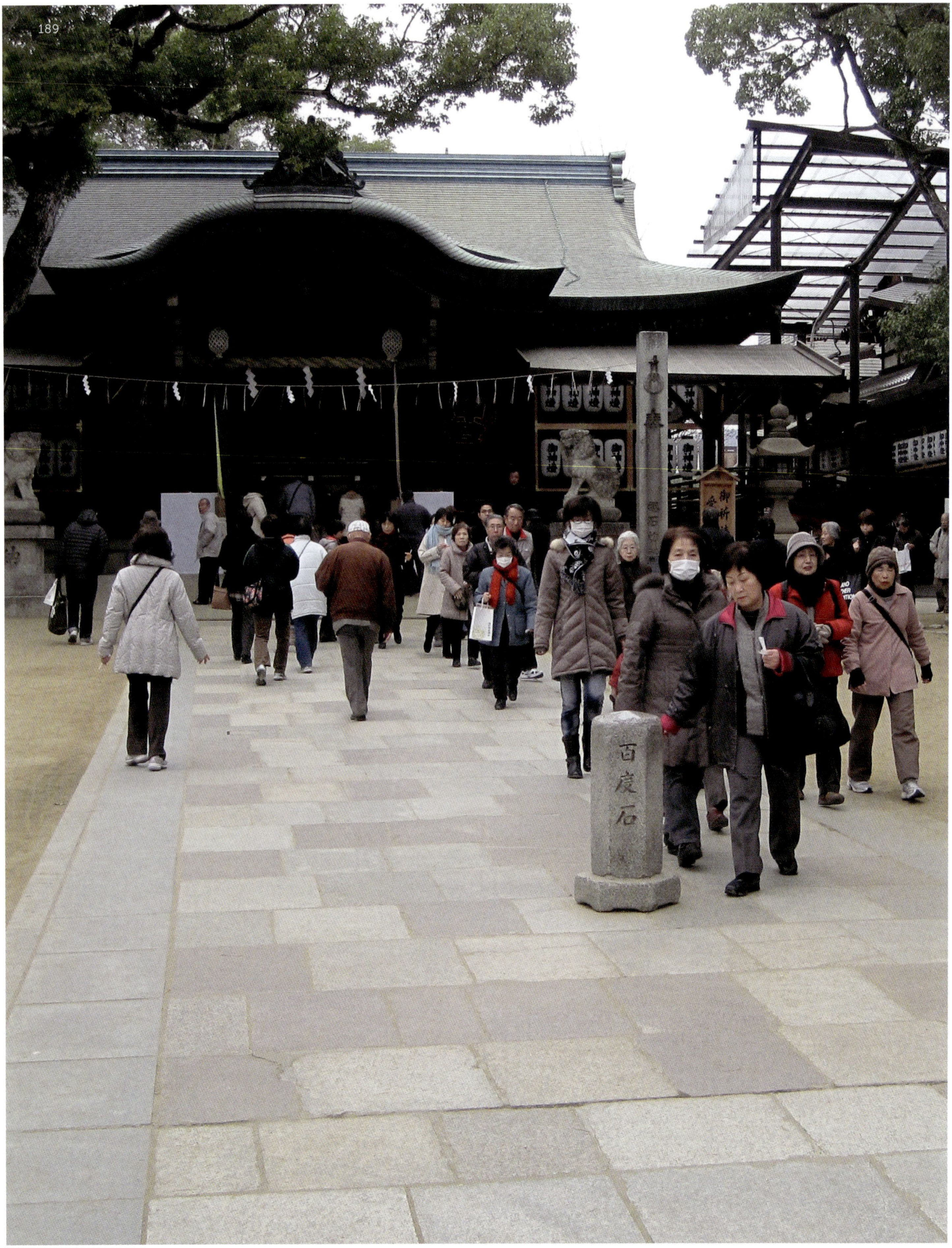
百度石

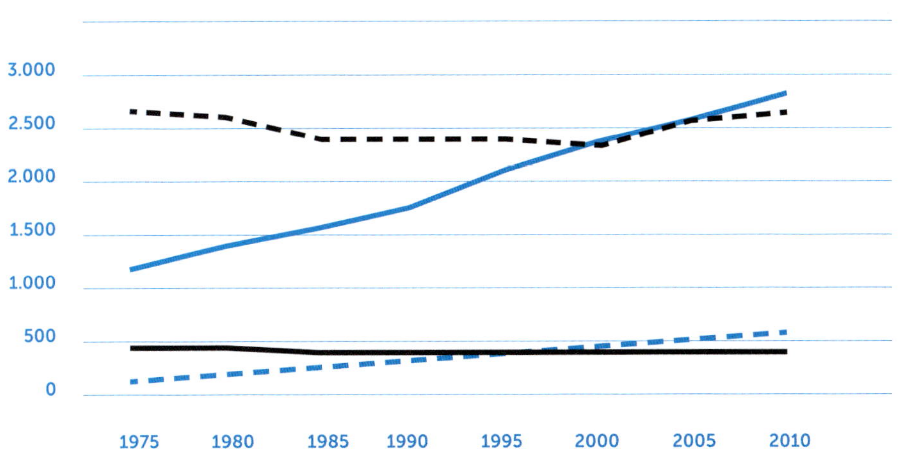

* Sum of hypertensive diseases, heart diseases, cerebrovascular diseases, and aortic aneurysm/ dissection

Figure 1 Leading causes of death in Japan: death rates per million inhabitants from 1975 to 2010. Based on Table 15 in Chapter 21 of the Japan Statistical Yearbook 2015 [SY15]

Neoplasms 新生物 (*shinseibutsu*)

Background

Around the turn of the last century, malignant neoplasms became the leading cause of death in Japan, taking over this top position from circulatory diseases. Around the same time, stomach cancer lost its number one ranking among cancers to lung cancer, primarily because the death rate for the latter increased almost fourfold in the late 20th century (Figure 1). Stomach cancer still occupies second place after lung cancer, however, and Japan continues to have one of the highest incidences of stomach cancer in the world. A type of cancer with a relatively low incidence compared to other well-developed countries is breast cancer [SY15; 1].

Several shrines and temples offer the benefit of *ganfūji* (prevention of cancer) or *gankiri* (removal of cancer). Among the figures of worship for these purposes are *Gankiri Jizō*, *Gankiri Kannon* (both at *Tsubakidō Henshōin*, Oita Prefecture) and *Gankiri Fudō-myō-ō* (*Nyoirinji*, Fukuoka Prefecture). Another figure of worship who is invoked not just for cancer, but for all kinds of ailments is *Yakushi Nyorai* (Medicine Buddha). Patients may first rub a selected part of his statue and then rub the same part of their own body, while asking to be cured of cancer, arthritis, headache and so on. This rubbing practice is also applied to statues of *Daikokuten* (one of the Seven Gods of Good Fortune), *Binzuru*, and *Fureai Kannon* [GG1-2014/04; MS]. Cf. p.113.

A shrine that is particularly famous for its benefits in cancer patients is *Ishikiri Jinja* (Higashiosaka, Osaka Prefecture). Its full name (*Ishikiri Tsurugiya Jinja*) literally means Stone-cutting Sword and Arrow Shrine, which reflects the enshrinement of a sharp sword and arrow (representing the grandson and great-grandson of the Sun Goddess *Amaterasu Omikami*). In the past, the shrine was visited particularly for cures for *dembo*, a local term for boils and tumours, but its major appeal today is the help that it offers to cancer patients and patients undergoing or about to undergo surgery of any type. There is an analogy between the sword and arrow enshrined and the surgical knife that cuts away tumours [EO-129,153].

189
Hundred times worship. 百度参り (*hyakudo mairi*). *Ishikiri Tsurugiya Jinja* 石切劔箭神社. Higashiosaka, Osaka Prefecture

Visitors of *Ishikiri Tsurugiya Jinja* who come to pray there because they or their loved ones have cancer must perform *hyakudomairi* (the hundred-round walking ritual): walking a hundred times between two stones in front of the shrine, thereby touching the stones each time [EO-126; RT-135].

190

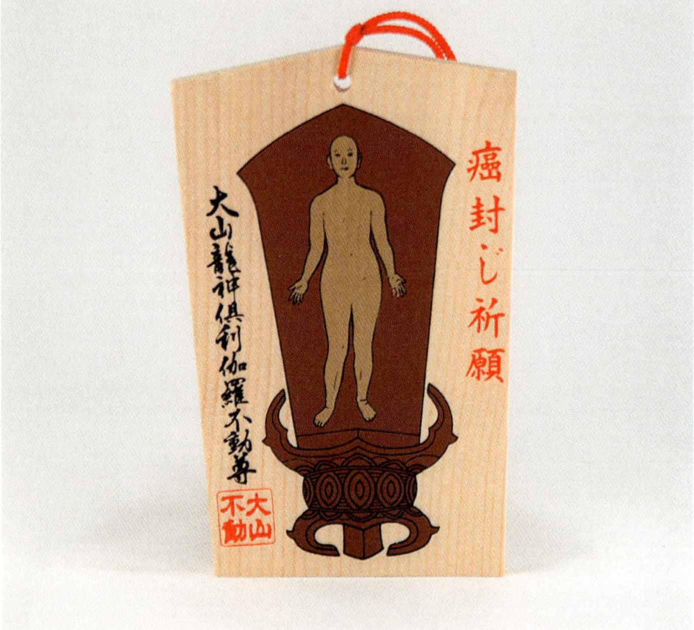

191

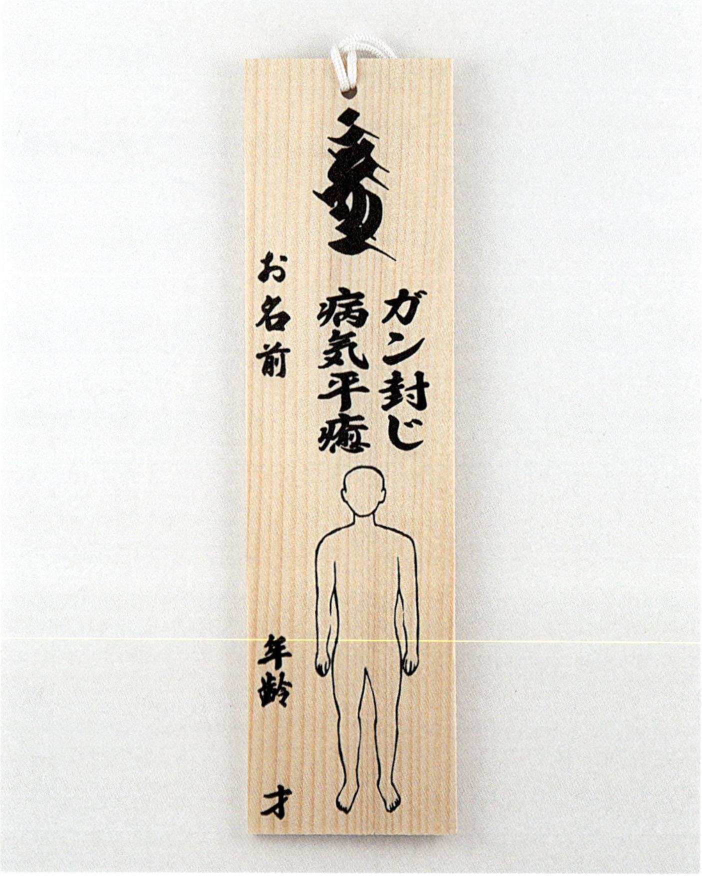

192

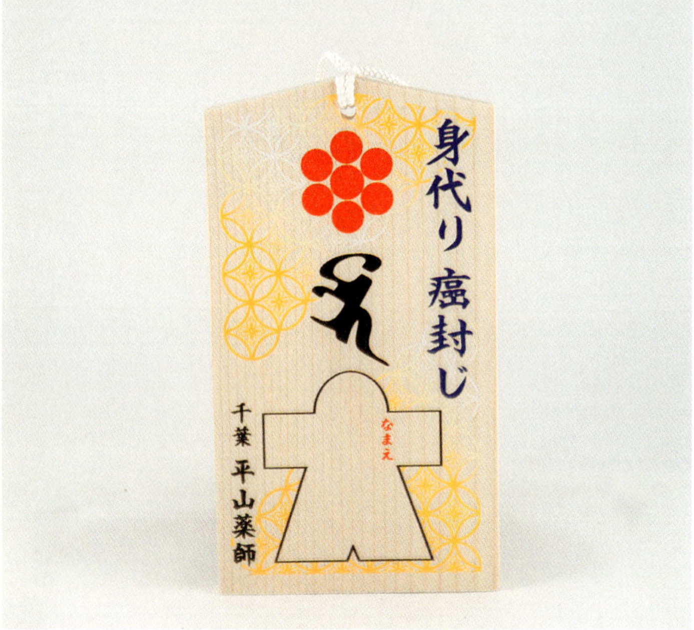

193

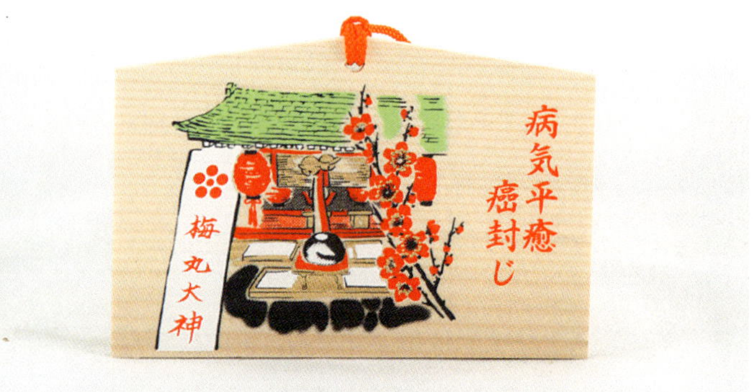

194

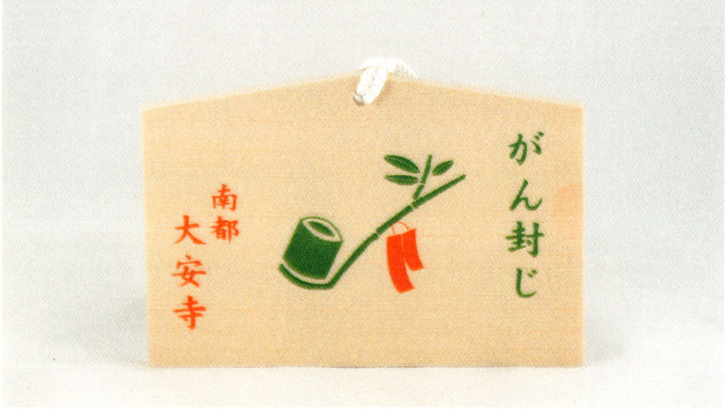

195

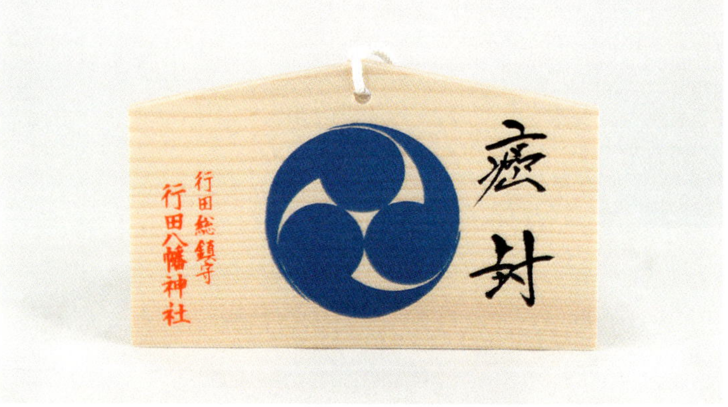

Ema designs

Human body 人体 *(jintai)*

Some *ema* for the prevention of *gan* (cancer) or for blocking the progression of *gan* have *jintai* (the human body) as their design. This allows the petitioner to mark on the *ema* which body part(s) are affected.

An *ema* design of the human body for cancer that is not illustrated here can be found at *Muryōji* 無量寺 (Gamagori, Aichi Prefecture). *Ema* with the human body have also been reported for *Kido Yakushidō* (Sasaguri, Fukuoka Prefecture) and *Hirahama Hachimangū/ Takeuchi Jinja* (Matsue, Shimane Prefecture), but these *ema* seem to serve more general purposes, such as *byōki heiyu* (recovery from illness). See p.105 for an example of an *ema* that is used more generally.

190
Ōyama Fudō Taisanji 大山不動 大山寺 (also known as *Ōyamadera*). Isehara, Kanagawa Prefecture. Early 21st century. W. 10.7 cm
The inscriptions read:
癌封じ祈願 = *ganfūji kigan* (prayer for prevention of cancer)
大山龍神倶利伽羅不動尊 = *Ōyama Ryūjin Kurikara Fudōson*

The temple enshrines *Tetsuzō Fudō-myō-ō*. His attribute is a *kongōsho* (= *vajra*) sword which is shown here as background in the *ema* design. *Vajra* is a Sanskrit word which means both diamond and thunderbolt (which symbolise indestructibility and irresistible force, respectively).

191
Tanukidaniyama Fudōin 狸谷山不動院. Sakyo Ward, Kyoto. Early 21st century. W. 5.0 cm
The inscriptions read:
ガン予防 = *gan yobō* (prevention of cancer)
病気平癒 = *byōki heiyu* (recovery from illness)
お名前 = *onamae* (your name)
年齢 = *nenrei* (age)
才 = *sai* (...years old)

192
Tōkōin 東光院. Chiba, Chiba Prefecture. Early 21st century. W. 9.0 cm
The inscriptions read:
身代り = *migawari* (substitute/scapegoat)
癌封じ = *ganfūji* (prevention of cancer)
なまえ = *namae* (name)
千葉 = *Chiba*
平山薬師 = *Hirayama Yakushi*

The inscription of *migawari* (substitute/ scapegoat) on the *ema* indicates that the enshrined Buddha (in this case *Yakushi Nyorai* = Medicine Buddha) prevents or heals cancer by substituting his body for the real human body, thereby absorbing any negative forces that would otherwise threaten or afflict the human body [RT-46].

Stone for recovery 平癒石 *(heiyu ishi)*

193
Ume Marusha 梅丸社 (subordinate shrine of *Sugawarain Tenmangū Jinja* 菅原院天満宮神社) Kamigyo Ward, Kyoto. Early 21st century. W. 13.4 cm
The inscriptions read:
病気平癒 = *byōki heiyu* (recovery from illness)
癌封じ = *ganfūji* (prevention of cancer)
梅丸大神 = *Umemaru Ōkami*

The *ema* design shows the large *heiyu ishi* (stone for recovery) in front of the subordinate shrine. Stones with healing properties can also be found at other Japanese sanctuaries.

Bamboo cup for bamboo grass liquor 笹酒 *(sasasake)*

Every year on 23 January a festival is organised at *Daianji* (Nara) to commemorate the former Emperor *Kōnin* (reigned 770-781). Rituals and prayers are offered for good health and to help fight cancer. *Sasasake* (bamboo grass liquor) is served from bamboo tubes into bamboo cups. This drink is believed to prevent and combat cancer.

194
Daianji 大安寺. Nara, Nara Prefecture. Early 21st century. W. 13.5 cm
The inscriptions read:
がん封じ = *ganfūji* (prevention of cancer)
南都 = *Nanto* (refers to Nara where the temple is located)
大安寺 = *Daianji*

Tomoe 巴

Tomoe is an abstract emblem that consists of one, two or three comma-like shapes and is generally regarded as a symbol of *Hachiman*. Its use is not confined to this God of War and *Hachiman* shrines may also use the pigeon as symbol (cf. the entry on *kannomushi* on p.161).

195
Gyōda Hachiman Jinja 行田八幡神社. Gyoda, Saitama Prefecture. Early 21st century. W. 14.2 cm
The inscriptions read:
癌封 = *ganfūji* (prevention of cancer)
行田総鎮守 = *Gyōda Sōchinju* (general protector deity of *Gyōda*)
行田八幡神社 = *Gyōda Hachiman Jinja*

The shrine also offers an *ema* with an orange-coloured *tomoe* emblem which has the same inscriptions except *ganfūji* (prevention of cancer).

Breasts 乳 *(chichi)*

The section on women's illnesses depicts an *ema* with three-dimensional breasts from *Karube Jinja* (Soja, Okayama Prefecture) (see p.191). This *ema* is used to pray not only for safe child birth, abundant lactation, or simply for large breasts, but also for the healing of *nyūgan* (breast cancer).

An additional *ema* design for neoplasms (not illustrated here) portrays *Gan Setsu Fudō Myō-ō* 癌切不動明王 (Cancer-Cutting *Fudō*). It is found at *Nyoirinji* 如意輪寺 (Ogori, Fukuoka Prefecture).

196

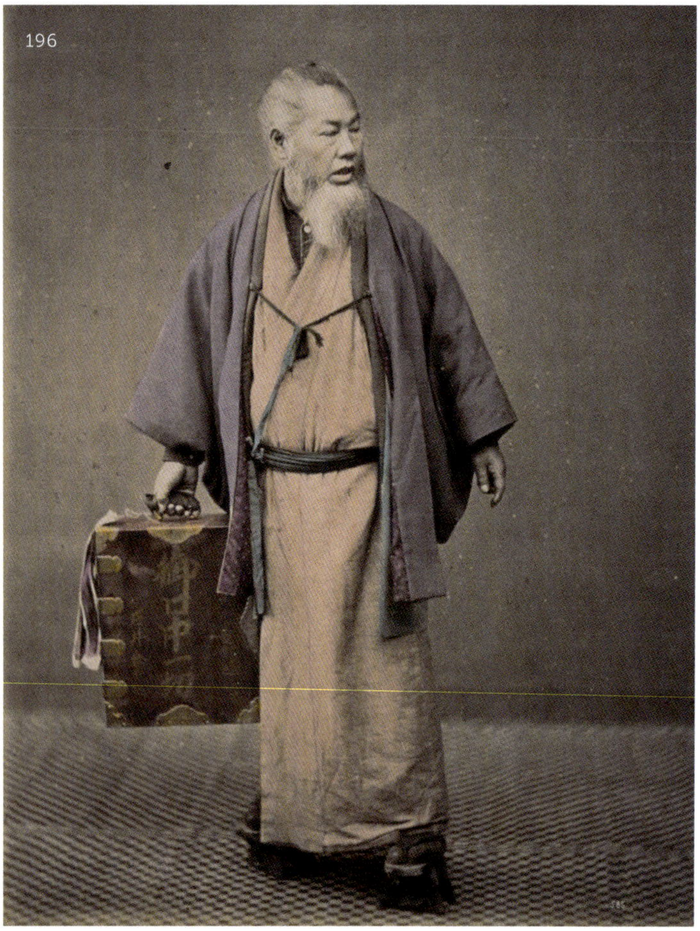

198

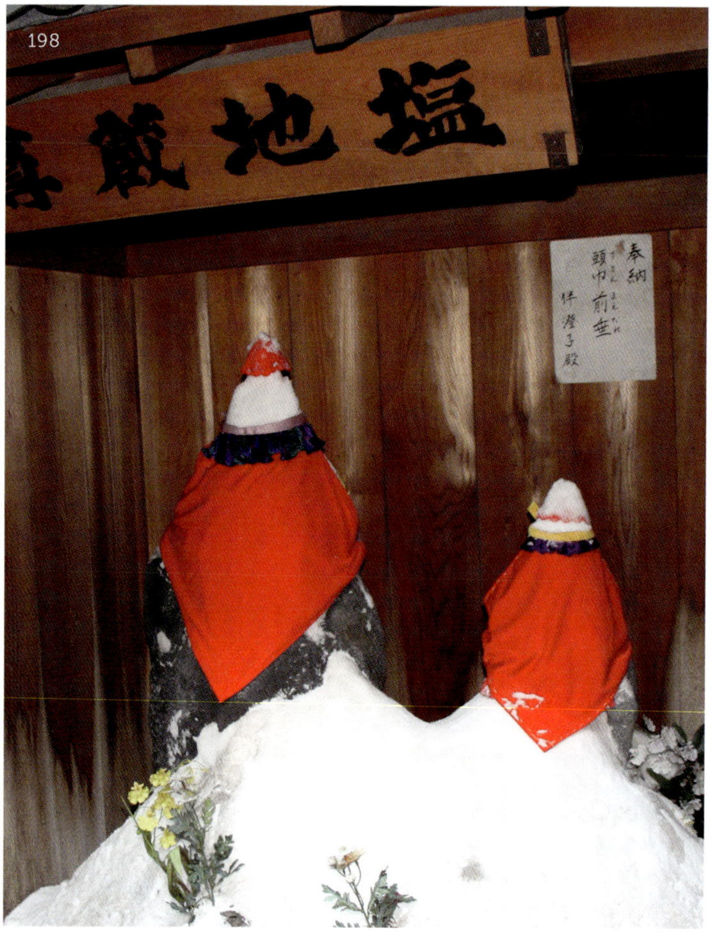

197

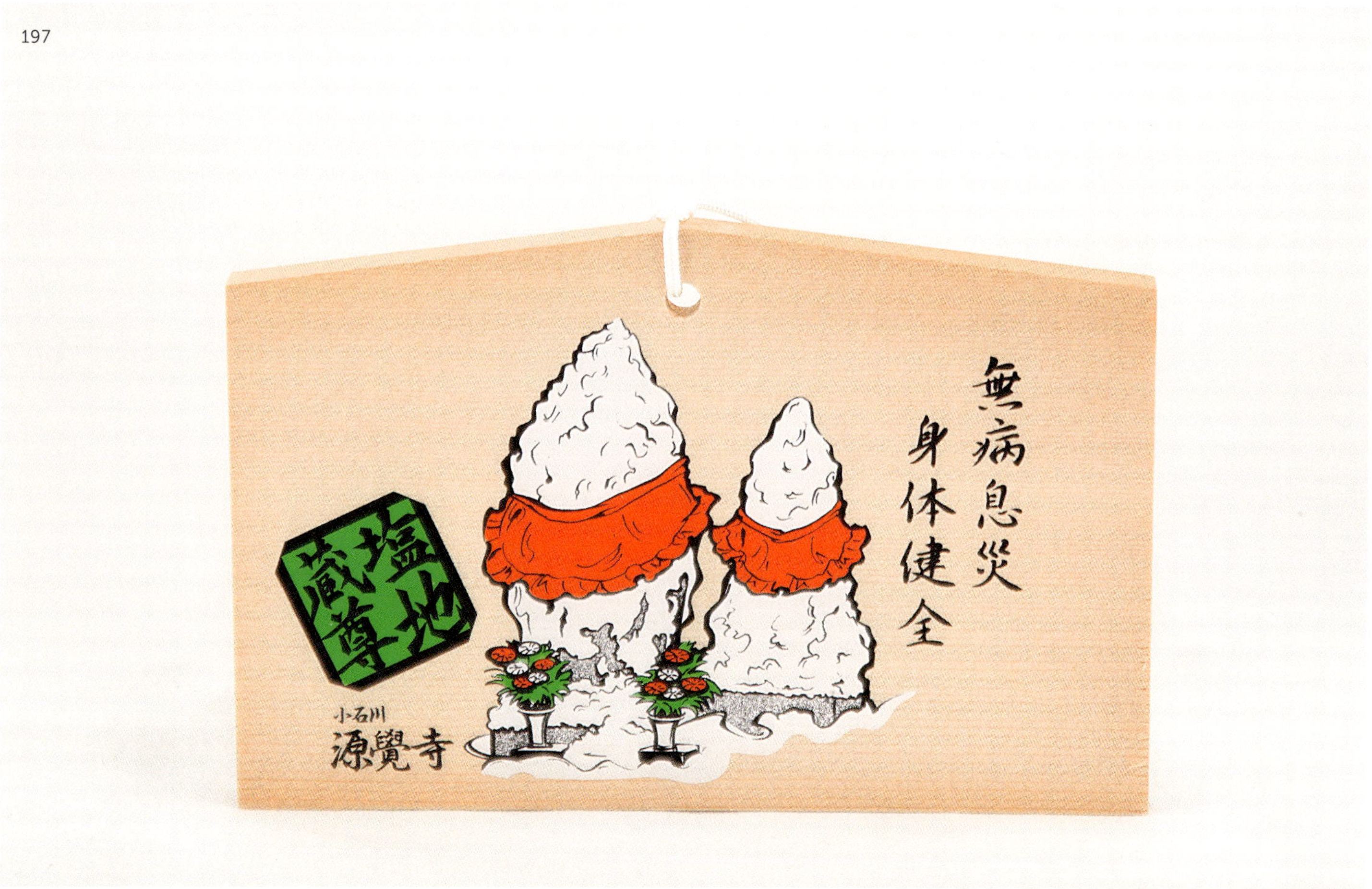

Tooth and mouth symptoms/complaints 歯と口の症状／愁訴 (*ha to kuchi no shōjō/ shūso*)

Background

Toothache as a result of dental decay (caries) has been a well-known problem in Japan since prehistoric times. One of the Japanese terms for caries (虫歯 = *mushiba*) is composed of the characters 虫 (*mushi* = worm) and 歯 (*ha* = tooth). This reflects the old Japanese belief that toothache was caused by a "tooth worm", which is also mentioned in texts from ancient Mesopotamia, Egypt, India and China. In the 1960s and 1970s, tooth decay increased in Japan due to rising sugar consumption, but it declined thereafter, even though Japan does not fluoridate its drinking water [2].

At *Hakami Jinja* (within the precincts of *Shitennōji*, Osaka), toothache sufferers would make a paste of soya beans, bury it in the ground at the shrine and pray to the tooth deity *Hakami* to release them from pain (at least until the bean paste sprouted). Another Shinto deity for toothache was *Genkurō Inari* in the *Genshōjizaka* area of Osaka. Calling on this deity was preceded by the tradition of praying to a local *tanuki* (raccoon dog) to cure toothache [3].

Today, there still are numerous shrines, temples and power spots where one can pray for the relief or prevention of dental ailments. Among the Buddhist figures of worship invoked for toothache are *Jizō*, *Yakushi*, and *Kannon* [GK; GG3-2007/07; MS]. Concrete examples include:

- *Nyoirin Kannon* 如意輪観音 at *Chōsenji* (Suginami Ward, Tokyo) This particular statue is holding its right hand against its cheek which seems to illustrate its relationship with toothache. However, this does not always apply. There are six-armed *Kannon* statues where each arm represents a vow to save beings in one of the six realms of rebirth. In these cases, the right hand touching the cheek represents a vow to save beings in hell [MS].
- *Shitsū Jizōbosatsu* (Toothache *Jizō*) 歯痛地蔵菩薩 at *Ryūfukuji* (Joyo, Kyoto Prefecture).
- *Agonashi Jizō* 腮無地蔵 (*Jizō* Without Jaw) at *Kōsaiji* (Kawagoe, Saitama Prefecture). This *Jizō* does not have toothache, because he does not have a lower jaw.
- *Shitsū Tome Yakushi* 歯痛止薬師 (Toothache-Stopping *Yakushi*). Wooden statue from the Heian Period (806-1184) at *Mibudera* (Nakagyo Ward, Kyoto) [GG3-2007/07].
- *Nurikobe Jizō* ぬりこべ地蔵 at a cemetery in Fushimi Ward, Kyoto

196
Dental practitioner from the Meiji Period. Photograph R. Stillfried. Nagasaki University Library (Nagasaki)

The writing on the box 御口中一切 = *o kōchū issai* (everything for the inside of your mouth) suggests that he was a *machiisha* (town doctor). Before Japanese dental law was established in 1906, traditional providers of dental care included [1]:

- *kōchū-i* (specialised mouth physicians) for the upper classes;
- *machiisha* (town doctors) for the middle classes, including *irebashi* (artisans fabricating wooden dentures) and *basshi-shi* (tooth pullers)
- *yashi* (showmen who would first perform acts in the street to attract an audience and then offered tooth drugs, tooth extraction or wooden dentures).

Ema designs

Shio Jizō 塩地蔵 (Salt *Jizō*)

At *Genkakuji* (Tokyo) two *Jizō* statues are enshrined, which are largely covered with *shio* (salt). Salt is thought to ward off evil and is sold at the temple in small packages as offerings. If a part of the body is ill, salt can be applied to the corresponding part of the statues. It is also possible to touch that part with the small *shakujō* (staff) hanging to the right of the statues. The statues are believed to be particularly helpful in the case of toothache. Cf. p.133 for the *Konnyaku Enma* enshrined at *Genkakuji*.

197
Genkakuji 源覚寺. Bunkyo Ward, Tokyo. Early 21st century. W. 16.0 cm
The inscriptions read:
無病息災 = *mubyō sokusai* (sound health)
身体健全 = *shintai kenzen* (healthy body)
塩地蔵尊 = *Shio Jizōson* (Salt *Jizō*)
小石川 = *Koishikawa* (locality in Bunkyo Ward)
源覚寺 = *Genkakuji*

198
Two statues of *Shio Jizō* (Salt *Jizō*) at *Genkakuji* (Bunkyo Ward, Tokyo).

199

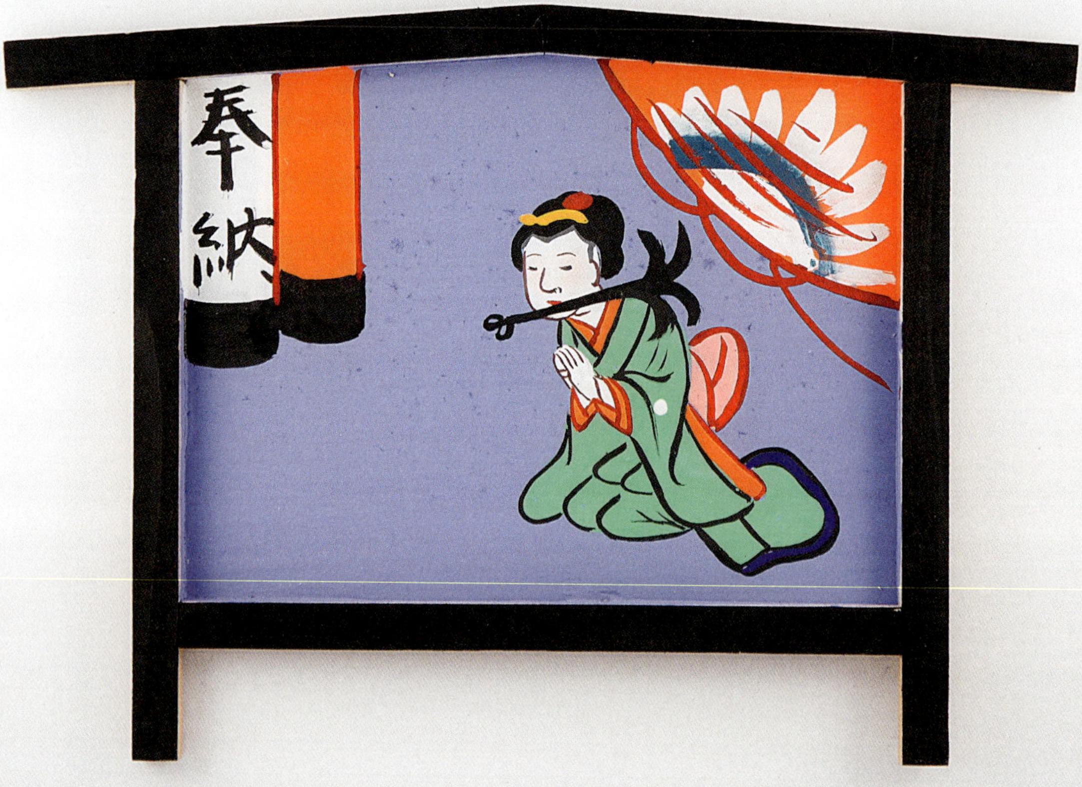

200

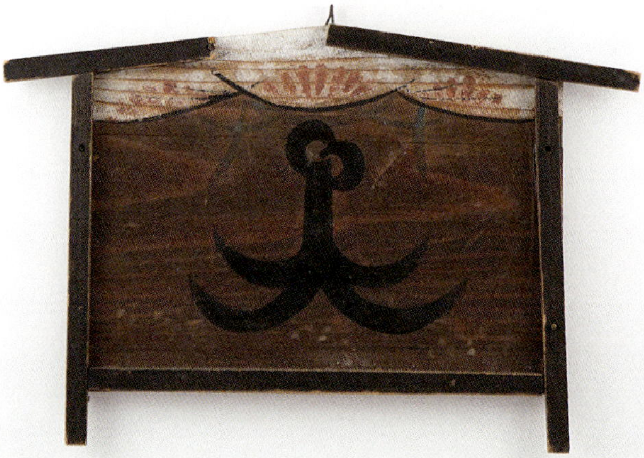

201

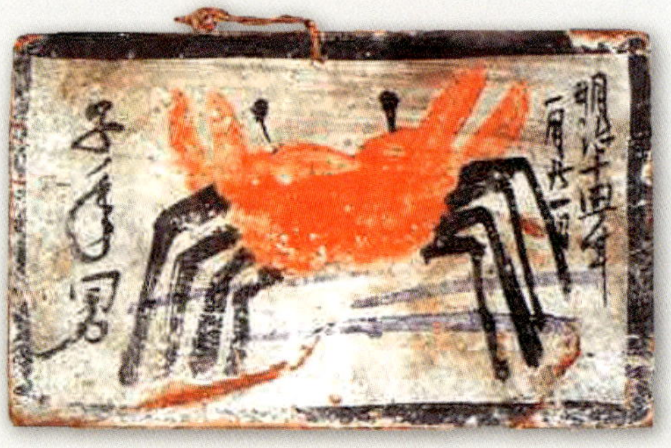

202

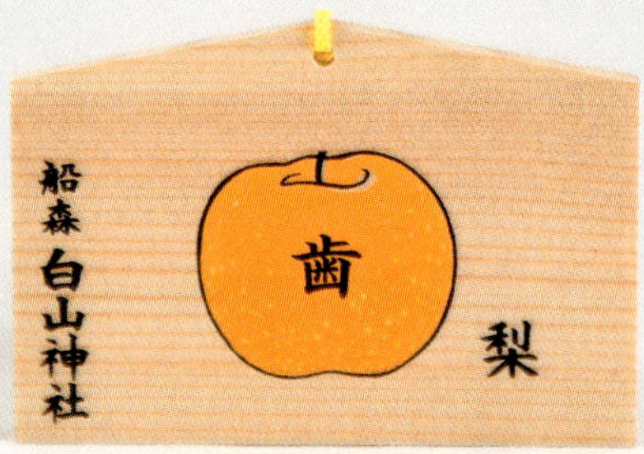

Anchor 錨 *(ikari)*
This design is sometimes represented as such, but more commonly as a human figure gripping an anchor in the mouth. It is recommended for *shitsū heiyu* (recovery from toothache). It refers to teeth that are so healthy and strong that they can even hold a very heavy object such as an anchor without pain [FS-16; IJ-132; IH2-78].

199
Hand-painted *ema*. From *Emaya Yoshidaya* (*ema* shop *Yoshidaya*), Senju, Adachi Ward, Tokyo (cf. p.23). Early 21st century. W. 20.6 cm
The inscription reads:
奉納 = *hōnō* (dedication, offering)

200
Hand-painted *ema*. Origin unclear.
Early or mid-20th century. W. 15.6 cm

Crab 蟹 *(kani)*
This *ema* design can be used for toothache and for teeth as strong as the shell of the crab [IH2-78].

201
Hinomine Jinja 日の峰神社. Komatsushima, Tokushima Prefecture. Image reproduced with permission of the publisher from Iwai H. *Ema ni negai o*. Tokyo: Nigensha, 2007:79

More recently, the shrine sold a hexagonal *ema* with a restyled monochromatic crab design.

Japanese pear 梨 *(nashi)*
This *ema* design is used for dental disorders (such as cavities). In former days, when one suffered from toothache, one was exhorted to drop a pear (known for its acid taste) into a river with an oath that one would not touch the fruit for a year in exchange for a cure for one's toothache [TS-9; 4].

202
Hakusan Jinja 白山神社 in precincts of *Kotohira Jinja* 金刀比羅神社 (commonly known as *Koyasu Jinja*). Hachioji, Tokyo Metropolis. Early 21st century. W. 13.0 cm
The inscriptions read:
梨 = *nashi* (Japanese pear)
歯 = *ha* (tooth)
船森 = *Funamori* (may refer to area in which the shrine is located)
白山神社 = *Hakusan Jinja*
Other shrines at *Kotohira Jinja* offer benefits for eye illnesses, musculoskeletal illnesses and respiratory illnesses (see p.171).

Additional *ema* designs for tooth and mouth symptoms/complaints (not illustrated here) are:

- **Mackerel 鯖 (*saba*). *Hibiya Jinja* 日比谷神社 (Minato Ward, Tokyo) used to sell an *ema* design of two mackerel for toothache. The person offering the *ema* promised to abstain from eating mackerel [FS-12; IH2-74; 5]. When we visited this shrine a few years ago the *ema* was no longer for sale there. See the section on skin illnesses on p.181 for another *ema* design with two mackerel.**
- **Catfish 鯰 (*namazu*). This *ema* design is often associated with skin illnesses (see the relevant section), but *Shirai Jinja* in Amagasaki offers a catfish design for toothache. The shrine is also known as the Catfish Shrine. In former days, many catfish lived in a large pond in its precincts, but the pond is no longer there.**

203

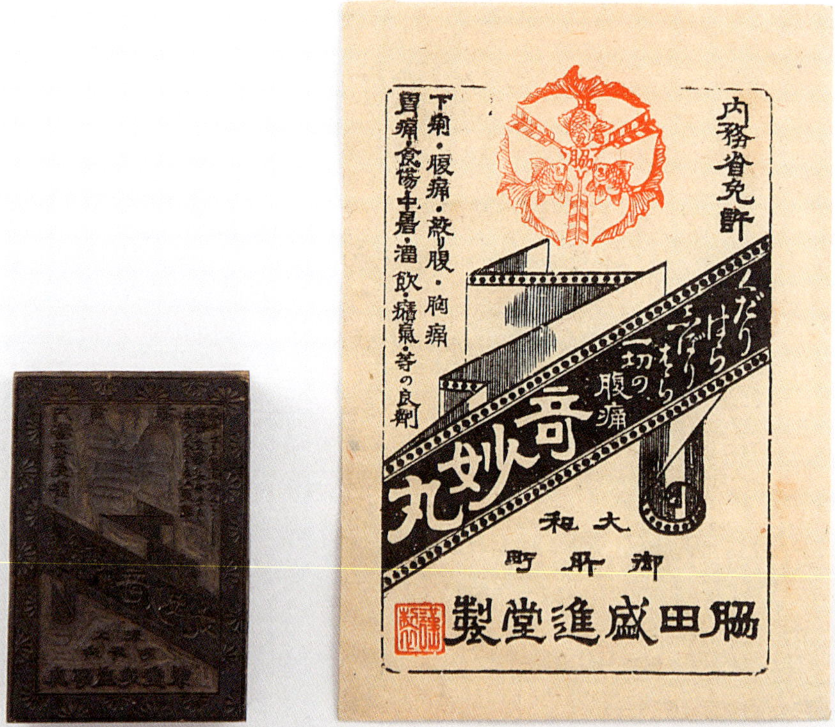
内務省免許
下痢・腹痛・澁り腹・胸痛
胃痛・食傷・中暑・溜飲・癪氣・等の良劑
くだりはら
しぶりはら
一切の腹痛
奇妙丸
大和
御所町
脇田盛進堂製

204

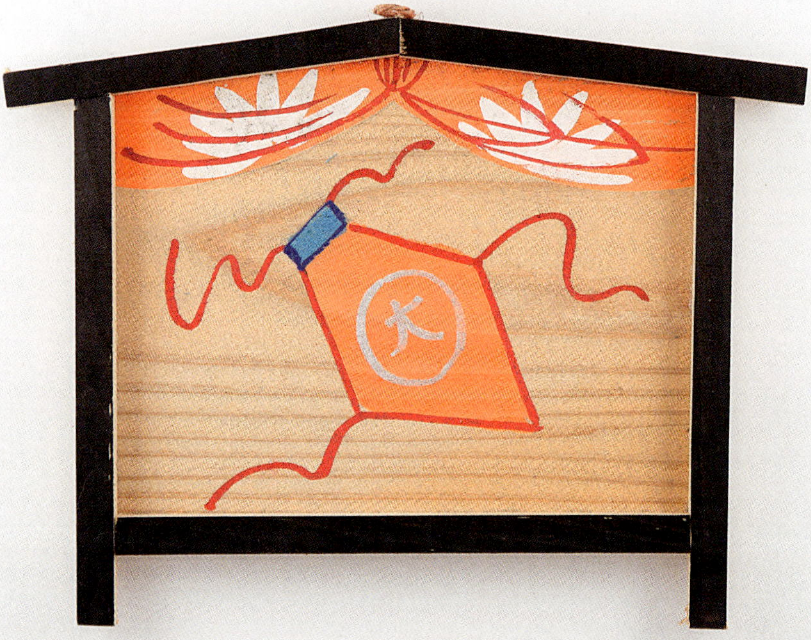

Digestive symptoms/complaints 消化器症状／愁訴 (*shōkaki shōjō/shūso*)

Background

Gastrointestinal symptoms are common in the Japanese population. Among the most frequent complaints are abdominal pain, diarrhoea, constipation, nausea, vomiting, dyspepsia and heartburn [IO; TT; 1].

The leading gastrointestinal causes of death in Japan have shifted from diarrhoeal diseases in the past to digestive tract neoplasms today. In 2008 stomach cancer was the number one cause of cancer in males and the number three in females. There is evidence that the high rate of stomach cancer in Japan is associated with the intake of salts and salted foods. Colorectal cancer is the second cause of cancer in females and the third cause in males [2].

In the past, the Japanese attributed special significance to the area of the stomach and abdomen (*hara*) because they considered it as the seat of the soul. The ritual act of *harakiri* (suicide) involved cutting into one's *hara* to remove the soul. The Japanese were most careful to keep the *hara* warm and therefore avoided cold drinks even in summertime. The *hara* of small children was often protected with a *haramaki* or *harakake* (stomach/abdominal band). In the 1980s, the number of stomach medicines on the Japanese market was higher than that of any other kind of medicine, and stomach specialists were the most common practising doctors. In view of this preponderance, one would have expected a plethora of nationwide and local figures of worship specialised in stomach/abdominal disorders. Yet the consulted sources have yielded only a small number of deities specialised in illnesses of the stomach (*Onaka no kamisama*, *Tsuri Tenjin* and *Shibari Jizō*) [EO-58,150].

Complaints such as stomach pain and diarrhoea were often attributed to *hara no mushi* (worms in the *hara*). These worms were also associated with emotional symptoms, such as anger. For instance, the Japanese expression *hara no mushi ga osamaranu* (the worm in the stomach/abdomen is not satisfied) means that one feels vengeful: since the worm will not stay quiet, one cannot get over what another person has done [GG1-2011/07; 3].

Examples of shrines that offer *goriyaku* (benefits) for digestive symptoms/complaints are:

- *Imakumano Jinja* 新熊野神社 (Higashiyama Ward, Kyoto) sells a *mamori* (charm) for health and longevity and especially for *fukutsū* (stomach ache, abdominal pain). There is a large old camphor tree at the shrine, which is worshipped as an abode of the shrine deities, in particular *Onaka no kamisama* (deity of the stomach) [GG2-2014/04].
- *Kuzuharaoka Jinja* 葛原岡神社 (Kamakura, Kanagawa Prefecture). Here one can perform *sara o nage*, i.e. throwing a dish against a special magical stone to pray for help for families that are especially prone to stomach illnesses and colds.
- *Kanazakura Jinja* 金櫻神社 (Kofu, Yamanashi Prefecture) offers *mushi kiri suzu* (earthenware bells) to stop *mushi* such as *hara no mushi* (worms in the stomach/abdomen) [GG1-2011/07].
- *Yakumo Hikawa Jinja* 八雲氷川神社 (Meguro Ward, Tokyo) offers *shakufūji* (prevention of *shaku* = spasms, cramps) [GK]. Cf. the *ema* design of a bamboo ladle below.

203
Medicine bag for digestive ailments.

On the right: prewar paper medicine bag for *Kimyōgan* (miraculous pills) for ailments in and below the stomach area, such as *fukutsū* (stomach pain) and *geri* (diarrhoea). Manufactured by *Wakita Seishindō*, Yamato Province (located in what is now Nara Prefecture).

On the left: wood printing block for smaller medicine bags of a similar product bearing the same product name but coming from another manufacturing company.

Ema designs

Apron 腹掛け *(haragake)*

Ema design for *fukubyō* (stomach/abdominal illnesses) such as *fukutsū* (stomach ache, abdominal pain) [TS-33; IH2-85; KM-17].

At *Umagami Jinja* (Otsu, Shiga prefecture), *haragake* for horses (or *ema* with a horse wearing such a garment) were presented to ward off *Daiba* (a god who could kill horses instantly by possessing them) [4].

204
Hand-painted reproduction for a Japanese club of *ema* collectors called *Nihon Ema Tomo no Kai* (Friends of Japanese Ema Society). No.338. Late 20th century. W. 17.6 cm. Original design from *Ōhara Jinja* 大原神社 (Ashikaga, Tochigi prefecture)

The kanji character on the *haragake* (大 = ō) is the first character in the name of the originating shrine. This shrine is believed to help people with stomach/abdominal illnesses because of the similarity between its name (*Ōhara*) and the Japanese word for stomach/abdomen (*hara*).

205

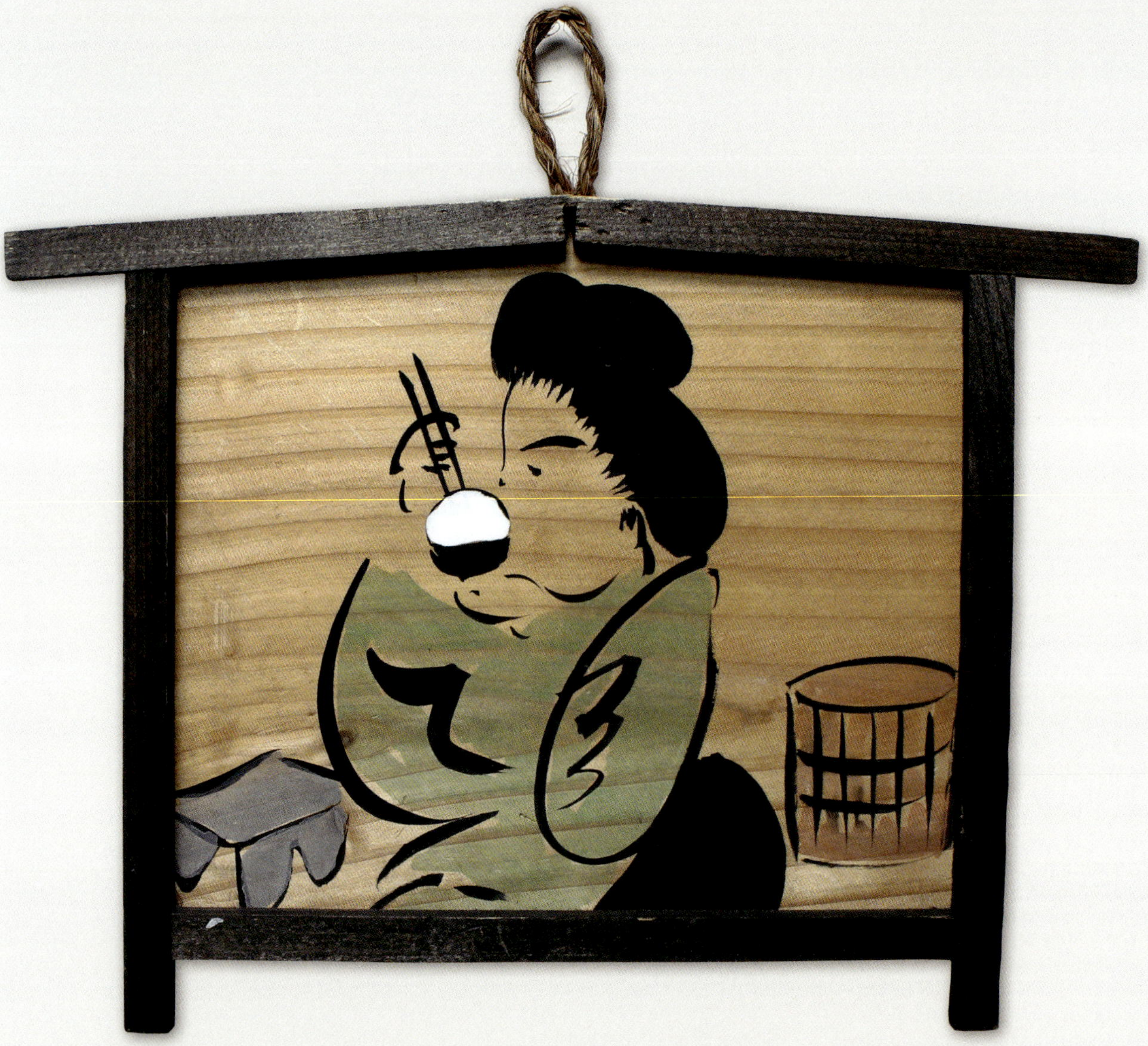

206

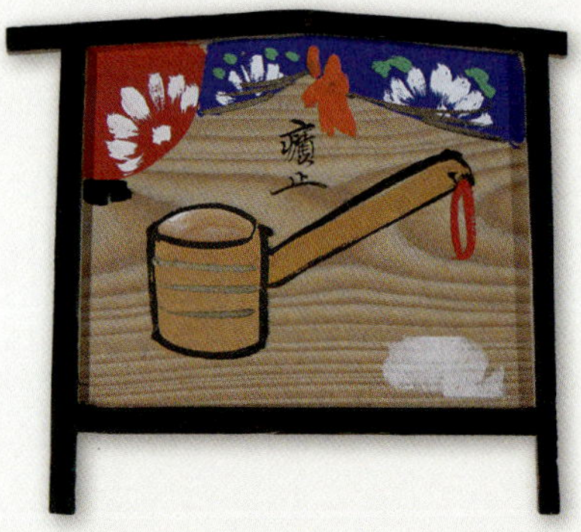

207

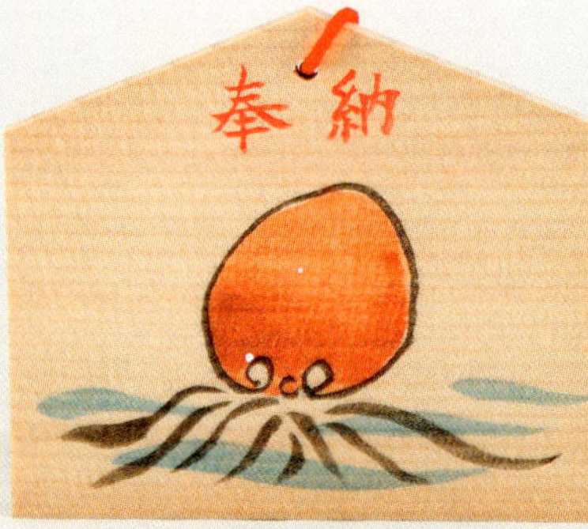

Serving of boiled rice 飯盛 *(meshimori)*

Japanese sources agree that this *ema* design was used for 胸のつかえ (*mune no tsukae*) [IH2-84; NM-Z22673]. It is somewhat ambiguous, however, what the best translation of this concept into English is. *Tsukae* literally means: load on one's chest; obstacle;hindrance. *Mune* has multiple meanings, including chest, breasts, heart, lungs and stomach. In accordance with this multiplicity, one source translates *mune no tsukae* as "obstruction in the chest" [5], while another source prefers "an upset stomach" [TS-26]. The latter interpretation seems to be the more common one, but perhaps it should not be forgotten that pulmonary tuberculosis was sometimes designated as *munenoke* (chest trouble) in premodern Japan [WF].

205

Ema hand-painted by *Norihito Yasuda* (Nagoya) on commission from the Naito Museum of Pharmaceutical Sciences and Industry (Kakamigahara, Gifu Prefecture). Museum inv.no. 22673. Late 20th century

Bamboo ladle 杓子 *(shakushi)*

There is an obvious word play between *shakushi* (bamboo ladle) and *shaku* (spasms, cramps). *Shaku* and *senki* are two ancient Japanese concepts of illness. While both refer to disorders causing stomach, intestinal or back pain, *shaku* seems to have been used for more acute problems and *senki* for more chronic conditions [AJ].

206

Originating sanctuary unclear.
Early or mid-20th century
The inscription above the ladle probably reads:
癪止 = *shakudome* (to stop *shaku* = spasms, cramps)

Nakano Ward Museum of History and Folklore, Nakano Ward, Tokyo

Octopus 蛸 *(tako)*

This *ema* design is used for abdominal hernias. These are a common problem in Japan, particularly among males. They show up as a visible bulge due to protrusion of abdominal content through an area of weakness or defect in the abdominal wall. Many are asymptomatic, but sometimes the hernia becomes strangulated or incarcerated, which can cause serious problems, if left untreated. In the 1930s, hernia and intestinal obstruction ranked 24th among the top 30 leading causes of death in Japan [US-67].

See p.183 for the use of this *ema* design for other symptoms/complaints, such as warts.

207

Tenshoji 天性寺. Kishiwada, Osaka Prefecture.
Early 21st century. W. 15.1 cm
The inscription reads:
奉納 = *hōnō* (dedication, offering)
The inscriptions on the reverse read:
蛸地蔵 = *Tako Jizō*
天性寺 = *Tenshoji*

Tenshoji accommodates a statue of *Tako Jizō* (Octopus *Jizō*). *Tako Jizō* is also the nickname of *Tenshoji*. According to legend, a local stone statue of *Jizō* came alive and saved Kishiwada Castle from falling into enemy hands with the aid of an army of *tako* (octopuses).

Tako Jizō can be addressed for illnesses in general, but especially for *dacchō* (abdominal hernia) [GK].

208

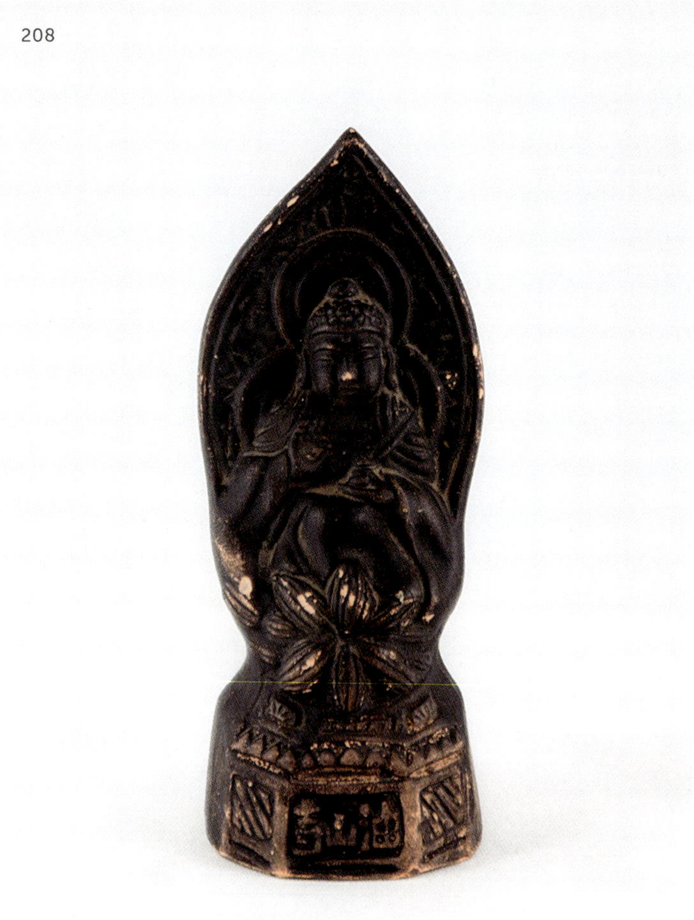

209

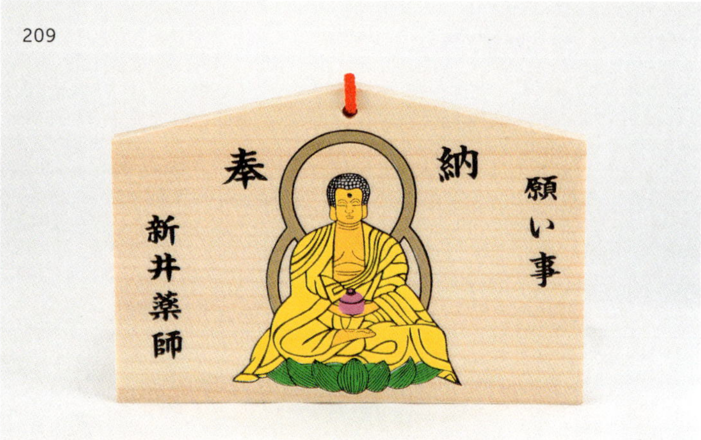

210

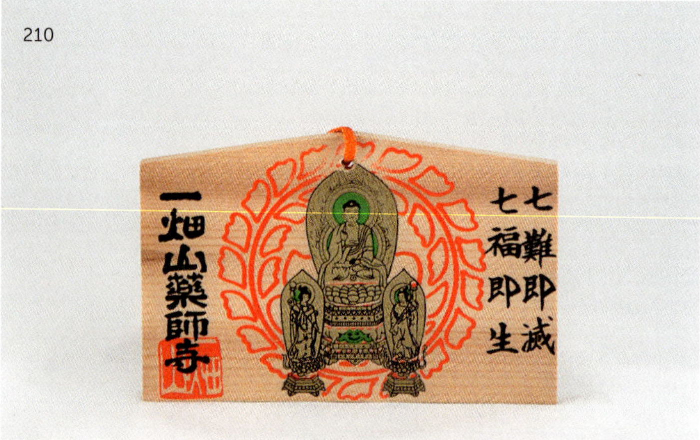

211

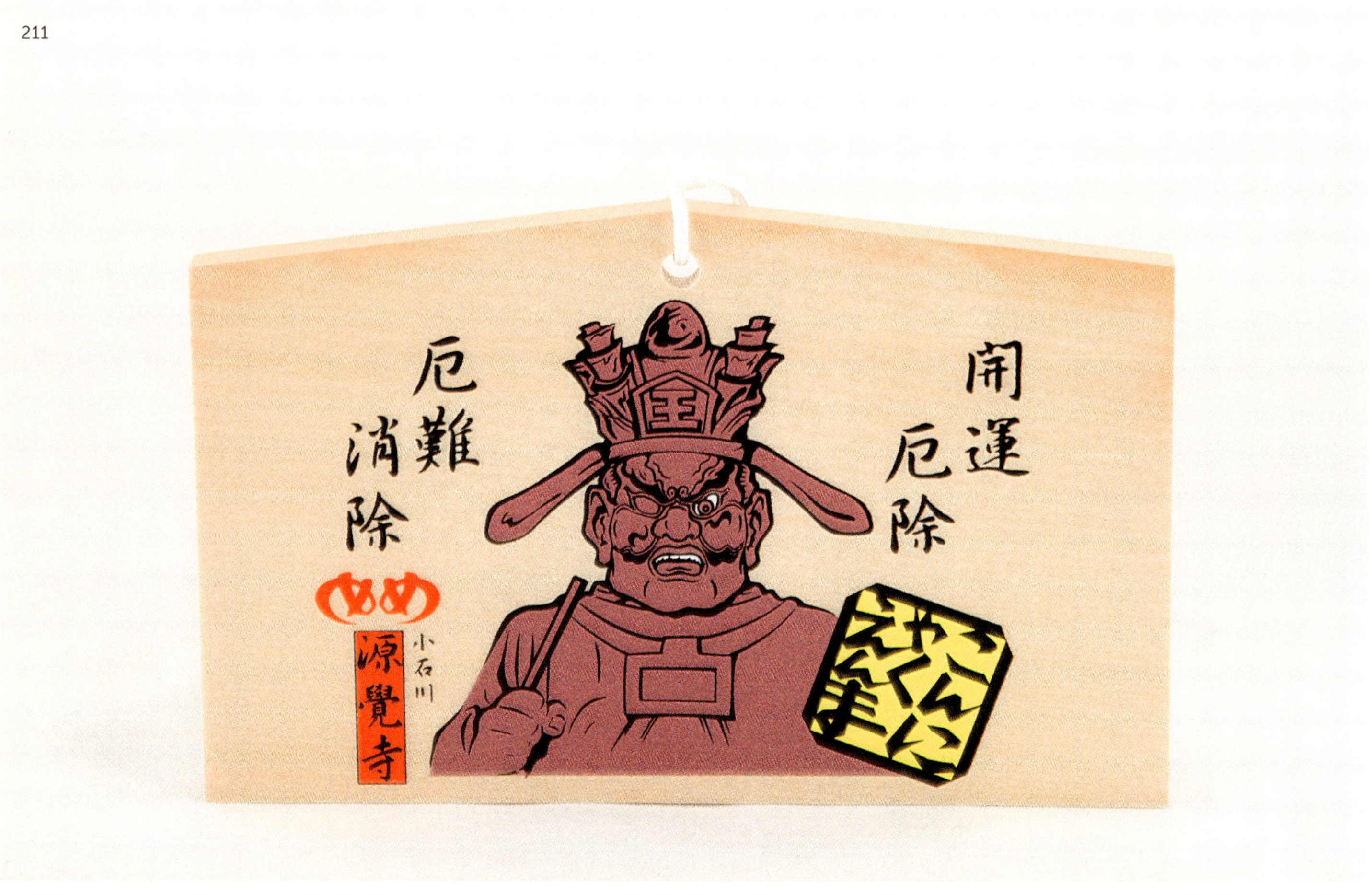

Eye symptoms/ complaints 眼 症状／愁訴 (*me shōjō/shūso*)

Background

In pre-war Japan, (i.e., before the arrival of antibiotics), bacterial eye infections (such as trachoma and gonorrhoeal ophthalmia) developed from early childhood on. In the 1920s, about 10% of the Japanese population was affected by trachoma. By the early 1950s, the incidence of trachoma had greatly decreased in urban areas, but it had remained high among the inhabitants of deprived rural settings, who were even called *akame* (*aka* = red and *me* = eyes) for this reason. Trachoma can gradually lead to inward folding of the eyelids (entropion) and to ingrown eyelashes (trichiasis). This can then lead to corneal abrasion (by the constant rubbing of the eyelashes against the cornea) and blindness (due to loss of corneal clarity). In the Edo and Meiji periods, another important cause of blindness must have been smallpox, since this epidemic disease often scarred the eyes [1].

Today, *ganbyō* (eye diseases) are especially seen in the aged. They include glaucoma, diabetic retinopathy, degenerative myopia and age-related macular degeneration cataracts [2].

The major Buddhist figure of worship for the healing of eye illnesses is *Yakushi Nyorai* (Medicine Buddha). Temples where *Yakushi* can be invoked for eye illnesses include *Arai Yakushi Baishōin* (Tokyo), *Ichibata Yakushi* (Izumo), *Chūsonji* (Hiraizumi), *Yamaya Yakushidō* (Aomori), and *Byōdōji* (Shikoku). According to legend, the 14th century monk *Seigan* discovered an influential text on the treatment of eye illnesses after *Yakushi* had appeared to him in a dream. According to the foundation legend of *Ichibata Yakushi*, an eye-healing miracle took place there as early as in the 9th century [MS; 3].

Another important Buddhist figure of worship for eye ailments is *Jizō* in his manifestations of *Mearai Jizō* (Eye washing *Jizō*), *Misoname Jizō* (Bean Paste Licking *Jizō*), *Kinomoto Jizō* (see the entry on *migawari kaeru* on p.137), and *Meyami Jizō* (Eye Illness *Jizō*) [MS; GG1-2011/07; 4].

208
Clay statue of *Yakushi Nyorai* (Medicine Buddha). *Yusanji* 油山寺. Fukuroi, Shizuoka Prefecture. Mid-20th century. H. 13.5 cm

The Medicine Buddha enshrined at *Yusanji* is especially known for recovery from eye illnesses. Cf. the entries on *Yakushi Nyorai* and on facing *me* characters below.

Ema designs

Yakushi Nyorai 薬師如来 *(Medicine Buddha)*

See also the entry on *hiragana* character for eye on p.137.

209
Baishōin Yakuōji 梅照院薬王寺. Nakano Ward, Tokyo. Early 21st century. W. 17.5 cm
The inscriptions read:
願い事 = *negaigoto* (wish, prayer)
奉納 = *hōnō* (dedication, offering)
新井薬師 = *Arai Yakushi*

The originating temple is commonly known as *Arai Yakushi*. This name is derived from *Yakushi Nyorai* (Medicine Buddha) who is the main enshrined deity.

210
Ichihatasan Yakushiji 一畑山薬師寺. Okazaki, Aichi Prefecture. Late 20th century. W. 13.8 cm
The inscriptions read:
七難即滅 = *shichinan sokumetsu*
(the death of the seven misfortunes)
七福即生 = *shichifuku sokushō*
(the birth of the seven good fortunes)
一畑山薬師寺 = *Ichihatasan Yakushiji*

The Medicine Buddha on this *ema* is called *Yakushi Rurikō Nyorai* (lit. Radiant Lapis Lazuli Medicine Buddha). He is flanked by *Gekkō Bosatsu* (Moonlight *Bosatsu*) and *Nikkō Bosatsu* (Sunlight *Bosatsu*).

Worshippers visit the temple for *ganbyō heiyu* (recovery from eye illnesses), *yakuyoke* (warding off evil) and *kōtsū anzen* (traffic safety).

Konnyaku Enma 蒟蒻閻魔

Konnyaku Enma is the king of the underworld and main judge of the dead (deciding whether someone has been good or bad). According to legend, an old woman with eye problems offered one of her own eyes to *Enma*, because she pitied his eyeless statue, whereafter she could see clearly again. To express her gratitude, she gave up her favourite food, *konnyaku* (konjac), and offered it to *Enma*. People still devote *konnyaku* in appreciation, when their wish for a cure for an eye illness has been granted. In another version of the legend, *Enma* gouged out one of his eyes and gave it to the old woman to restore her eyesight [JM-229; RT-250; GG1-2011/07].

211
Genkakuji 源覺寺. Bunkyo Ward, Tokyo. Early 21st century. W. 16.1 cm
The inscriptions read:
開運 = *kaiun* (opening up good luck)
厄除 = *yakuyoke* (warding off evil)
こんにゃくえんま (in yellow seal) = *Konnyaku Enma*
王 (on helmet of *Enma*) = *ō* (king)
厄難消除 = *kinan shōjo* = eradication of peril
め = *me* = eye (also in reverse)
小石川 = *Koishikawa* (locality within Bunkyo ward)
源覺寺 = *Genkakuji*

This *ema* depicts a one-eyed statue of *Konnyaku Enma*.

212

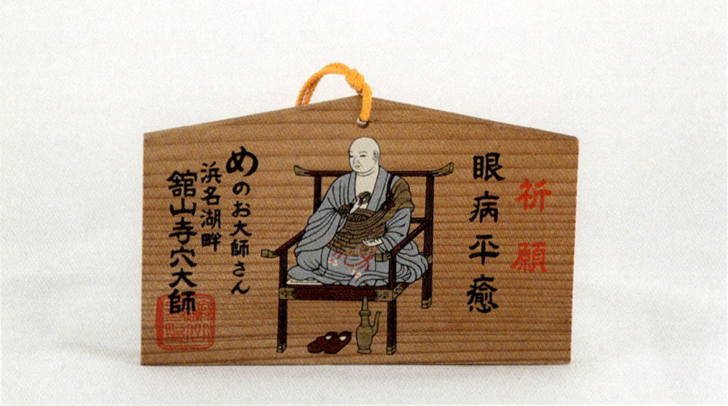

213

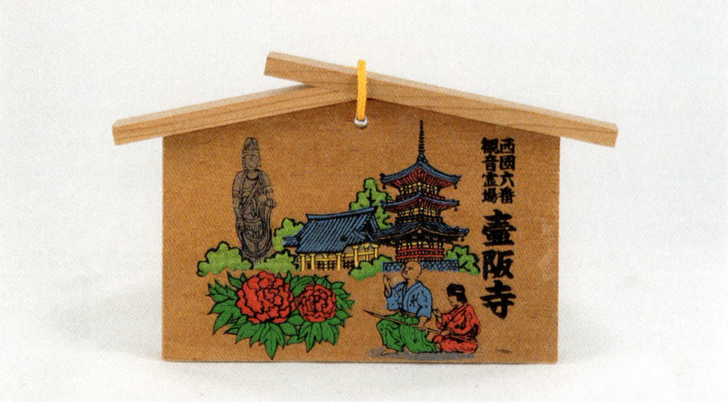

214

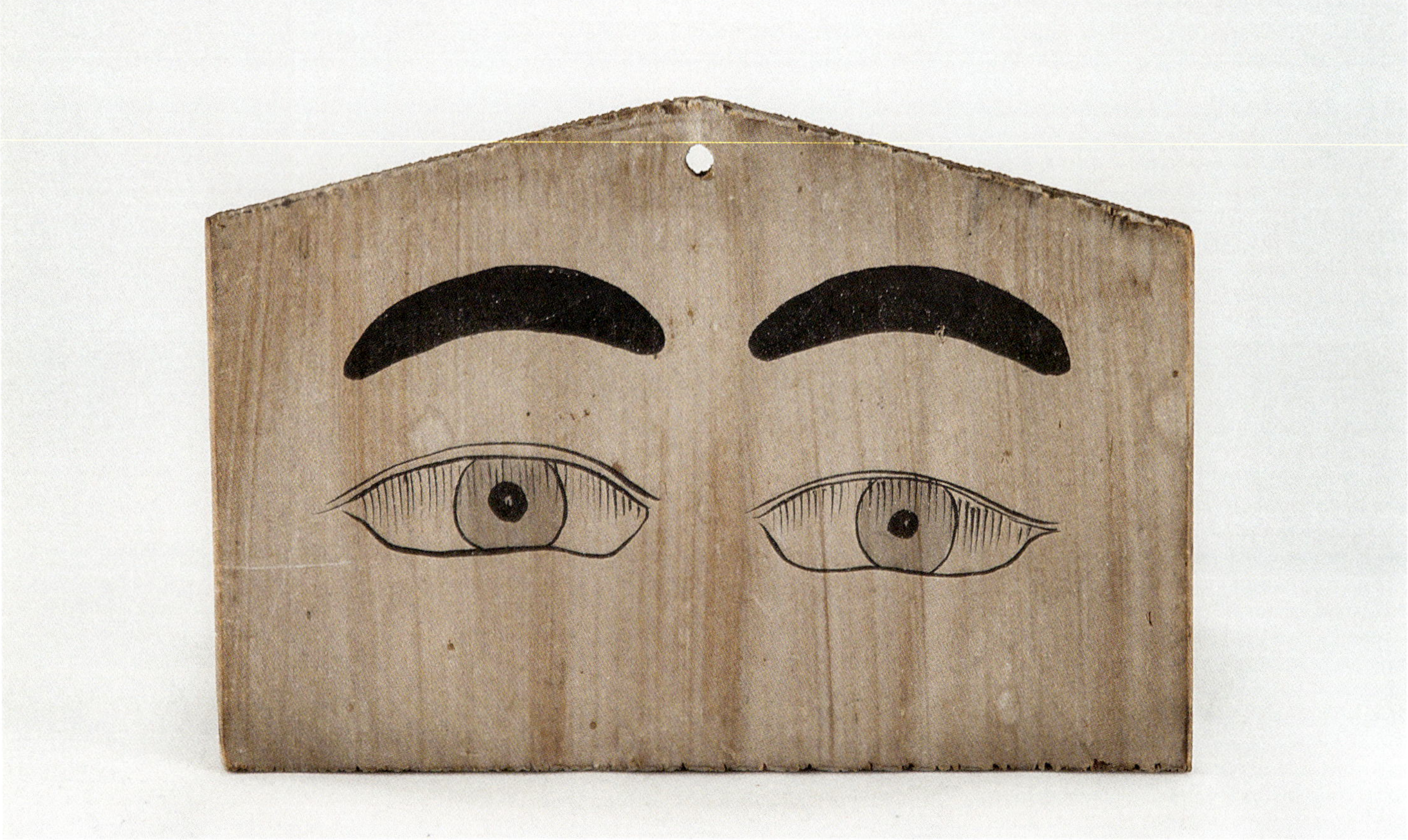

215

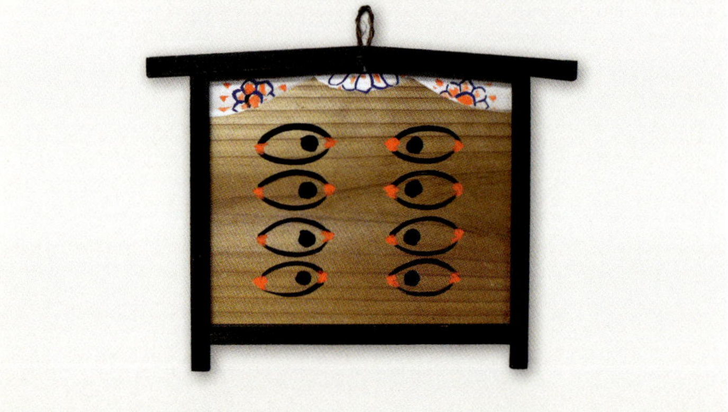

216

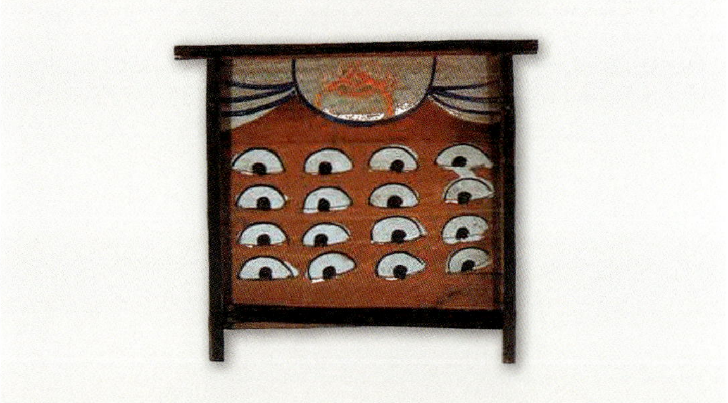

Ana Daishi 穴大師

It is said that *Ana Daishi* (lit. great master of the hole) stayed in a hole at *Kanzanji* for 21 days and carved stone buddha statues there. According to legend, there once was a farmer living near this temple who was not so religious. One day, a piece of grass stuck in his eye during farming and he started to lose his sight. He then began to visit the temple every day to pray to be healed, even though it was difficult for him to go to the temple because of his growing blindness. Then, a black kite dropped a towel on him while he was farming. He wiped his eyes every morning with this towel and regained his eyesight.

212
Kanzanji 舘山寺. Hamamatsu, Shizuoka prefecture. Late 20th century. W. 14.4 cm
The inscriptions read:
祈願 = *kigan* (prayer)
眼病平癒 = *ganbyō heiyu* (recovery from eye illness)
めのお大師さん = *me no o daishi-san* (honourable great teacher of the eyes)
浜名湖畔 = *Hamanakohan* (shore of Lake Hamana)
舘山寺 = *Kanzanji*
穴大師 = *Ana Daishi*

Sawaichi 沢市 *and Osato* お里

The blind masseur *Sawaichi* and his beautiful wife *Osato* are a legendary couple who once lived near *Tsubosakadera*. When *Sawaichi* noticed that his wife secretly went out every night, he accused her of meeting with a lover. In reality, however, she was going to the temple to pray to the Goddess *Kannon* for the restoration of his eyesight. When *Sawaichi* discovered this real reason, he felt so ashamed that he threw himself off a cliff. *Osato* followed his example, but *Kannon* rescued both and gave *Sawaichi* his vision back.

213
Tsubosakadera 壺阪寺. Takatori, Nara Prefecture. Late 20th century. W. 13.0 cm
The inscriptions read:
西国六番 = *Saikoku Rokuban* (no.6 of the *Saikoku* [Pilgrimage])
観音霊場 = *Kannon Reijō* (*Kannon* sacred ground)
壺阪寺 = *Tsubosakadera*

Pair(s) of eyes 双眸 *(sōbō)*

Ema depicting one, four or eight pairs of eyes were intended for the healing of *ganbyō* (eye illnesses) [TS-26; IH2-72]. *Ema* with four pairs of eyes were known as *yamume* which consists of *yamu* (ill) and *me* (eyes) [NM-Z04982]. There may be possible wordplays between *yamume* and *ya* (the Japanese word for eight) and between *yamu* (to become ill) and *yamu* (to stop, cease).

In Ashikaga (Tochigi Prefecture), *ema* with eight pairs of eyes were called *yame*. They were offered to *Yakushi* for the healing of an eye illness also called *yame* [FS-21]. The underlying play on words was that *yame* consists of *ya* (eight) and *me* (eyes).

At *Atago Jinja* (Sendai, Miyagi Prefecture), *ema* with a *yatsume* (lamprey eel) were offered for eye illnesses. Since the lamprey has seven gill pores and one eye (making a total of eight) on each side, *yatsume* not only means lamprey in Japanese but also "having eight eyes" [FS-20].

214
Originating sanctuary unclear.
Early to mid-20th century. W. 18.5 cm

215
Ema hand-painted by *Norihito Yasuda* (Nagoya) on commission from the Naito Museum of Pharmaceutical Sciences and Industry (Kakamigahara, Gifu Prefecture). Museum inv.no. Z22684. Late 20th century.

216
Ema from a *Yakushidō* in Tochigi Prefecture
Image reproduced with permission of the publisher from Iwai H. *Ema ni negai o*. Tokyo: Nigensha, 2007 p.73

217

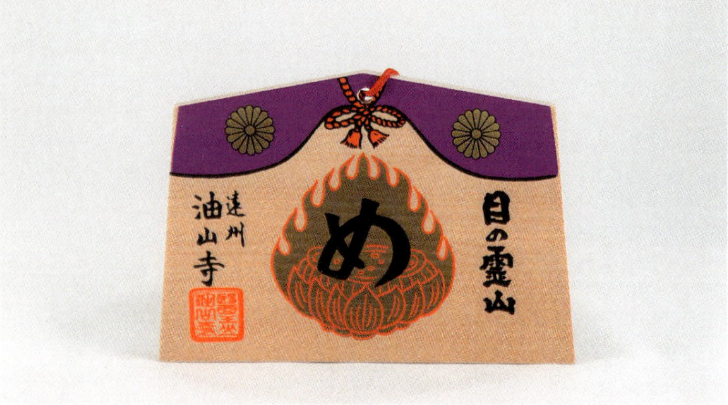

218

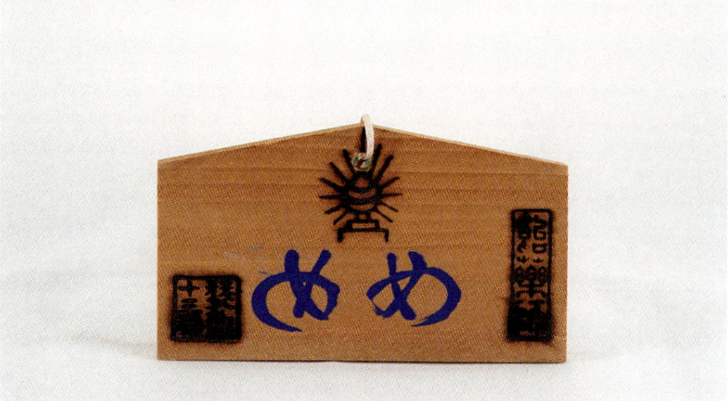

219

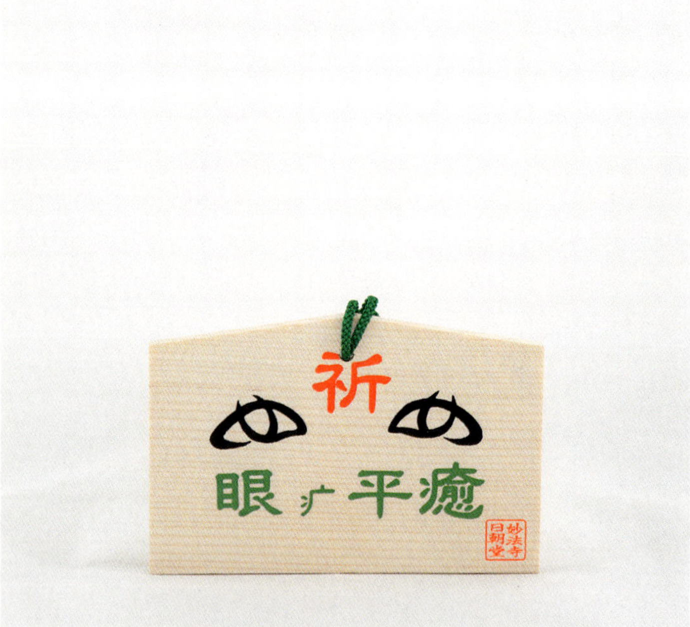

220

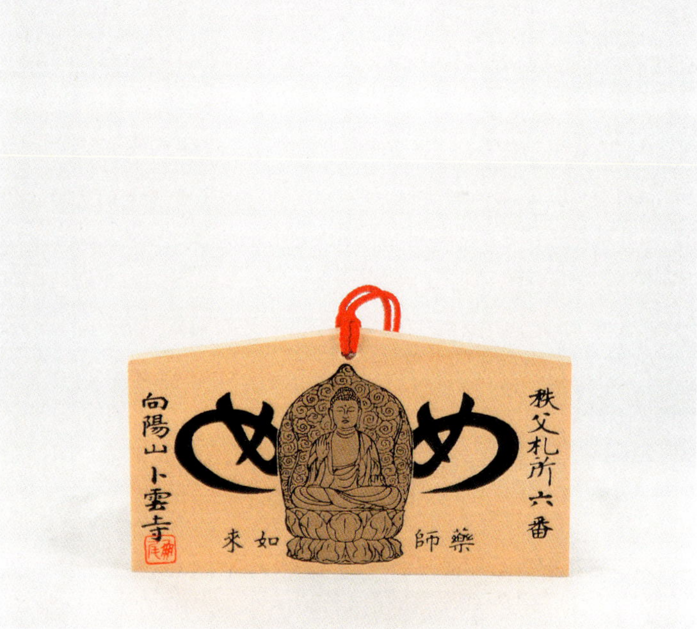

221

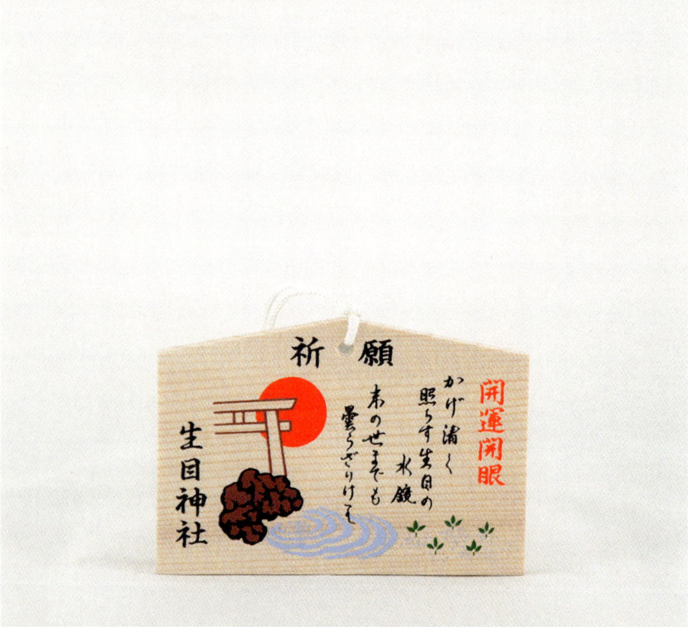

222

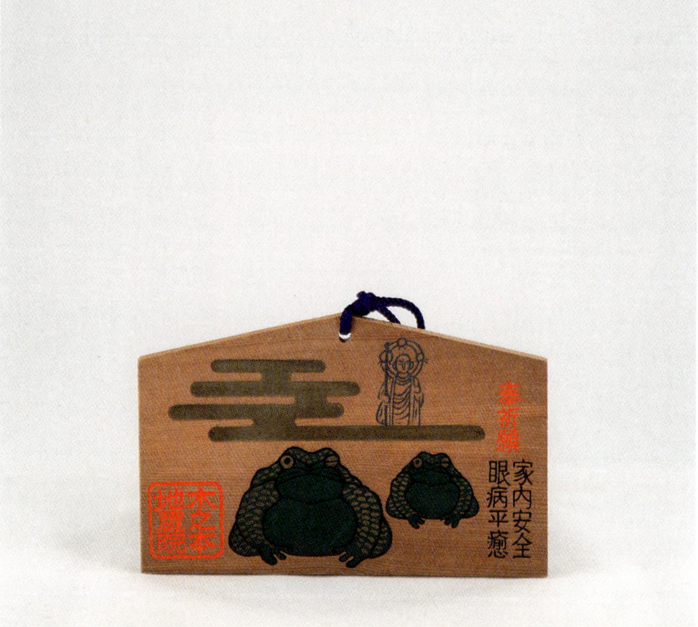

Hiragana character for eye め *(me)*

Ema with one or two *hiragana* characters for *me* (meaning eye or eyesight) are used in various places for *ganbyō* (eye illnesses). When two *me* characters are displayed, the left one is usually shown in reverse (*mukai me* = facing *me*) [FS-16; AE; TS-26; IH2-72].

217
Yusanji 油山寺. Fukuroi, Shizuoka Prefecture. Early 21st century. W. 13.7 cm
The inscriptions on the *ema* read:
目の霊山 = *me no reizan* (sacred mountain for eyes)
遠州 = *enshū* (refers to three distinguished temples in Fukuroi)
油山寺 = *Yusanji*

The *Yakushi Nyorai* (Medicine Buddha) enshrined at *Yusanji* is especially known for recovery from *ganbyō* (eye illnesses). According to legend, Empress *Kōken* was cured of an eye illness in the 8th century after her eyes had been rinsed with water from the Ruri Falls in the temple precincts.

218
Jigenji 慈眼寺. Chichibu, Saitama Prefecture. Late 20th century. W. 13.5 cm
The inscription on the right reads:
飴薬師 = *Ame Yakushi*

There is a radiant *hōju* (wish granting jewel) above the two *me* characters.

Jigenji is the 13th sanctuary of the *Chichibu* pilgrimage and is also known as *Ame Yakushi*. *Ame* means candy and refers to special sweets that are believed to heal eye illnesses and that are sold at the annual temple fair on 8 July. The sweets contain a Japanese maple tree species called *megusurinoki* that grows locally. The temple also offers a herbal tea with this ingredient for eye illnesses. The Japanese word *megusuri* means eye drops or eyewash.

219
Myōhōji 妙法寺. Suginami Ward, Tokyo. Early 21st century.
The inscriptions read:
眼疒平癒 = *gan* [radical no.104] *heiyu* (recovery from eye sickness)
祈 = *inori* (prayer)

This *ema* design constitutes a hybrid between a pair of *me* characters and a pair of actual eyes.

220
Kōyōsan Bokūnji 向陽山卜雲寺. Yokoze, Saitama Prefecture. Early 21st century. W. 15 cm
The inscriptions read:
秩父札所六番 = *Chichibu fudasho Rokuban* (amulet-issuing temple no.6 of the *Chichibu* [Pilgrimage])
薬師如来 = *Yakushi Nyorai*
向陽山卜雲寺 = *Kōyōsan Bokūn-ji*

The facing *me* characters on this *ema* are flanking *Yakushi Nyorai* (Medicine Buddha).

Water from Kamei Mountain 亀井山から水 *(Kamei Yama kara mizu)*

At *Ikime Jinja* (situated on Kamei Mountain), one can be cured of eye illnesses if one rinses one's eyes with local water (御神水 = *gojinzui*; lit. honourable deity water) and if one drinks tea prepared by boiling this water. In former days, the *ema* of this shrine depicted either eight pairs of eyes or a circle of eight eyes in the middle with a *torii* (Shinto shrine archway) on the right and flowing water on the left.

221
Ikime Jinja 生目神社. Miyazaki, Miyazaki Prefecture. Early 21st century. W. 13.0 cm
The inscriptions read:
開運 = *kaiun* (opening up good luck)
開眼 = *kaigen* = opening one's eyes to the truth; also a Buddhist ceremony to "open the eyes" of a statue so that it becomes a living Buddhist figure)
祈願 = *kigan* (prayer)
生目神社 = *Ikime Jinja*

Substitute frog 身代わり蛙 *(migawari kaeru)*

Migawari kaeru (substitute frog) takes on the suffering of patients with an eye illness (cf. the entry on *Migawari Jizō* on p.47). According to legend, there once lived a frog in the temple compound of *Kinomotojizōin* (Nagahama, Shiga Prefecture). When it saw countless patients coming for a cure of their eye illness, it vowed that it would close one eye to experience their pain and that it would ask *Jizō* to heal them. The *Jizō* in question was *Kinomoto Jizō*, the main figure of worship of the temple. Only when all people have been cured of eye illnesses will the frog open its eye again [GG1-2012/05].

222
Kinomotojizōin 木之本地蔵院. Nagahama, Shiga Prefecture. Late 20th century. W. 14.0 cm
The inscriptions read from right to left:
奉祈願 = *hō kigan* (prayer of dedication/offer)
家内安全 = *kanai anzen* (prayer for household safety)
眼病平癒 = *ganbyō heiyu* (recovery from an eye illness)

The *ema* design depicts *Migawari kaeru* as well as *Kinomoto Jizō*.

223

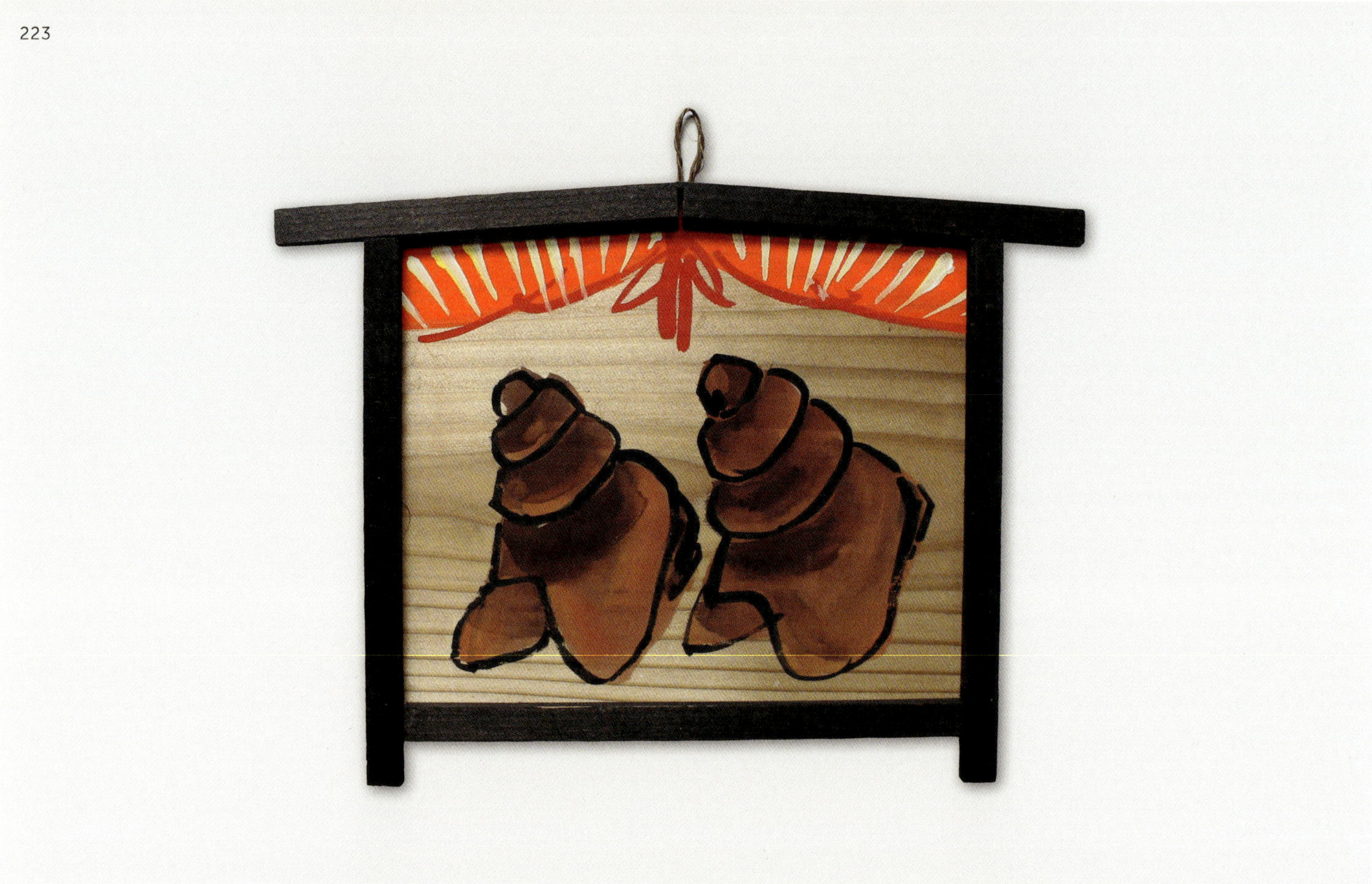

224

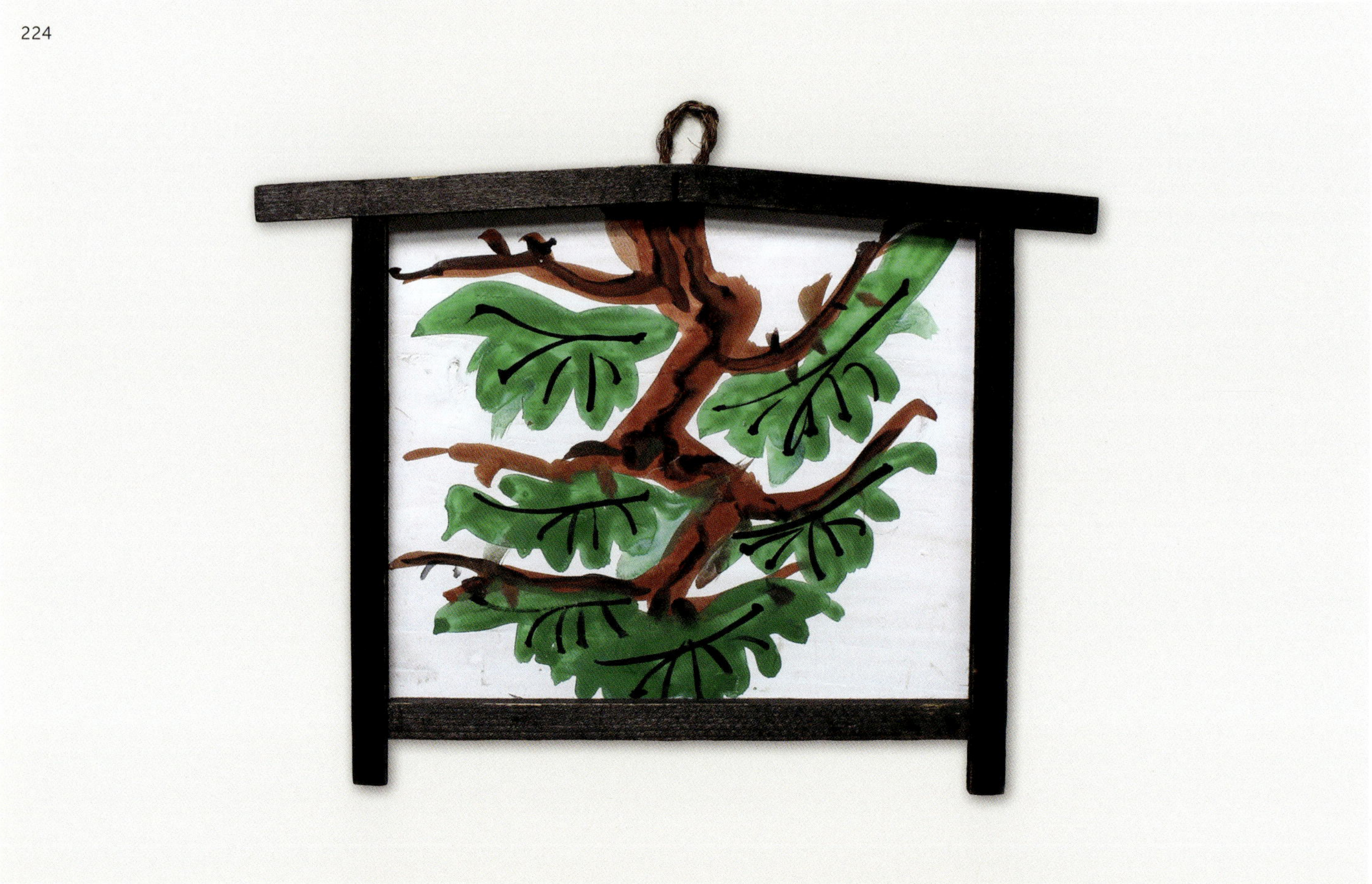

Mud snails 田螺 *(tanishi)*

Tanishi is a type of river snail that is eaten by some people in Japan. *Ema* with this design were used for *ganbyō heiyu* (recovery from eye illness) and could also serve as a charm against harmful *mushi* (worms – cf. the entry on *kannomushi* on p.161) [TS-7; IH2-74; NM-Z03685; NM- Z22651].

In the mid-20th century, there was a hall on the outskirts of Satte (Saitama Prefecture) that was dedicated to *Fudō* (Buddhist figure of fire with the power of keeping down evil spirits). This *Fudō* was commonly known as *Tanishi Fudō*. People who prayed to him for a cure did not eat *tanishi* and offered him an *ema* with the picture of *tanishi*. There was also a *Fudō* sanctuary in Shinano Province (now Nagano Prefecture) where petitioners could pray for a cure for an eye illness and would promise to refrain from eating *tanishi* [AE; JM-156].

223
Ema hand-painted by *Norihito Yasuda* (Nagoya) on commission from the Naito Museum of Pharmaceutical Sciences and Industry (Kakamigahara, Gifu Prefecture). Museum inv.no. Z22651. Late 20th century.

Inverted pine tree 逆松 *(sakamatsu)*

The *ema* design of *sakamatsu* is used for the healing of ingrown eyelashes (trichiasis) because the Japanese word for the latter sounds almost the same (*sakamatsuge*) [AE; IH2-75; NM-Z22695]. Ingrown eyelashes can lead to serious corneal scarring and blindness. In prewar Japan, the underlying cause was frequently trachoma.

224
Ema hand-painted by *Norihito Yasuda* (Nagoya) on commission from the Naito Museum of Pharmaceutical Sciences and Industry (Kakamigahara, Gifu Prefecture). Museum inv.no. Z22695. Late 20th century

Additional designs for eye symptoms/ complaints (not illustrated here) are:

- **Chickens 鶏 (*niwatori*). Among the medical purposes of this *ema* design were night blindness and eye illnesses [IH1-168; IH2-70]. The Japanese word for night blindness (鳥目 = *torime*) can be read as composed of 鳥 (*tori* = chicken) and 目 (*me* = eye). Cf. the entry on chickens on p.171.**
- **Octopus 蛸 (*tako*). *Ema* with this design have been recommended for a variety of medical problems, including *ganbyō* (eye illnesses) [IH2-90]. Cf. the entry on octopus on p.183.**

225

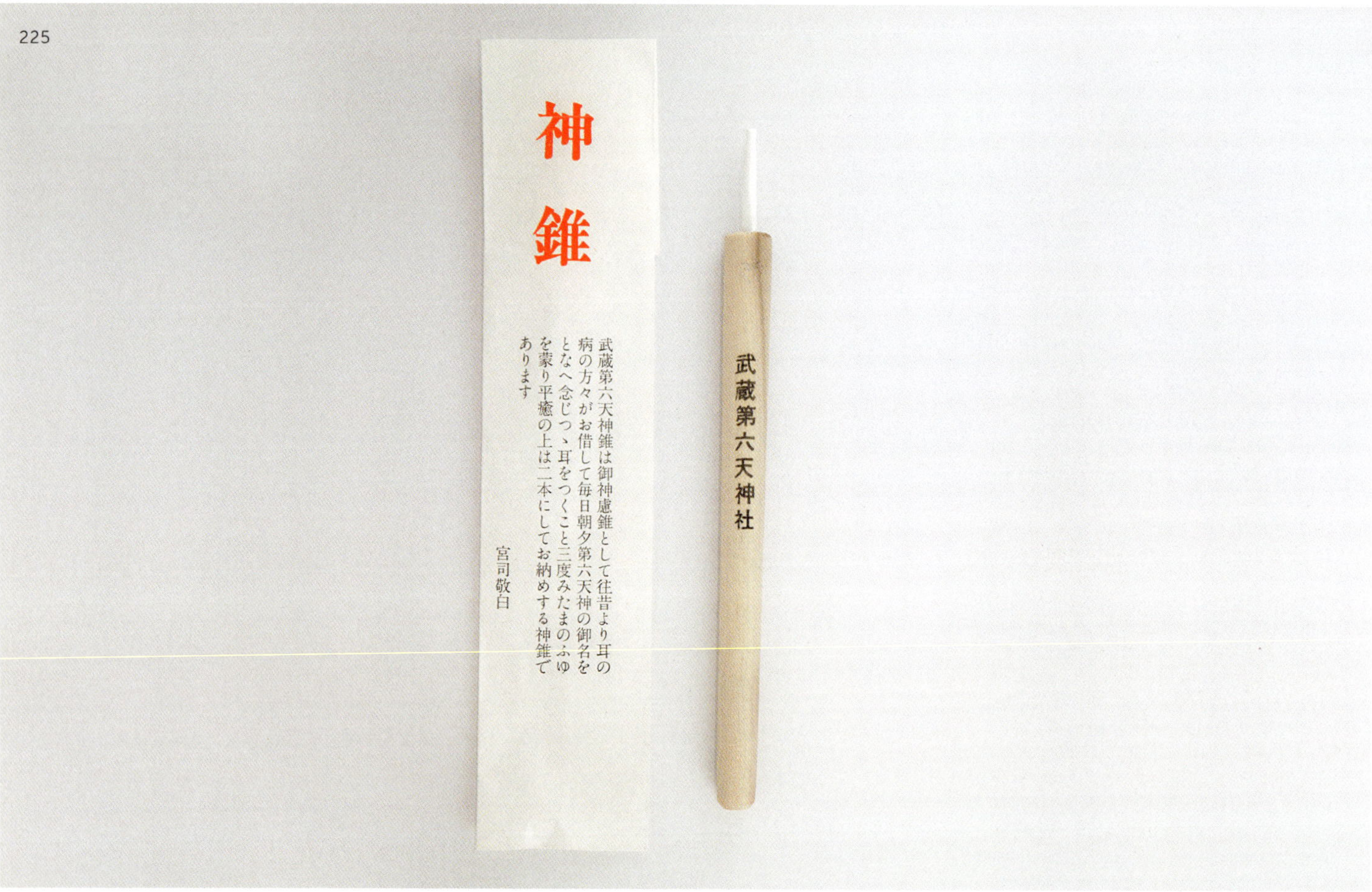
神錐
武蔵第六天神錐は御神慮錐として往昔より耳の病の方々がお借して毎日朝夕第六天神の御名をとなへ念じつゝ耳をつくこと三度みたまのふゆを蒙り平癒の上は二本にしてお納めする神錐であります
宮司敬白
武蔵第六天神社

226

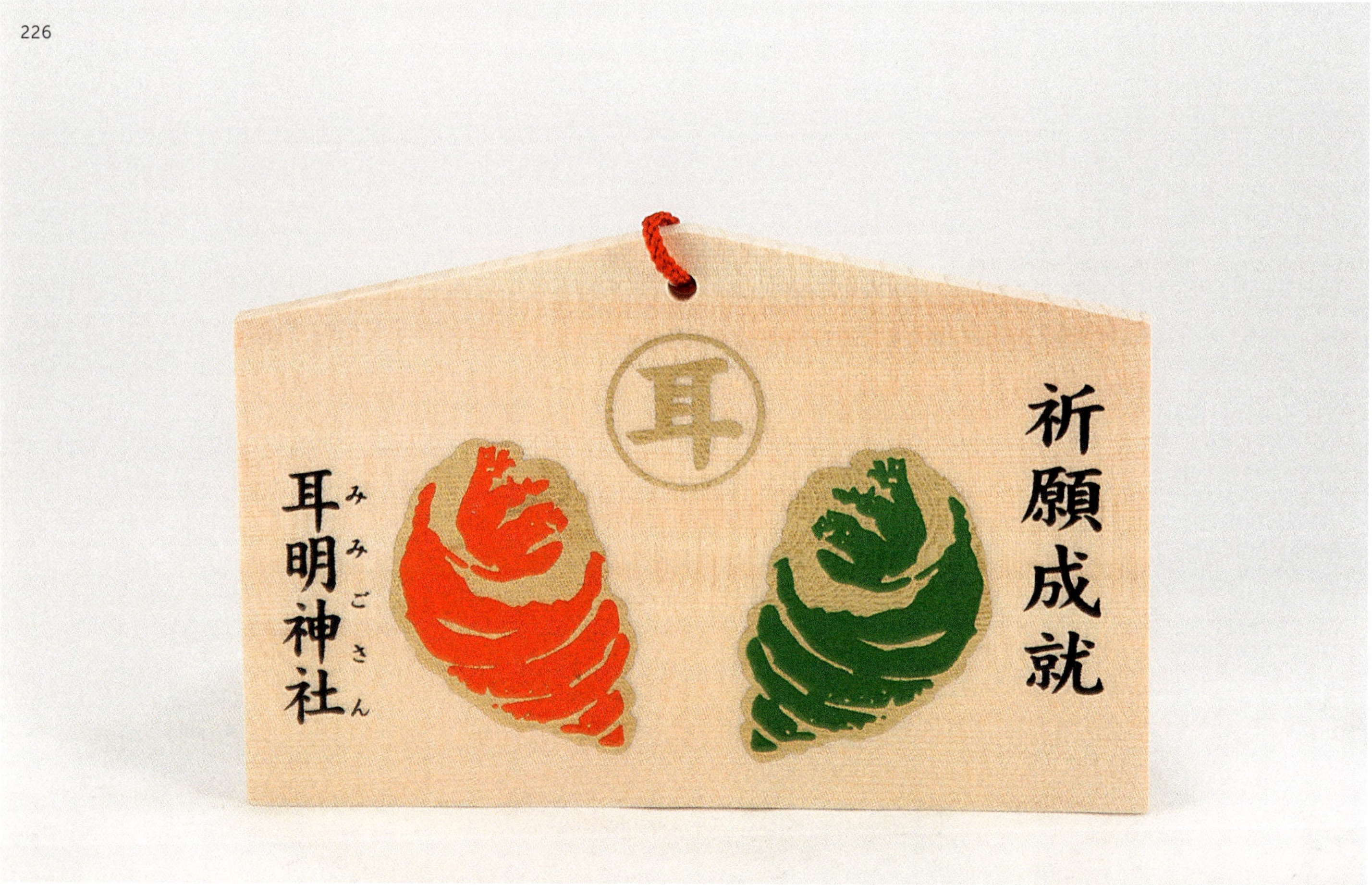
耳
祈願成就
耳明神社
みみごさん

Ear symptoms/ complaints 耳症状／愁訴 (*mimi shōjō/shūso*)

Background

Common ear problems in the Japanese population include excessive earwax, ringing in the ears (tinnitus) and ear infections [EO-130; IO; 1]. Examples of sanctuaries that offer recovery from ear symptoms/complaints are:

- *Mitsumine Jinja* 三峰神社 (Arakawa Ward, Tokyo). People can offer a rice bowl with a hole to a statue of *Miminashi* (Earless) *Fudō* to ask for the healing of an ear illness [RT-249].
- *Muryōsan Saifukuji* 無量山 西福寺 (Izumi, Osaka Prefecture) offers *kiri* (gimlets which are tools for drilling small holes) for the healing of ear illnesses. *Kiri* for ear illnesses or headache can also be found at *Musashi Dairokuten Jinja* (see illustration 225).
- In the early to mid-20th century, *kiri* (gimlets) were also employed for ear illnesses at the *Mine Yakushidō* of *Hōryūji* (Ikaruga, Nara Prefecture). If one desired a cure, one took home a drill that had been offered, prayed and made an offering. If this resulted in a cure, ten drills tied together were returned with or in place of the one borrowed [FS-16; AE].

225
Drill of the deity 神錐 (*kami kiri*). *Musashi Dairokuten Jinja* 武蔵第六天神社. Saitama, Saitama Prefecture. Early 21st century. L. 24.1 cm. Wood, metal, paper.
The inscription reads:
武蔵第六天神社 = *Musashi Dairokuten Jinja*

This charm is used for the healing of ear illnesses. It has the form of a *kiri* (gimlet, which is a tool for drilling small holes). Its metal tip is wrapped with a *fuda* (paper charm) which is not to be removed. After the ear illness has been cured, one has to return the gimlet to the shrine and add an additional gimlet. The shrine will then purify and bury the gimlets.

Ema designs

Turban shells 栄螺 *(sazae)*

This *ema* design is found at *Mimigo Jinja*. The *kami* (deity) enshrined there can be invoked for ringing ears, deafness, and other ear complaints. According to legend, people started to believe in his healing powers, after a grandmother had successfully petitioned at the shrine for her grandson to be cured of an ear illness.

226
Mimigo Jinja 耳明神社. Onomichi, Hiroshima Prefecture. Early 21st century. W. 15.1 cm
The inscriptions read:
祈願成就 = *kigan jōju* (fulfilment of prayer)
耳 = *mimi* (ear/ears)
耳明神社 = *Mimigo Jinja*

Additional *ema* for ear symptoms/complaints (not illustrated here) are:

- Gimlets 錐 (*kiri*) which are tools for drilling small holes. One source on small *ema* presents three gimlets attached to an *ema* that was used for the healing of ear illnesses and hearing difficulties [TS-4]. *Musashi Dairokuten Jinja* and *Muryōsan Saifukuji* still offer gimlets as such for ear problems (see the information above).
- There is a small shrine near *Ishikiri Tsurugiya Jinja* (Osaka), where one can offer a blank rectangular prayer tablet or prayer pebble for ringing ears or ear wax. The belief that stones can cure excessive discharge of ear wax was found throughout Japan [EO-129]. Prayer pebbles may not only be used for offering votive messages concerning ear illnesses but also for other reasons, such as good business and fishery [MK-31].

227

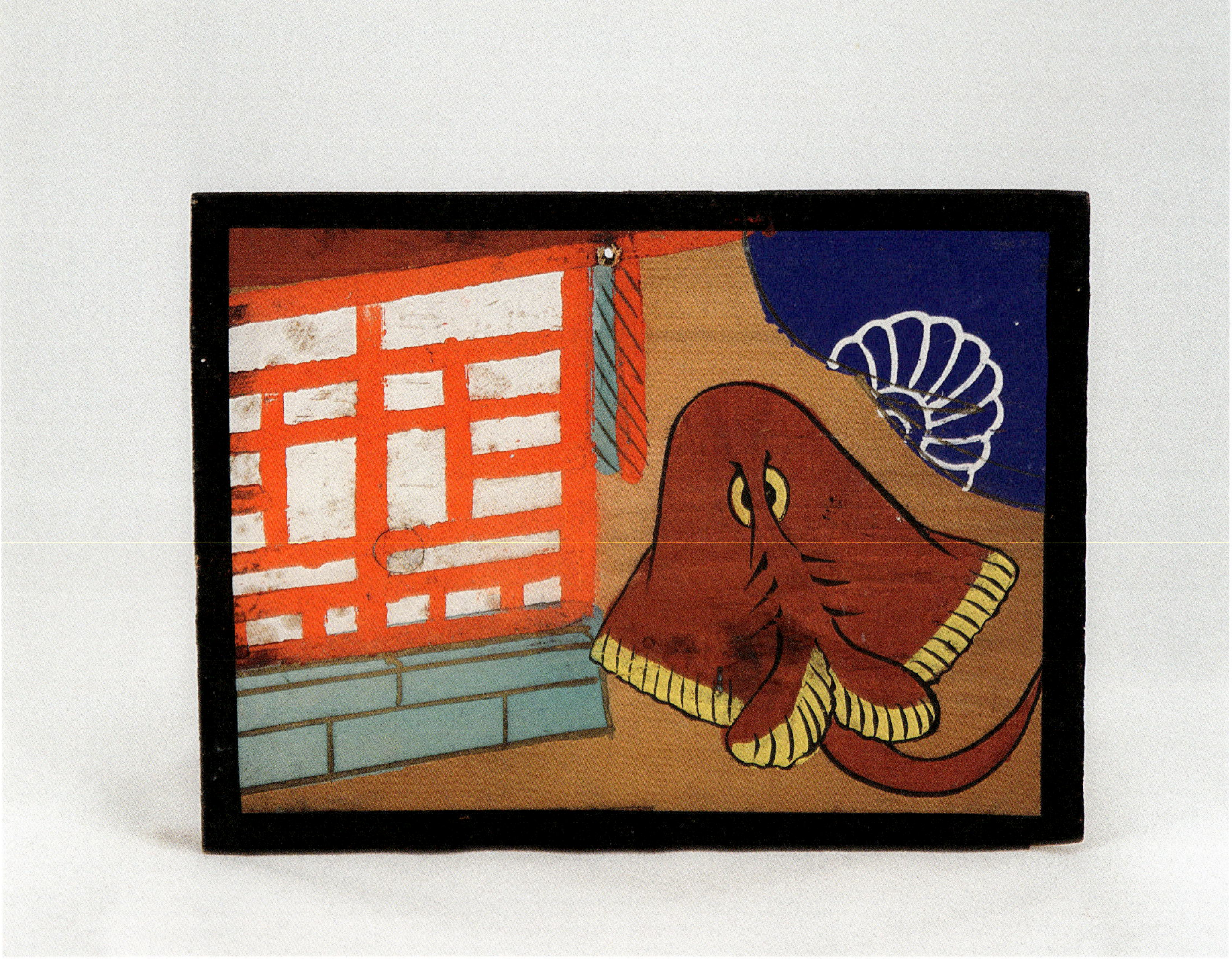

228

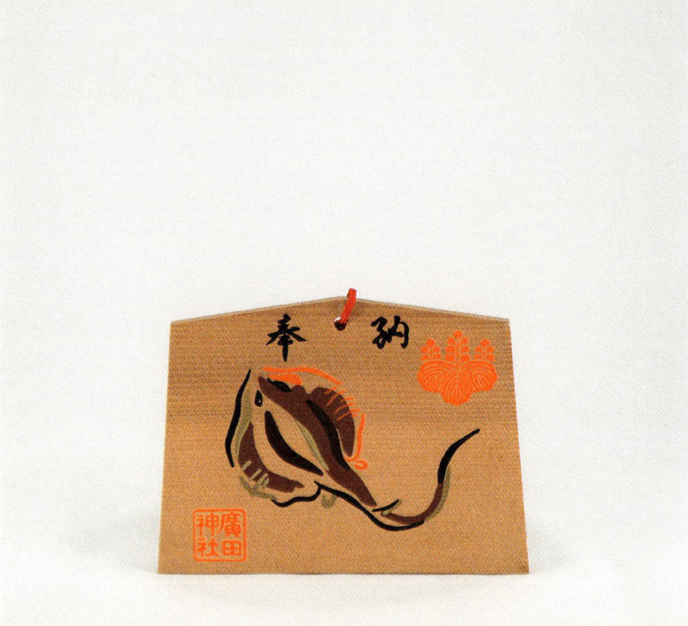

229

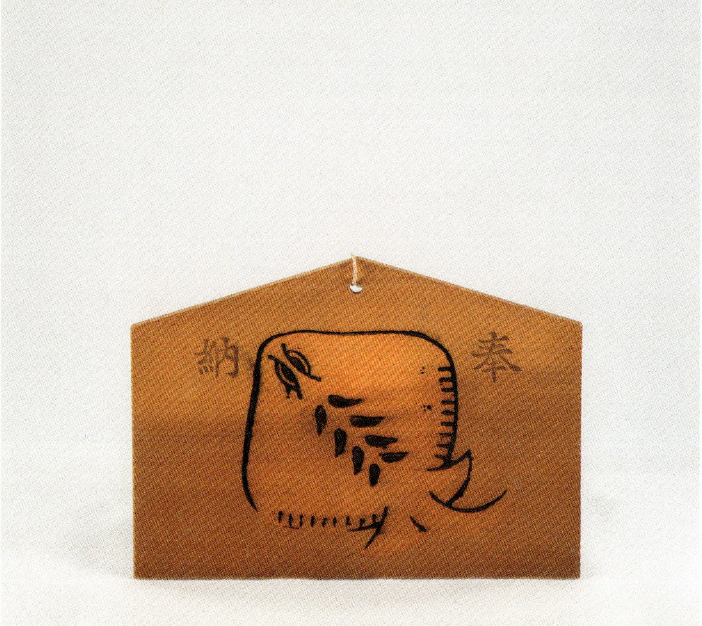

Circulatory symptoms/ complaints 循環器症状／愁訴 (*junkanki shōjō/shūso*)

Background

Outpatients sometimes manifest circulatory symptoms or signs (such as palpitations, chest pain or hypertension) [IO; TT] and circulatory diseases are only outranked by malignant neoplasms in the current death rate figures for Japan (see Figure 1 on p.121). Yet the only *ema* design that has emerged unequivocally for specific circulatory complaints is that of the red stingray for *ji* (haemorrhoids) (see the discussion on *ema* designs below). The main symptoms of haemorrhoids (rectal itching, pain, and bleeding) occur regularly in the adult population of Japan [EO-53,124]. Advertisements for haemorrhoidal ointments are common in Japanese newspapers. Haemorrhoids were also a problem in Buddhist (Zen) temples where monks meditated for hours in *zazen* (the seated cross-legged position for Zen meditation) and had sparse diets without much fibre. The kanji for haemorrhoids (痔 = *ji*) is composed of two parts – the radical for illness (疒) plus the phonetic 寺 (*ji* = temple) – that read "illness of the temple" in combination. In his famous work called *Shōbōgenzō*, *Eihei Dōgen* (the 13th century founder of *Sōtō Zen*) praises a monk who continued to sit in meditation even though he suffered from haemorrhoids [1].

A Shinto deity specialised in the curing of haemorrhoids is *Ji no Kami* (Deity of Haemorrhoids). He can be invoked at *Hirota Jinja* in Osaka. This shrine was in earlier times located within the *jiryō* (temple estate) of *Shitennōji*. When *jiryō* is written differently, it can be read as healing (*ryō*) haemorrhoids (*ji*). In addition, the shrine's deity was a protector of the local area (*ji no kami*). When the sound *ji* is written differently, *ji no kami* becomes the god of haemorrhoids. One can also pray to *Ji no Kami* at *Kusumiya Inari Sha* (Kobe, Hyogo Prefecture) and at *Honshōji* (Taito Ward, Tokyo). The latter temple harbours the tomb of *Magoemon Okada*, a sake merchant from the Edo period. *Okada* suffered from haemorrhoids for years on end. His dying wish was for the salvation of people suffering in the same way. Rumours spread after his death that a friend suffering from haemorrhoids had been cured after praying for recovery at his gravestone [RT-237; 2].

At *Kunigami Jinja* (Haga District, Tochigi Prefecture), there is a special ritual for the healing or prevention of haemorrhoids. First, one has to cleanse oneself by bathing naked in a local holy river. Then one must crouch down with one's backside to a stone holy egg, while saying a special prayer. Finally, one must consume boiled egg offerings. This kind of unusual ritual is known as a *kisai* (strange festival) and was particularly designed to amuse the *kami*. The festival ceased in 1988, but was revived in 2012. Instead of cleansing themselves in the river, participants now turn their backsides to a "butt washing stone" at the shrine, while they chant to be relieved [3].

Ema designs

Red stingray 赤エイ (*akaei*)

There are two reasons why the major *ema* design for wishes concerning *ji* (haemorrhoids) is the *akaei* (the red stingray). Firstly, the stingray can cause severe wounds with its sharp spines. Both the stingray and haemorrhoids are associated with a sting at the rear end, and the red colour of the stingray may be associated with an inflamed condition. Secondly, patients may promise to give up eating stingray while praying for recovery or they may present an *ema* after recovery. To give up eating stingray is expressed in Japanese as *akaei o tatsu*. As the verb *tatsu* means to break with, *akaei o tatsu* implies a radical break with haemorrhoids [FS-21; AE; TS-5; IR; IH2-89].

227
Hand-painted *ema* depicting a red stingray at a shrine. Origin unclear. Early to mid-20th century. W. 18.1 cm

228
Hirota Jinja 広田神社. Naniwa Ward, Osaka. Late 20th century. W. 13.6 cm
The inscription reads 奉納 = *hōnō* (dedication, offering)

229
Kusumiya Inarisha 楠宮稲荷社 in compound of *Nagata Jinja* 長田神社. Kobe, Hyogo Prefecture. Late 20th century. W. 16.0 cm
The inscription reads 奉納 = *hōnō* (dedication, offering)

Pumpkin 南瓜 (*kabocha*)

This *ema* design serves not only for the prevention of *boke* (senility) but also as protection against *chūfū* (paralysis). It can thus be indirectly aimed at the prevention of strokes/cerebrovascular accidents. See the entry on senility on p.167 for background and illustrations.

An additional *ema* design (not illustrated here) portrays the two statues of Deva Kings (*Niō*) that are standing guard at the entrance of *Manmanji* 萬満寺 (Matsudo, Chiba Prefecture). As is usual, one statue is depicted with its mouth open (*ah*) and the other one with its mouth closed (*un*). These two sounds are the first and the last in the Japanese alphabet and symbolize beginning and end, respectively [MS]. Three times a year (at New Year, the spring festival in March and the autumn festival in October), visitors are allowed to crawl through the small gap between the legs of the *Ah* statue. This practice is believed to keep illness and other misfortune away. It may have started in the old days to ask for protection against *ekibyō* (epidemics). According to some websites, the practice is nowadays associated with the prevention of *kumomakukashukketsu* (subarachnoid haemorrhage), *nōsocchū* (stroke) and *mahi* (paralysis).

The temple offers an *ema* showing its two *Niō* statues, but the actual crawling under the *Ah* statue is not depicted [4] and the inscription on the *ema* refers to the much broader concept of *shintai kenzen* (bodily health). Hence it cannot be inferred that this *ema* is only or specifically for cerebrovascular afflictions.

231

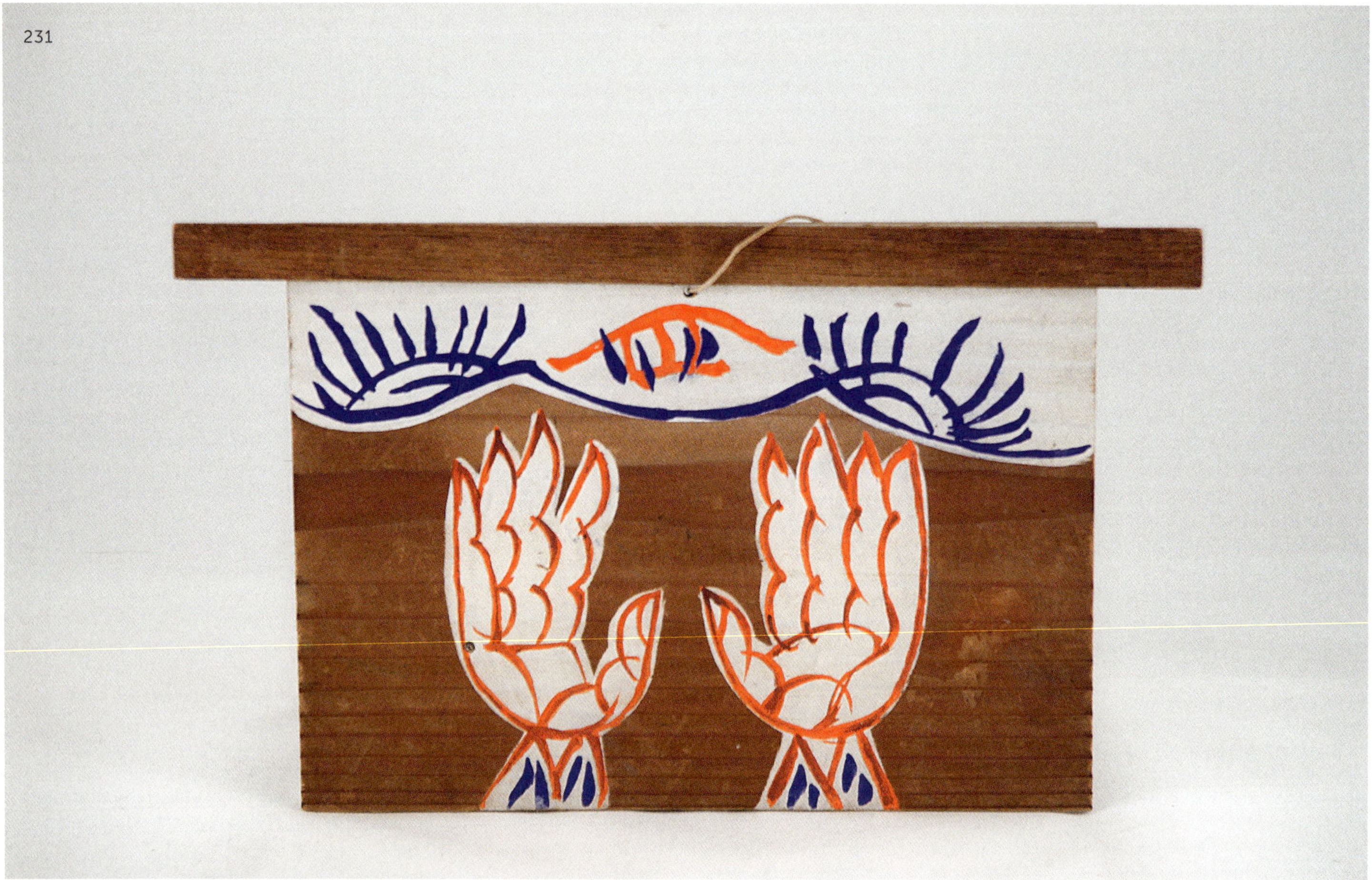

230

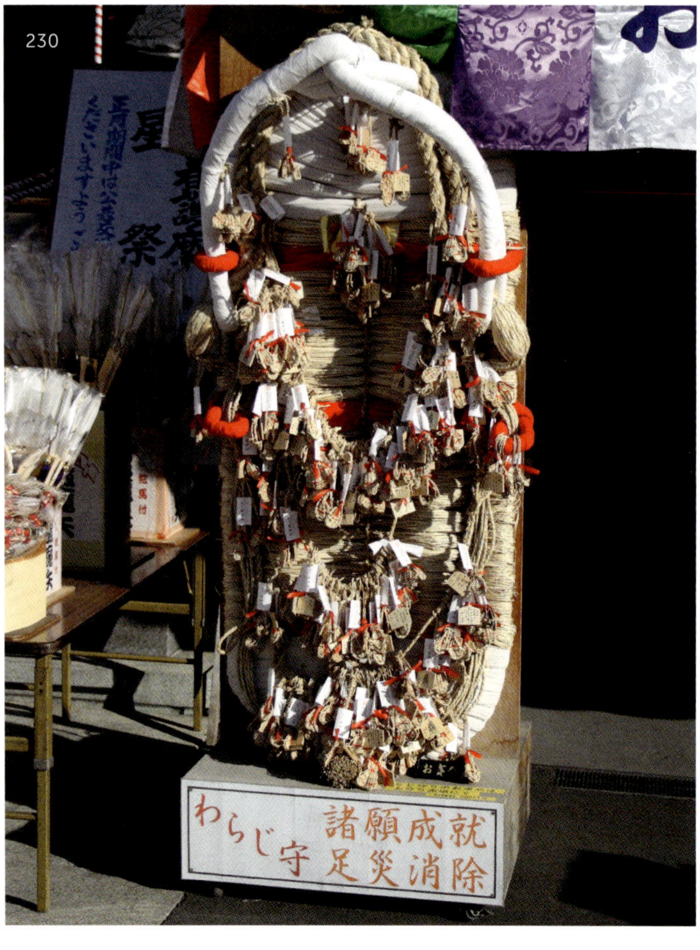

232

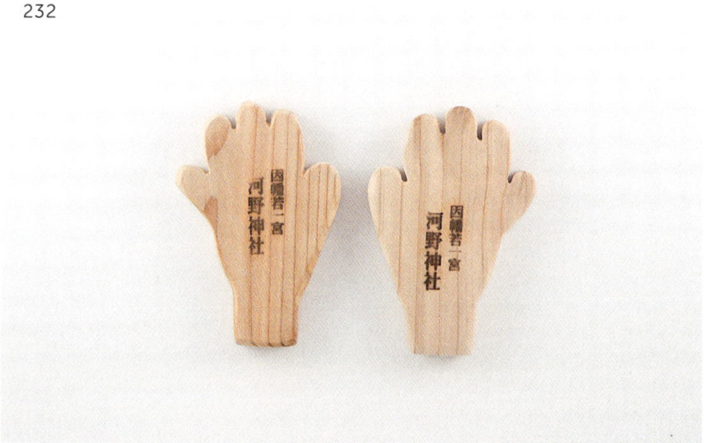

233

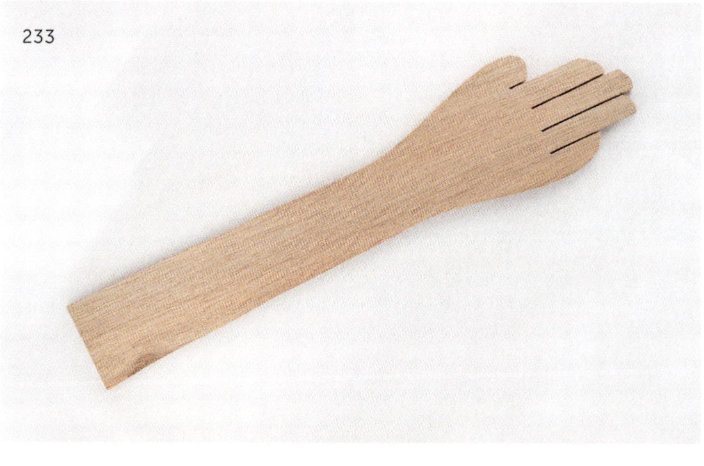

Musculoskeletal symptoms/complaints 筋骨格 症状／愁訴 (*kinkokkaku shōjō/ shūso*)

Background

In the past, common musculoskeletal complaints included *ryūmachi* (rheumatism), *yōtsū* (lower back/hip pain, lumbago) and *katakori* (stiff shoulders/neck) [JE; EO-53]. An important cause of leg problems was beriberi, which resulted from deficiency of vitamin B1 due to the consumption of white rice that had been dehusked to extend its shelf life. The disease would begin with weakness and loss of feeling in the legs, which commonly proceeded to swelling or dropsy, and could end in heart failure and death. Another underlying cause must have been the crippling effect of syphilis [1].

Since the last century, life expectancy has continued to rise and Japan's population has continued to age, and this has meant that the prevalence of musculoskeletal complaints has remained high [IO; TT]. Lower back and knee pains appear to be particularly common. In a recent large study, both symptoms were reported by more than one-third of the respondents (most of whom were aged ≥ 60 years) [2].

Figures of worship for the healing of musculoskeletal symptoms/complaints (e.g., *Ashi Jizō* = leg/foot *Jizō*) are presented in the entries on specific *ema* designs for this purpose.

Konoshima Jinja (Ukyo Ward, Kyoto) can be especially visited for *shimoyake* (frostbite, chilblains). The shrine organises an annual *Mitarai* Festival where one can immerse one's hands and feet in the water of *kamiike* (lit. pond of the deity) to be cured of *shimoyake* and other afflictions [GK].

230
Enormous *waraji* 草鞋 (straw sandal) at *Narita-san Fukagawa-Fudō-dō* (Koto Ward, Tokyo). It is packed with pairs of small *waraji* with a small *ema* attached to them that portrays the Buddhist figure of worship *Fudō Myō-ō*. Cf. the entry on straw sandals on p.151.

Ema designs

Arm/hand 手 (te)

The Japanese word *te* means arm as well as hand. Its exact translation into English depends on the context. Several *ema* designs depicting *te* are used for illnesses of the arms/hands.

231
Ōte Jinja 大手神社. Ashikaga, Tochigi Prefecture. Mid-20th century. W. 19.0 cm

This *ema* design is called *sōte* (pair of hands) and comes from the Ashikaga region, which was renowned for its weaving industry. It was offered for skilled and strong hands in weaving and other crafts, *sōba ni seikō* (successful market) and for recovery from *te no byō* (illnesses of the hand), such as arthritic fingers. The main deity of the shrine is *Ameno-Tajikara-Onokami*. This literally means a man with very strong hands and he is worshipped as a deity of hands. According to Japanese mythology, he brought the sun goddess *Amaterasu* back to the world after she had retreated to a cave and had thereby deprived the world of its sunlight [FS-15; OT; TS-11; KM-26; IH2-81]. In the past, not only were *ema* portraying a pair of hands presented at *Ōte Jinja*, but also *ema* with a single hand (*katate*) painted on them. One source states that wooden hands were also offered there as votive objects [FS-15; OT; IH2-81]

232
Kōno Jinja 河野神社. Chizu, Tottori Prefecture. Early 21st century. H. 10 cm
The inscriptions read:
因幡若一宮 = *Inaba Waka Ichinomiya*
河野神社 = *Kōno Jinja*

This type of wooden votive is called *katashiro* (representation of a sacred object). The shrine offers votives not only in the shape of a hand, but also in the shape of a foot (see p.147).

The origin lies in a legend of a benevolent giant named *Sanbutarō*, who once lived in Mimasaka province (now in the north of Okayama Prefecture). He was so large that he could reach Kyoto in three strides. After his death, his head was buried in Okayama, while his hands, feet and shoulders were buried at *Kōno Jinja*.

233
Kai Jinja (*Ashite Kōjin*) 甲斐神社 (足手荒神). Kashima, Kumamoto Prefecture. Early 21st century. H. 44.5 cm

This type of wooden votive is called *kata* (model) and can be presented for recovery from an illness of the arm/hand. The shrine offers votives not only in the shape of an arm, but also in the shape of a leg (see p.147).

234

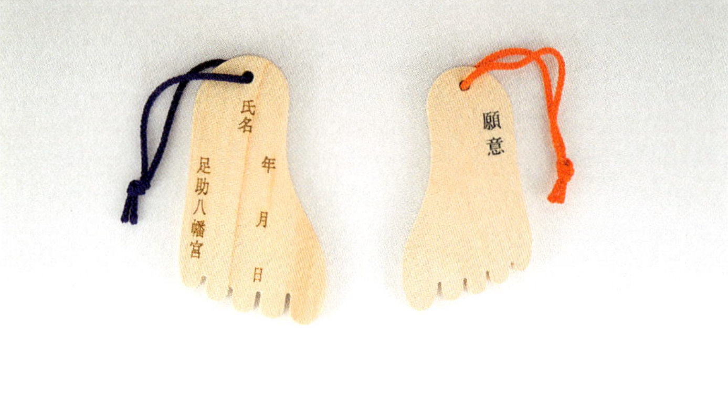

235

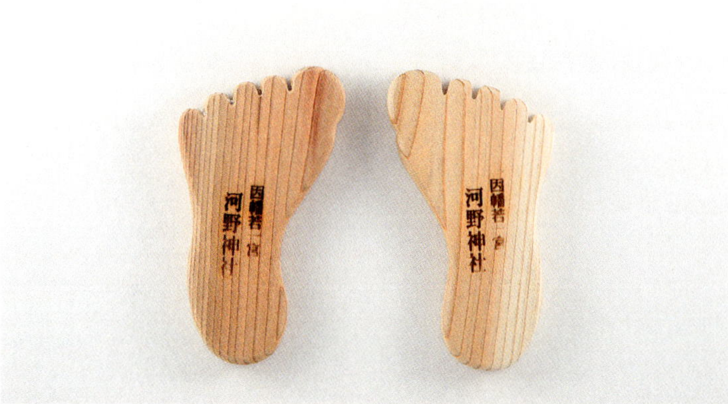

236

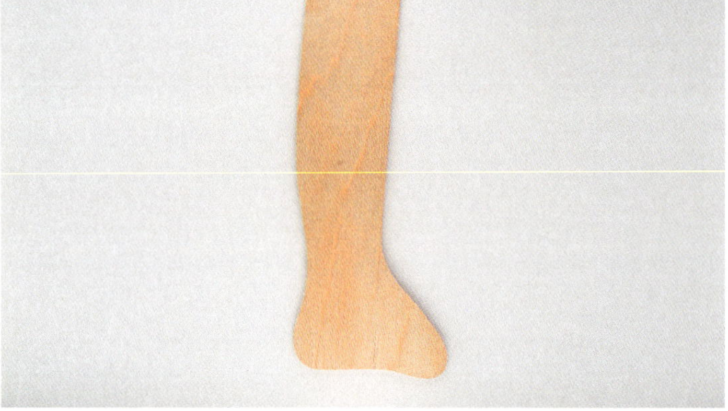

237

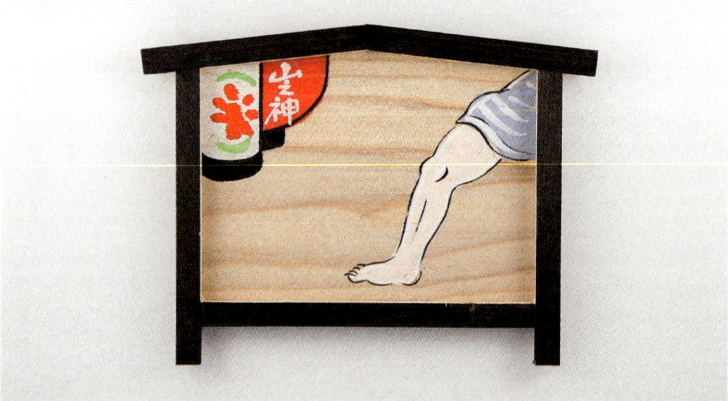

238

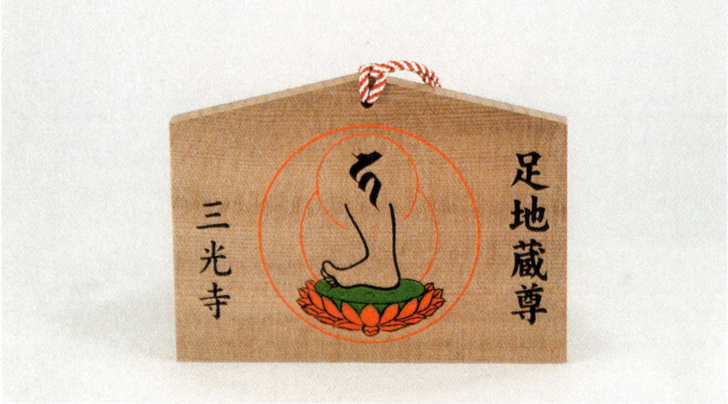

239

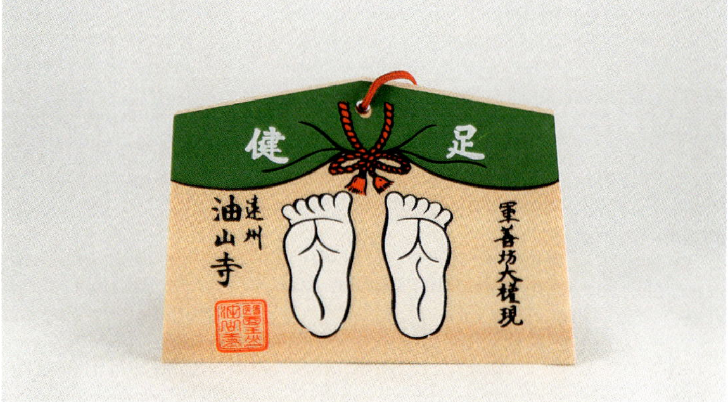

240

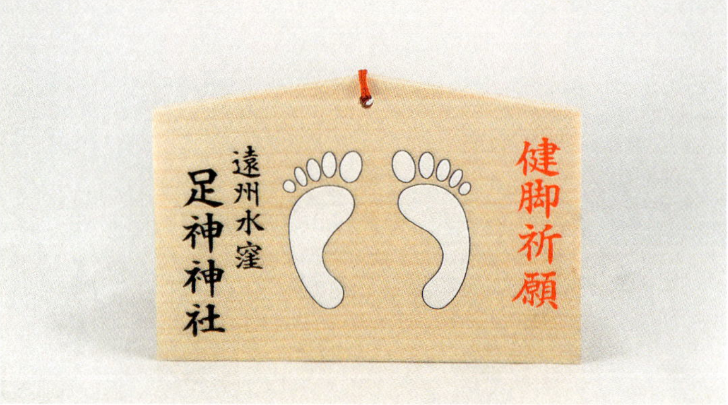

241

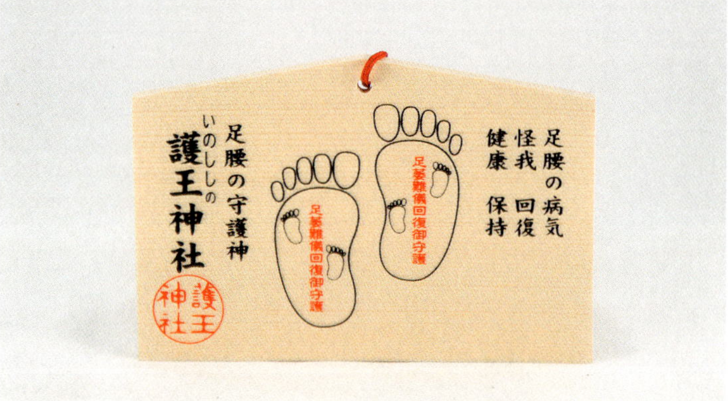

Leg/foot 足 *(ashi)*

The Japanese word *ashi* means leg as well as foot. Its exact translation into English depends on the context. Several *ema* designs depicting *ashi* are used for illnesses of the legs/feet.

234
Asuke Hachimangū 足助八幡宮. Toyota, Aichi Prefecture. Early 21st century.
The inscriptions read:
平成 = *Heisei*
年 月 日 = *toshi getsu nichi* (year month day)
氏名 = *shimei* (name)
足助八幡宮 = *Asuke Hachimangū*
The shrine is visited for foot problems, e.g. by football players. The enshrined deity is *Ashi no Kamisama* (Deity of the Foot).

235
Kōno Jinja 河野神社. Chizu, Tottori Prefecture. Early 21st century. H. 11 cm
The inscriptions read:
因幡若一宮 = *Inaba Waka Ichinomiya*
河野神社 = *Kōno Jinja*
This type of wooden votive is called *katashiro* (representation of a sacred object). The shrine offers votives not only in the shape of a foot, but also in the shape of a hand (see p.145).

236
Kai Jinja (Ashite Kōjin) 甲斐神社 (足手荒神). Kashima, Kumamoto Prefecture. Early 21st century. H. 35 cm
This type of wooden votive is called *kata* (model) and can be presented for recovery from an illness of the leg/foot. The shrine offers votives not only in the shape of a leg, but also in the shape of an arm (see p.145).

237
Hand-painted reproduction for a Japanese club of *ema* collectors called *Nihon Ema Tomo no Kai* (Friends of Japanese Ema Society). No.373. Late 20th century. W. 18.2 cm

238
Sankōji 三光寺. Shimada, Shizuoka Prefecture. Early 21st century. W. 13.0 cm
The inscriptions read:
足地蔵尊 = *Ashi Jizōson* (leg/foot *Jizō*)
三光寺 = *Sankōji*
The enshrined figure of worship is *Ashi Jizō* (leg/foot *Jizō*) who is believed to cure disorders of the legs/feet.

239
Yusanji 油山寺. Fukuroi, Shizuoka Prefecture. Early 21st century. W. 13.8 cm
The inscriptions read:
軍善坊大権現 = *Gunzenbō Daigongen* (guardian deity of *Yusanji*)
健足 = *kensoku* (healthy feet/legs)
遠州 = *Enshū* (former name of Shizuoka Prefecture)
油山寺 = *Yusanji*
The main figure of worship of *Yusanji* is *Yakushi Nyorai* (Medicine Buddha). The temple is famous for curing eye illnesses, which goes back to a legend about the healing of an eye illness of the Emperor *Kōken*. However, the temple guardian *Gunzenbō-Daigongen* is known as a protector of strong healthy feet. Although originally revered by travellers and pilgrims, the temple has lately been popularised by athletes and elderly people.

240
Ashigami Jinja 足神神社. Hamamatsu, Shizuoka Prefecture. Early 21st century. W. 14.1 cm
The inscriptions read:
健脚祈願 = *kenkyaku kigan* (prayer to be able to walk well)
遠州水窪 = *Enshū Misakubo (now part of* Hamamatsu City in Shizuoka Prefecture)
足神神社 = *Ashigami Jinja*

241
Goō Jinja 護王神社. Kamigyo Ward, Kyoto. Early 21st century. W. 15.0 cm
The inscriptions read:
足腰の病気 = *ashikoshi* no *byōki* (illness of the legs and loins)
怪我 回復 = *kega kaifuku* (recovery from injuries)
健康 保持 = *kenkō hoji* (preservation of health)
足萎難儀回復御守護 (on each of the two feet) = *ashinae nangi kaifuku o shugo* (protection/recovery from the affliction of lameness)
足腰の守護人 = *ashikoshi no shugojin* (guardian deity of the legs and loins)
いのししの 護王神社 = *inoshishi no* (wild boar of)
護王神社 = *Goō Jinja*
The figure enshrined at *Goō Jinja* is *Wake no Kiyomaro*. He was a high-ranking official living in the 8th century A.D. who was once sent to *Usa Hachimangū* to receive an oracular message. This message refuted the previous message that someone named *Dōkyō* was to be the successor of the reigning empress. *Dōkyō* then arranged the exile of *Kiyomaro* and had the sinews of his legs cut. Yet *Kiyomaro* managed to escape, because hundreds of wild boar appeared to defend him. When he reached the destination of his flight, his injuries had miraculously healed. The following year, the empress died and was succeeded by a new emperor, who recalled *Kiyomaro* and exiled *Dōkyō*. In the wake of this legend, *Kiyomaro* became a figure of worship for the healing of foot/leg illnesses. As indicated by one of the inscriptions (*kega kaifuku*), the *ema* can also be used for recovery from injuries (such as wounds and sprains).

242

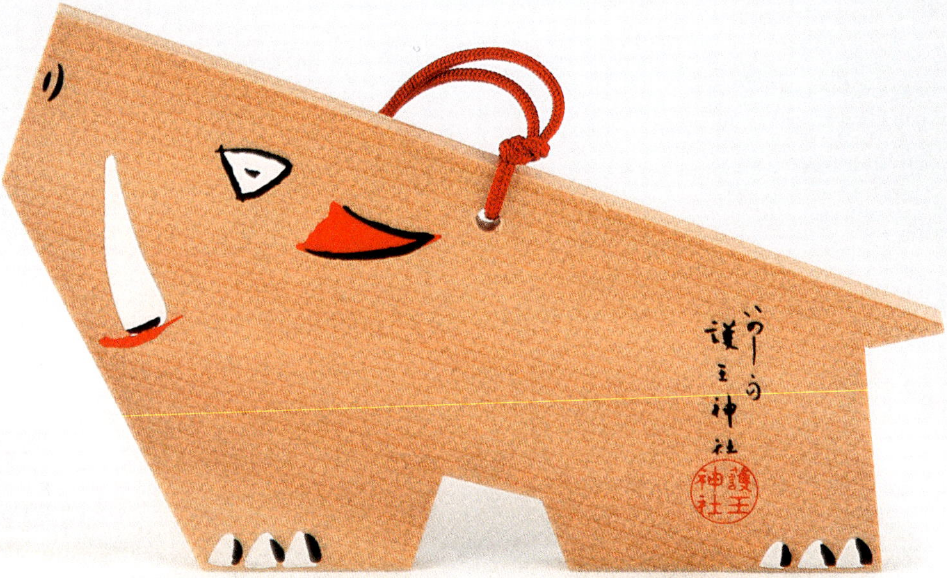

243

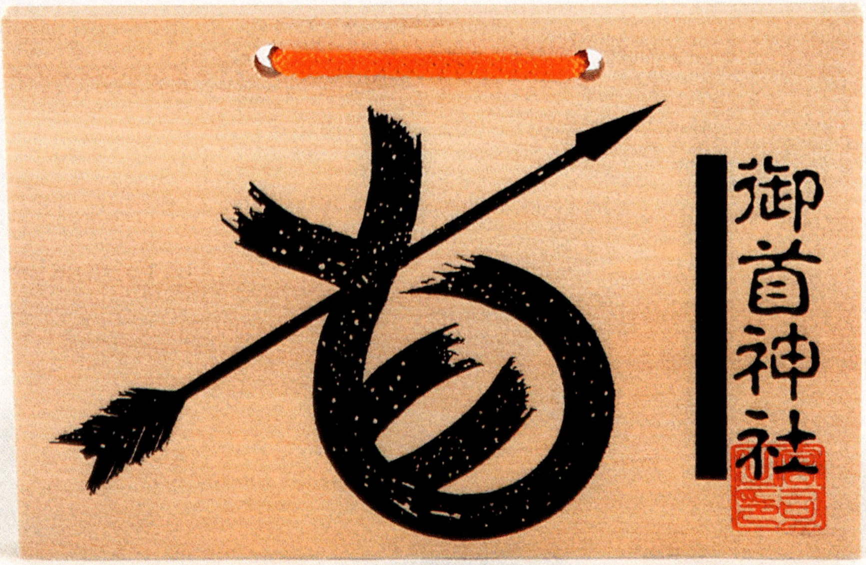

Wild boar 猪 (inoshishi)

242
Goō Jinja 護王神社. Kamigyo Ward, Kyoto.
Early 21st century. W. 15.3 cm
The inscriptions read:
いのししの = *inoshishi* no (wild boar of)
護王神社 = *Goō Jinja*

The figure of worship enshrined at *Goō Jinja* is *Wake no Kiyomaro*, who was once saved by hundreds of wild boar (see p.147). The shrine is therefore famous for its relation with the wild boar. The *ema* design of this animal is used for *ashikoshi no kenkō anzen* (health and safety of the legs and loins) and for *supōtsu jōtatsu hisshō* (sport progress and victory). The shrine also offers an *ema* with the soles of two feet for illnesses of the legs and loins (see p.147).

Character for neck/head 首 (kubi)

243
Mikubi Jinja 御首神社. Ogaki, Gifu Prefecture.
Early 21st century. W. 13.5 cm
The inscription reads:
御首神社 = *Mikubi Jinja*

The second character in the name of the shrine also reads *kubi* (首). This *ema* design is especially used for 首から上の病気 = *kubi kara ue no byōki* (illnesses from the neck up).

244

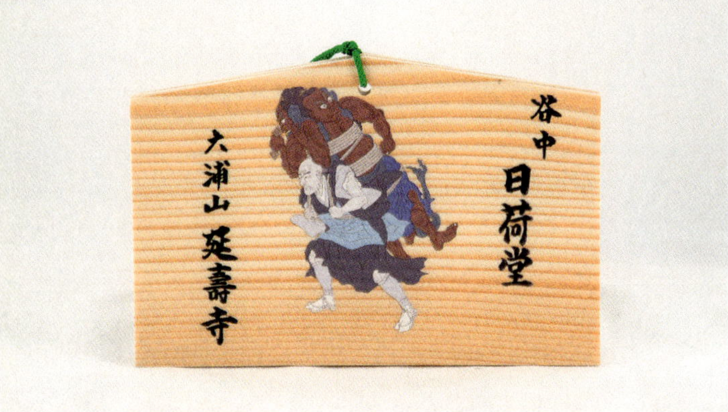

245

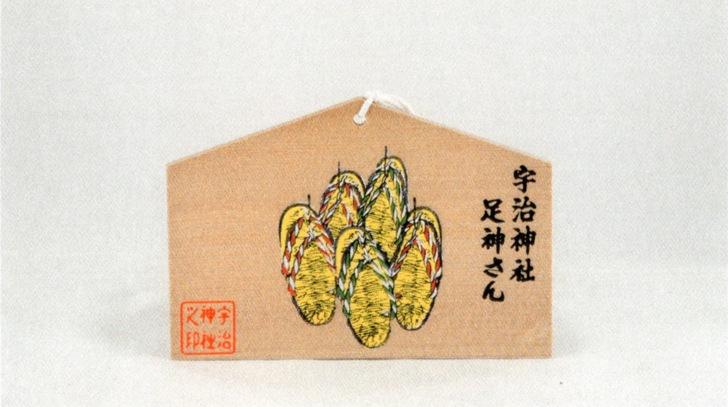

246

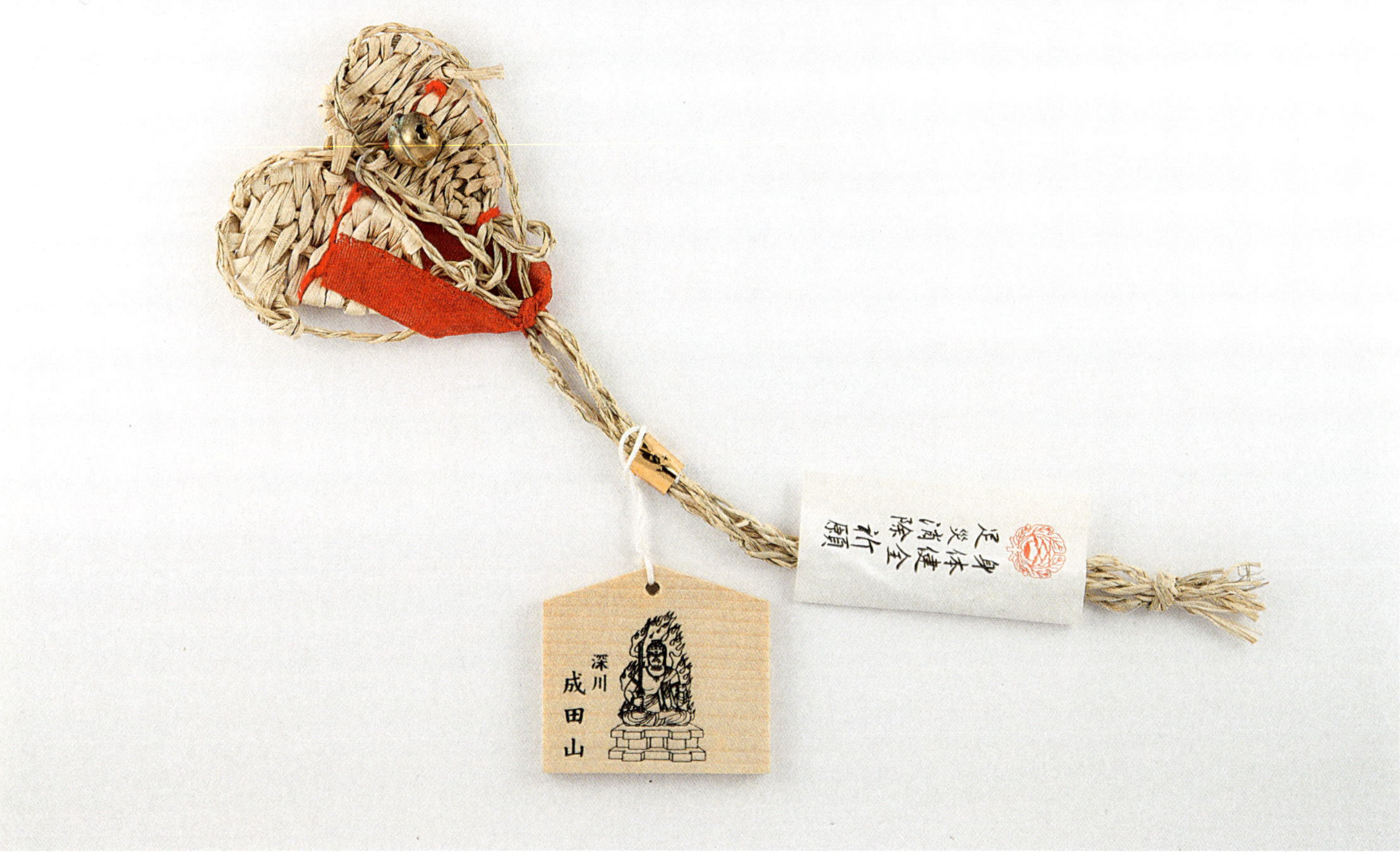

247

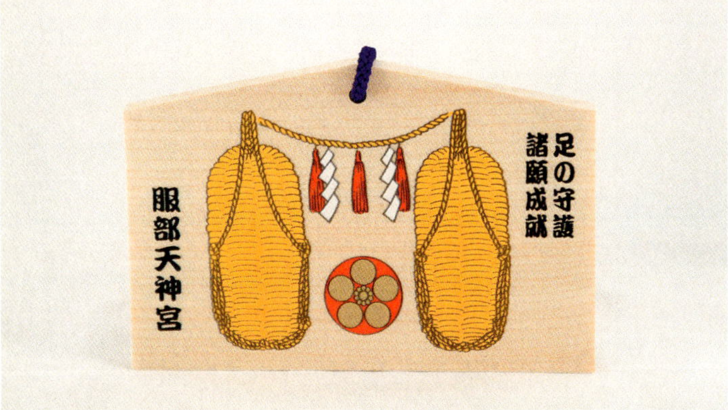

248

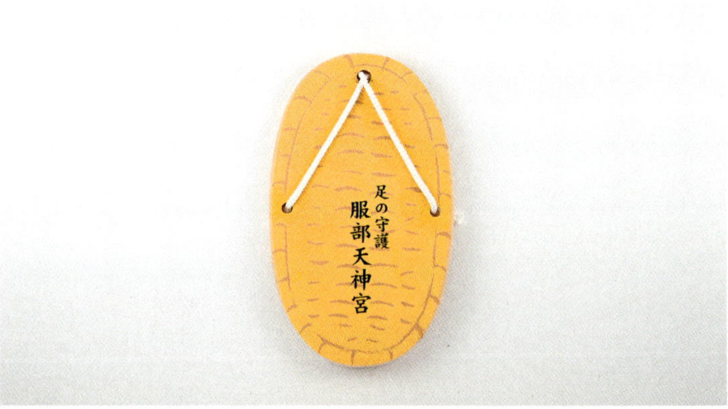

Nichika 日荷

This *ema* design is used for *ashibyō shugo* (protection against illnesses of the legs/feet). It is based on the legendary story of the holy monk *Nichika* who carried two very heavy statues on his back for about 100 kilometres after winning them in a game of *go*.

244
Nichikadō (*Mutsūrasan Enjūji*).
日荷堂「六浦山延壽寺」. Taito ward, Tokyo. Early 21st century. W. 17.5 cm
The inscriptions read:
谷中 = *Yanaka* (location of the temple)
日荷堂 = *Nichikadō*
六浦山延寿寺 = *Mutsūrasan Enjūji*
In former days, the ailments of the legs/feet for which the temple was visited also comprised beriberi (cf. p.185).

Straw sandals 草鞋 (*waraji*)

Waraji or their images on *ema* are offered for the prevention or treatment of foot and leg illnesses, and for travel safety. In former days, these uses also included beriberi (see p.185). Small *ema* with small sandals attached to them are used for similar purposes [FS-17; HD; TS-4,26].

245
Uji Jinja 宇治神社. Uji, Kyoto Prefecture. Early 21st century. W. 14.5 cm
The inscriptions read:
宇治神社 = *Uji Jinja*
足神さん = *Ashikamisan*

Ema design for *kenkyaku* (being able to walk well). *Ashikami* literally means deity (*kami*) of the legs/feet (*ashi*).

246
Narita-san Fukagawa-Fudō-dō
成田山 深川不動堂. Koto Ward, Tokyo.
Late 20th century. W. 5.6 cm (*ema*)
The inscriptions on the *ema* read:
深川 = *Fukagawa* (region in Koto ward)
成田山 = *Narita-san*
The inscriptions on the paper above the *ema* read:
身体健全 = *shogan jōju* (fulfilment of various wishes)
足災消除 = *ashi sai shōjo* (eradication of problems of the feet/legs)
祈願 = *kigan* (prayer)

The purpose of this small *ema* (healthy feet/legs) is evident from the small pair of *waraji* attached to it. The *ema* itself portrays the Buddhist figure of worship *Fudō Myō-ō* who is a principal protector of Buddhism and a destroyer of delusion. He is popularly depicted as an angry figure surrounded by flames, holding a rope and a sword. The originating temple is famous for *kōtsū anzen* (traffic/road safety). See also the picture on p.144.

Sandals 草履 (*zōri*)

Zōri are sandals made of grass, straw, iron or copper which resemble flip-flops. Their depiction on *ema* serves the same foot/leg-related purposes as *waraji* (straw sandals) on *ema*. In the past, *ema* with small *zōri* were used to pray for strong legs, for health and for the prevention of beriberi (see the section on nutritional/metabolic complaints) [TS-4].

247
Hattori Tenjingū 服部天神宮. Toyonaka, Osaka Prefecture. Early 21st century. W. 17.5 cm
The inscriptions read:
足の守護 = *ashi no shugo* (protection of the feet/legs)
諸願成就 = *shogan jōju* (fulfilment of various wishes)
服部天神宮 = *Hattori Tenjingū*

248
Hattori Tenjingū 服部天神宮. Toyonaka, Osaka Prefecture. Early 21st century. W. 9.0 cm
The inscriptions read:
足の守護 = *ashi no shugo* (protection of the feet/legs)
服部天神宮 = *Hattori Tenjingū*

In the past, *Hattori Tenjingū* was visited to pray for recovery from beriberi and other problems of the legs/feet. Nowadays, it is still visited for problems with the legs/feet (inter alia by sportsmen) [GK].

249

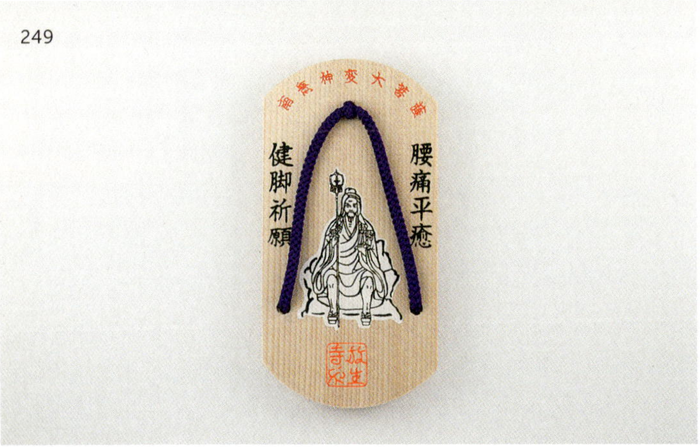

251

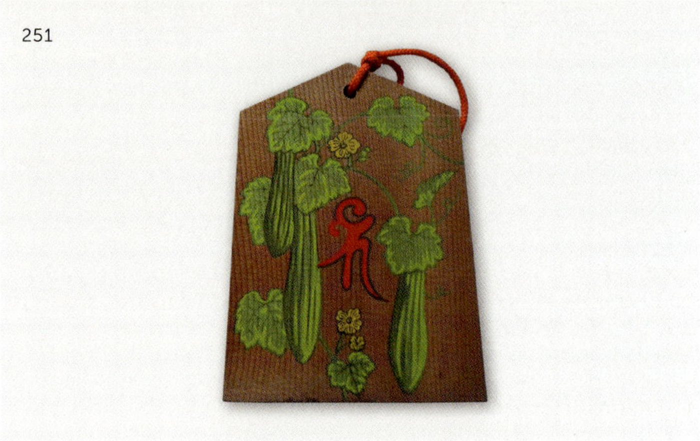

250

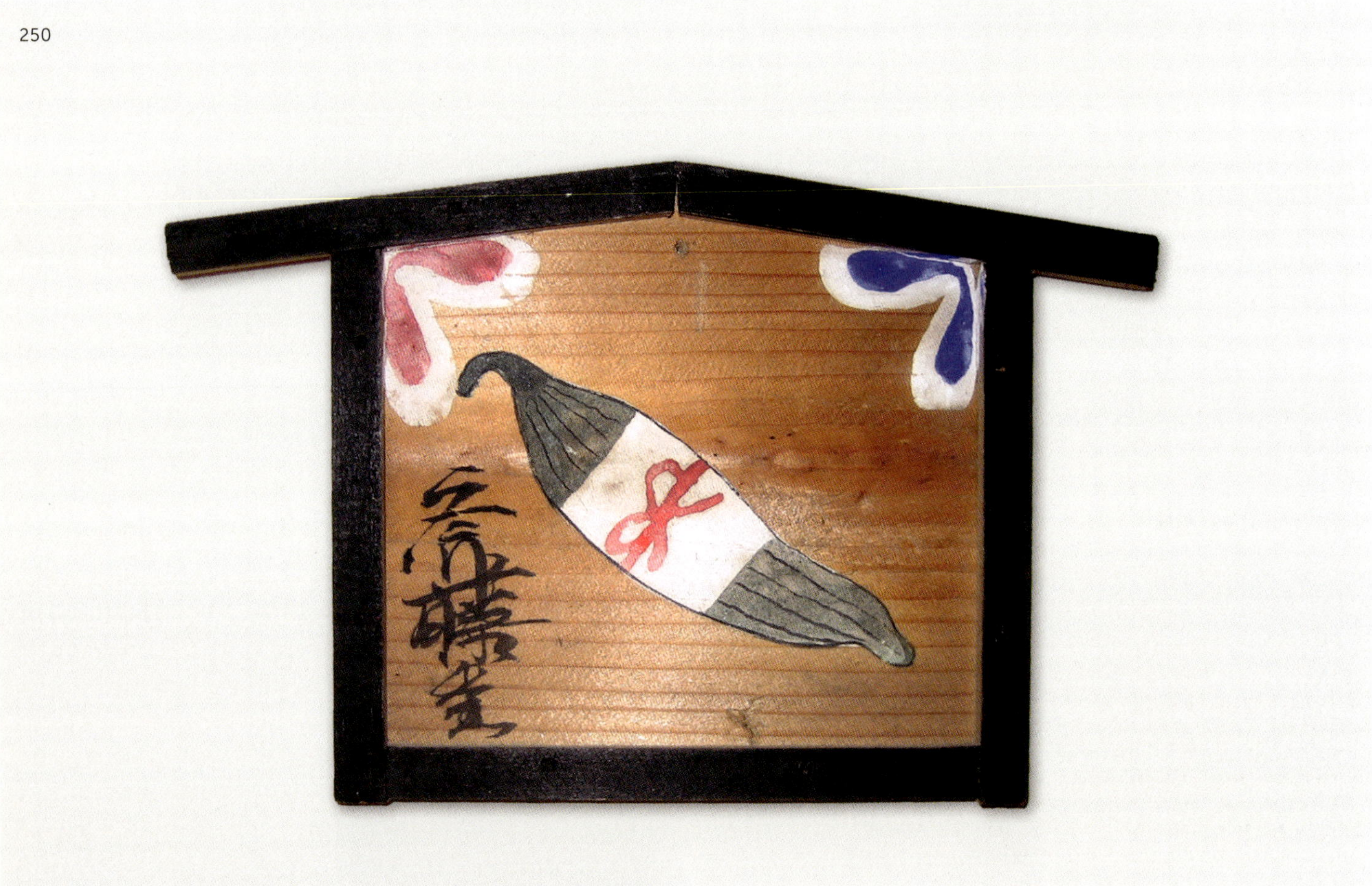

252

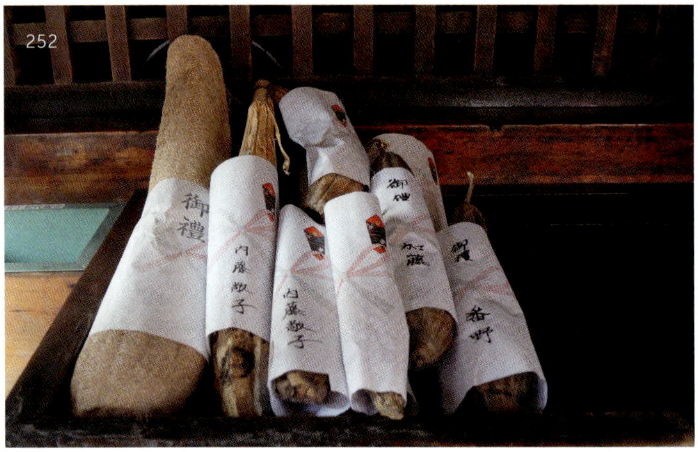

253

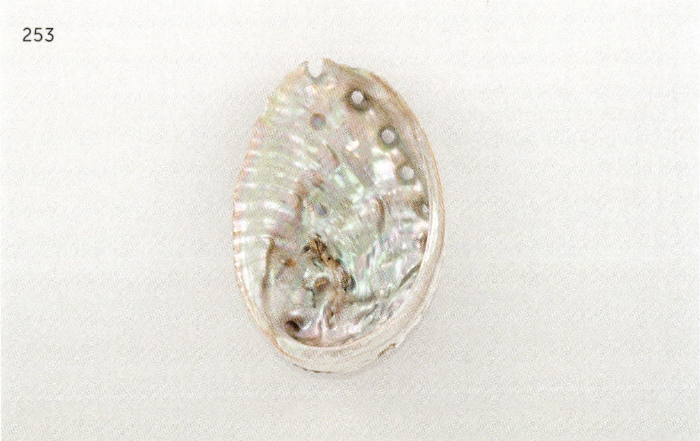

Wooden clog 下駄 *(geta)*

Ema in the shape of a *geta* (traditional wooden footwear resembling both clogs and flip-flops) are used for healthy legs and for *yōtsū* (lower back pain).

249
Geta-shaped *ema* depicting *En no Gyōja* 役行者. *Hōshōji* 放生寺. Shinjuku Ward, Tokyo. Early 21st century. W. 8.3 cm
The inscriptions read:
腰痛平癒 = *yōtsū heiyu* (recovery from lower back pain)
南無神変大菩薩 = *Namu Jinben Dai Bosatsu* (hail to *Jinben Dai Bosatsu*)
健脚祈願 = *kenkyaku kigan* (prayer to be able to walk well)

Jinben Dai Bosatsu is an honorary title of *En no Gyōja* (lit. *En* the Ascetic), who probably was a real person living in the 7th century. Many legends accumulated around him and he is traditionally considered to be the founder of *Shugendō*, the path of ascetic training practised by *yamabushi* (mountain priests).

Sponge gourd 糸瓜 *(hechima)*

At *Hechima Yakushi Tōjūji* (Nagoya, Aichi Prefecture), people offer real *hechima* (a type of gourd) for *byōki heiyu* (recovery from illness). When they first make their request, they take home a small gourd amulet, rub it on an ailing spot on their bodies, place it on their home altars, plant a gourd seed, raise the plant, and, if their wish is fulfilled, pluck a gourd and return it to the shrine with a pasted slip of paper saying "in gratitude for the fulfilment of my wishes". The gourd literally represents fruition and the importance of thanksgiving after the harvest [RT-120].

250
Hechima Yakushi Tōjūji へちま薬師東充寺. Nagoya, Aichi Prefecture. Early or mid-20th century. W. 20.3 cm. The inscription may refer to *Hechima Yakushi* [TS-9].

Tenri University Sankokan Museum (Tenri, Nara Prefecture) inv.no. 18208E982.
In the past, this *ema* design was presented to *Hechima Yakushi* for *kinnikutsū* (muscle pain) and *shinkeitsū* (nerve pain).

251
In 1990, *Hechima Yakushi Tōjūji* issued a special souvenir *ema* with a *hechima* design to commemorate the reconstruction of its temple gate.

252
Hechima gourds waiting to be offered at *Hechima Yakushi Tōjūji*.

Abalone shell 鮑 *(awabi)*

In the 1950s, the picture of an *awabi* (abalone shell) was offered at *Atago Hanazono Jinja* (Iwaki, Fukushima Prefecture) to pray for prevention of *aretate* (splits in one's hands) or for the cure of *seibyō* (venereal diseases). The parishioners of that shrine refrained from eating *awabi* [AE].

Today, *awabi* shells serve as an *ema* to pray for *anzan* (easy childbirth) at *Shinmeisha* (Yokohoma, Kanagawa Prefecture). It is said that one will be blessed with children with big and beautiful eyes, because the inside of the *awabi* shell sparkles so brightly. The website of the shrine cautions that the shells (which are procured from *sushi* shops in Yokohama) are not always available because the consumption of abalone (an expensive food) has declined due to the effects of recession in contemporary Japan.

253
Abalone shell. W. 9.9 cm

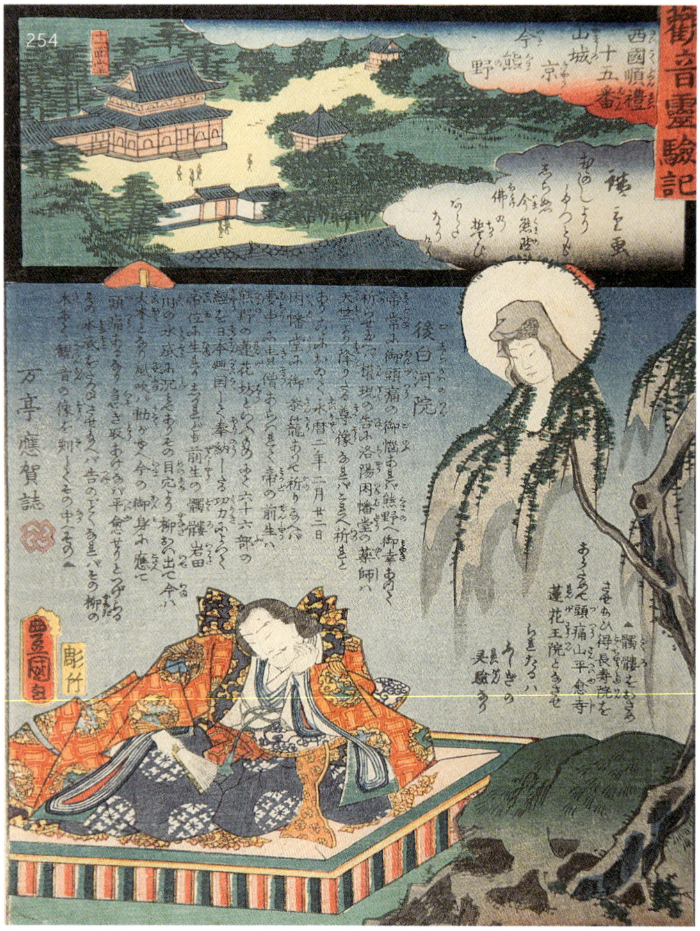

254

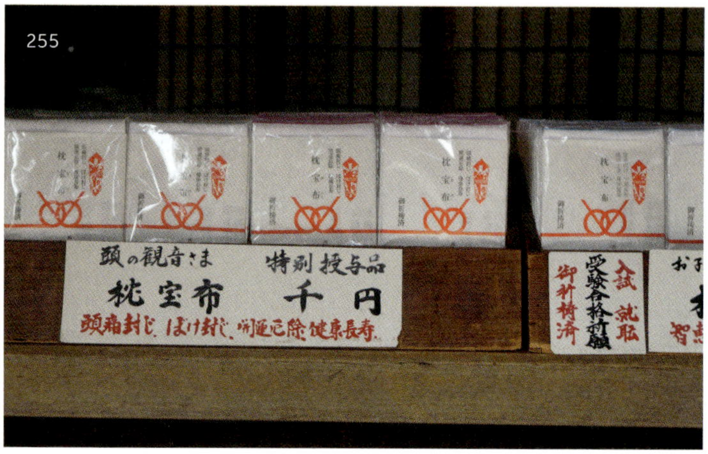

255

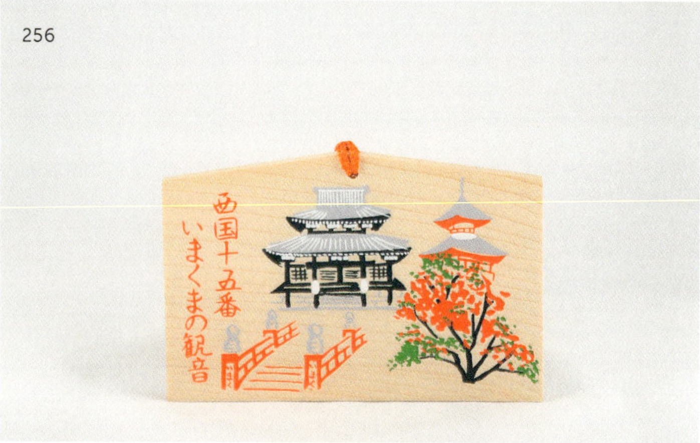

256

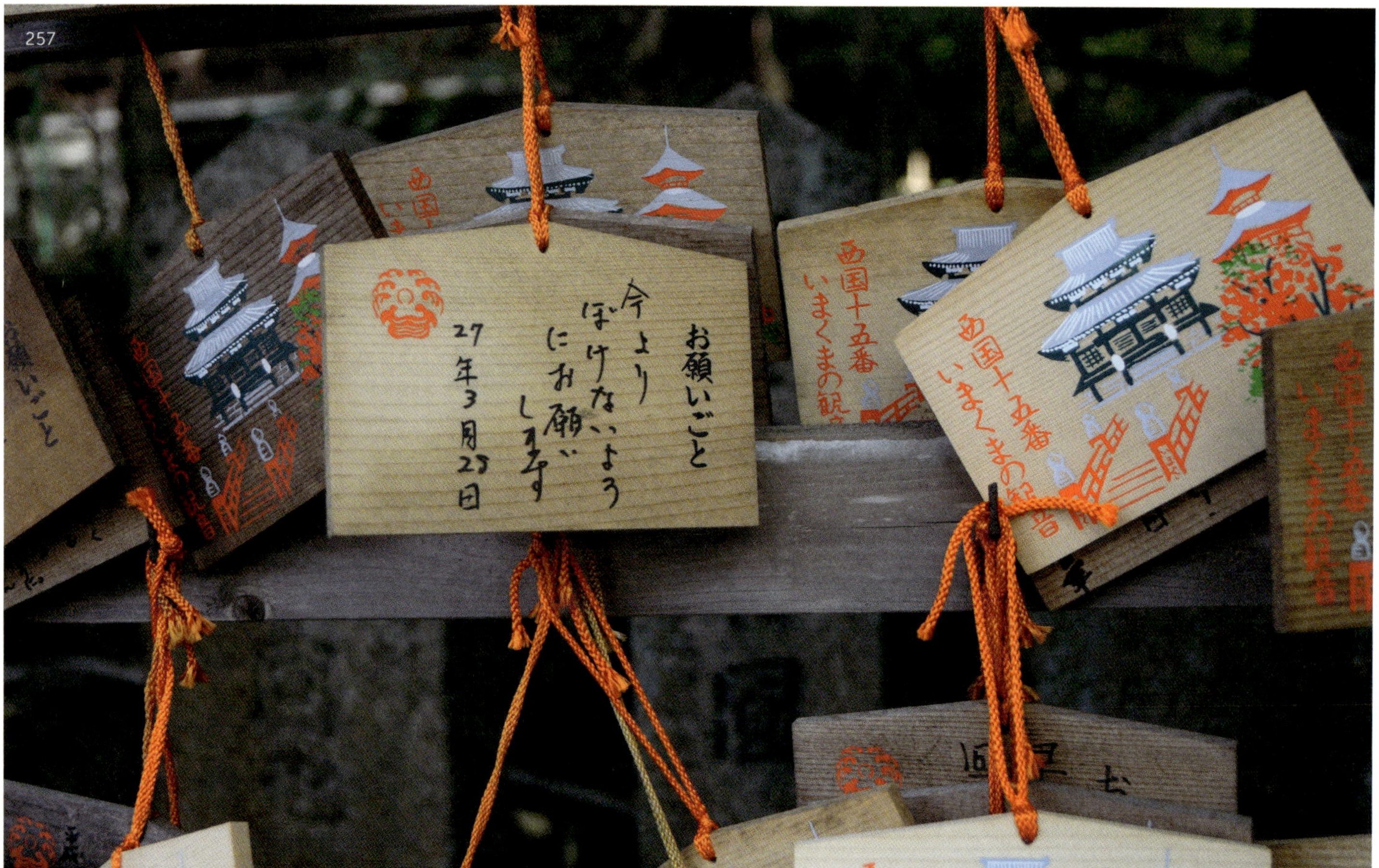

257

Nerve symptoms/ complaints 神経症状／愁訴 (*shinkei shōjō/shūso*)

Background

Common neurological disorders in Japanese outpatients are *zutsū* (headache) and *memai* (dizziness) [IO; TT]. A common complaint in small children has been febrile convulsions [1]. This condition was called *kyōkan* or *kyōfū* in the 19th century.

Examples of *goriyaku* (benefits) concerning headache 頭痛 (*zutsū*) are:

- *Hōroku Jizō* ほうろく地蔵 (Earthenware *Jizō*) for the prevention or curing of headaches. Worshippers offer *hōroku* (earthenware plates) to him to be relieved from headaches and other head ailments. They write their prayer on a plate and then present it to his statue or place it on top of his head. A well-known example of such a *Hōroku Jizō* statue is found at *Daienji* 大円寺 (Bunkyo Ward, Tokyo) [MS].
- The annual rite of *yōryū* (willow branch), which is closely associated with *Yōryū Kannon* (Willow Branch *Kannon*), is held at *Sanjūsangendō* 三十三間堂 (formally known as *Rengeōin* 蓮華王院) in the Higashiyama Ward of Kyoto. Devotees are touched on the head with a sacred willow branch to cure and prevent headaches, and to pray for another year of good health.
- *Yasaka Kōshindō* 八坂庚申堂 (Higashiyama Ward, Kyoto) sells *zutsū noke suribachi* (a mortar to remove headache by burning moxa). The Science Museum in London has a comparable clay device (inv.no.2002-472) which is described as having been used in a process known as Dream or Earthern Mortar moxibustion. This goes back to the legend of a Samurai warrior who was experiencing a terrible headache, but could not remove his helmet during battle. After moxibustion had been applied on top of his helmet, his headache vanished and he went on to claim victory [2].
- *Imakumano Kannonji* 今熊野観音寺 (Higashiyama Ward, Kyoto) sells special pillowcases that adults can use (while sleeping) for *zutsū fūji* (the prevention of headache), *yakuyoke* (warding off evil), *kenkō* (health), *boke fūji* (the prevention of senility), and *chōju* (longevity) [RT-193].

254
Ukiyo-e (woodblock print). Mid-19th century. W. 24 cm

This print shows how *Jūichimen Kannon* (eleven-headed *Kannon*) appeared in a dream to the emperor *Goshirakawa* at *Kannonji* (original name of *Imakumano Kannonji* in Kyoto). The famous *Kōbō Daishi* is said to have founded *Kannonji* in the 9th century, after a divine instruction to enshrine a wooden image of *Jūichimen Kannon* there. In the 12th century, the emperor *Goshirakawa* visited the temple in the hope that he would be cured of his terrible headaches. His headaches indeed ceased after he had dreamt about a radiant image of *Jūichimen Kannon* at his bedside. News of this miracle spread rapidly and from that time on people would travel to pray to *Jūichimen Kannon* at *Kannonji* for relief from headaches and for protection from illness and disaster in general.

255
Pillowcases for sale at *Imakumano Kannonji* (Higashiyama Ward, Kyoto).

256
Imakumano Kannonji also offers an *ema* with its own image (W. 13.5 cm).

This *ema* is generic in nature, citing no specific prayer requests it is to be used for. It simply gives the temple's name and says that this is the 15th temple on the *Saikoku* 33 temple pilgrimage. Such generic types of *ema* can be used for any request that the petitioner seeks and are common at Japanese shrines and temples.

257
It is possible, of course, to provide a generic *ema* design with a request concerning a specific illness. In this case, a wish for the prevention of *boke* (ぼけ = senility) has been written on a nonspecific votive tablet from *Imakumano Kannonji*.

258

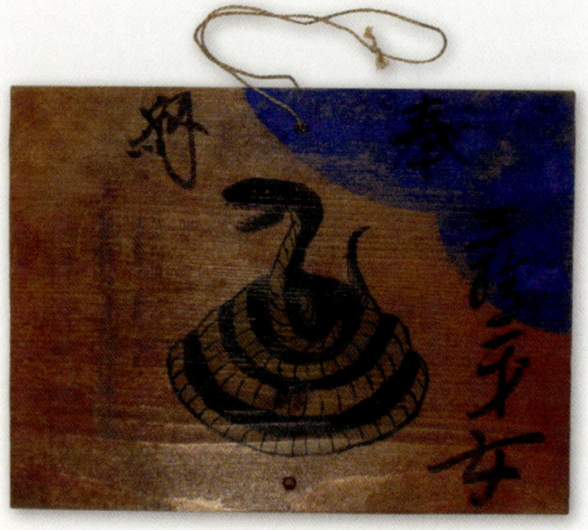

259

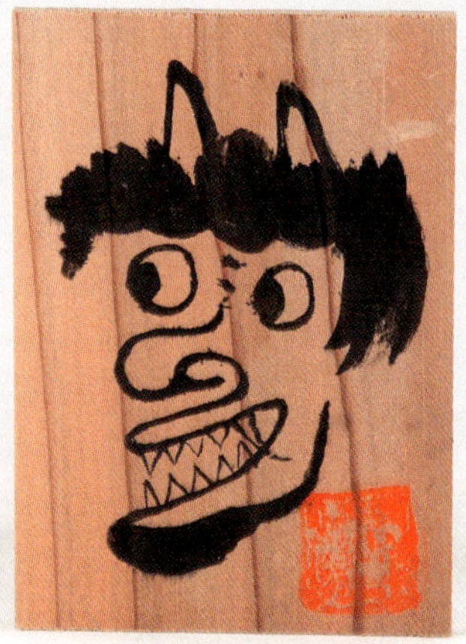

260

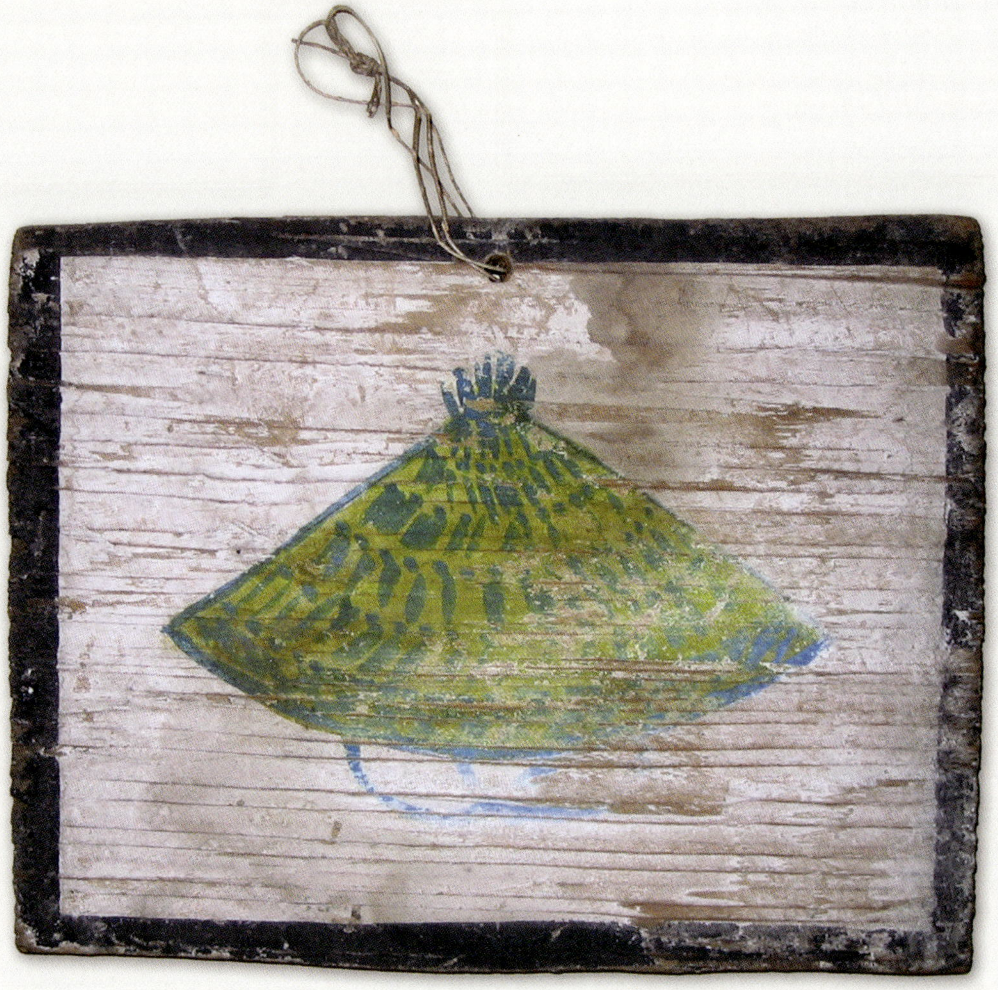

Ema designs

***Ema* designs for nerve symptoms/complaints particularly concern headache 頭痛 (*zutsū*).**

Coiled snake 蜷蛇 (toguro hebi)

258
Precincts of *Sumadera* 須磨寺. Kobe, Hyogo Prefecture. Early 20th century. W. 16.8 cm
Tenri University Sankokan Museum (Tenri, Nara Prefecture). Museum inv.no.16040E59 [acquired in 1916]

This *ema* design was offered to a snake tomb in the precincts of *Sumadera*, which was said to provide miraculous cures for headache and toothache [TS-21].

Demon 鬼 (oni)

259
Oni Jinja 鬼神社 (in precincts of *Tenmansha* of *Shirakihama* 白木浜の天満社). Oita, Oita Prefecture. Early 21st century. W. 10.0 cm

This *ema* is recommended for *zutsū* (headache) and *atama no byōki* (illnesses of the head). When hung at the entrance to one's home, it wards off evil [GG1-2011/10].

Braided hat 編笠 (amigasa)

This *ema* design was used for headache [TS-11].

260
Tokushima Prefecture. Precise origin unclear. Early or mid-20th century. W. 13.7 cm
Tenri University Sankokan Museum (Tenri, Nara Prefecture). Museum inv.no. 16322E336.

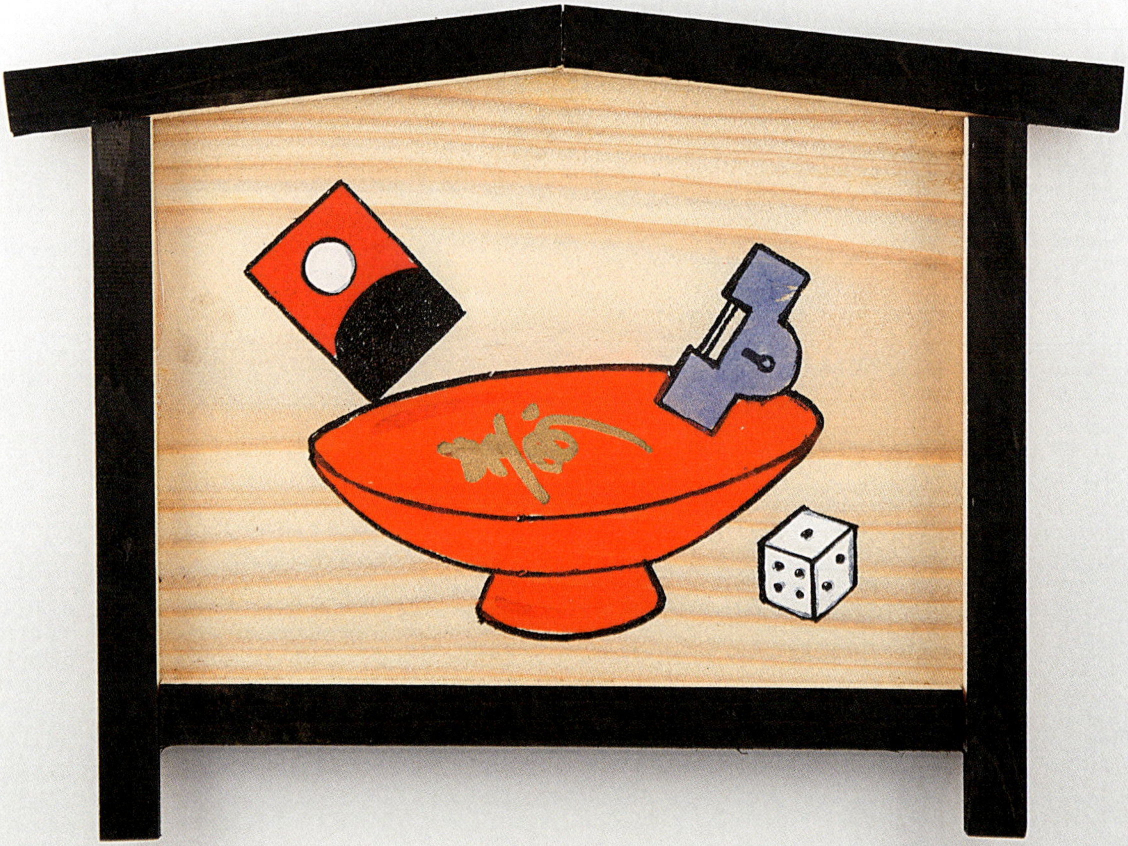

Mental/behavioural symptoms/complaints 精神的／行動的 症状／愁訴 (*seishinteki/kōdōteki shōjō/shūso*)

Background

Mental disorders may be more open to cultural interpretations than physical disorders. It should therefore come as no surprise that the Japanese literature on mental disorders includes diagnostic entities that are distinct from Western psychiatric labels. Notable examples are *shinkeishitsu* (constitutional neurasthenia) and its subtype *taijin kyōfushō* (anthropophobia). *Shinkeishitsu* is no longer important in Japanese psychiatry, but historically it formed the basis for Morita therapy, a Japanese model of psychotherapy. From a biomedical view, *shinkeishitsu* is a complex disorder, which corresponds to anxiety disorders, but can also embody mood disorders and personality disorders. *Taijin kyōfushō* comes under the category of social anxiety disorders, as it is centred around the concern for offending others with inappropriate behaviour or offensive appearance [1].

A large household survey of mental disorders in Japanese communities in 2002-2003 showed that 4.8% of the subjects had experienced an anxiety disorder in the preceding year, and 2.9% had suffered a major depression. These percentages were lower than corresponding figures in Western countries [2]. Japanese mental patients are more likely to describe their condition in somatic terms than their Western counterparts. One of the reasons may be the stigma (which is still stronger in Japan than it is in Western societies) that mental disorders indicate a personal weakness of character. Another factor may be that mind and body are not thought of as a duality in traditional Japanese thought but are seen as forming a unified mind-body entity. An illness is interpreted as an imbalance of *ki* (universal energy) in the human body and its symptoms are not divided into psychological and physical problems. In a cross-cultural study of depressed patients in primary care, Japanese patients reported psychological complaints less frequently and physical complaints more frequently than American patients. The Japanese mentioned abdominal symptoms, headache and *katakori* (neck/shoulder pain) significantly more often, perhaps because these body sites had a special cultural significance for them. Digestive complaints are the most common reason why Japanese outpatients visit a doctor (cf. the section on digestive symptoms/complaints on p.129). The abdominal area (*hara*) is associated with emotions, and it is an important diagnostic site in *kanpō* medicine [3].

In the 19th and early 20th centuries, several shrines and temples offered therapies for the mentally ill in the form of incantations, prayers and bathing (in waterfalls, at the seaside, or in hot springs). For instance, many mental patients stayed, together with their families, at *Nissekiji* (Kamiichi, Toyama Prefecture). The water from the waterfalls around the temple was believed to be holy water, which could heal mental illnesses as well as eye illnesses. This is reminiscent of ascetic *Shugendō* practices, which included praying and bathing under waterfalls. Through such training, *Shugendō* practitioners were thought to have healing powers, and they would sometimes conduct exorcisms for the ill [4].

In Japanese folk medicine, mental illnesses were commonly attributed to possession by an evil spirit. Consequently, treatment consisted of driving out the evil spirit responsible (which could have come from either a dead or living person or from an animal, such as a fox or a raccoon dog). In medieval times, possession by *mononoke* (vengeful ghosts) was particularly common, while *kitsunetsuki* (possession by a fox spirit) became more important in the Edo period. One reason may have been that the fox was the messenger of the rice deity *Inari* and was thus endowed with supernatural power. In addition, foxes were seen as cunning and greedy. According to Japanese folklore, they were able to possess people and then demand their favourite food (fried tofu). Such traditional concepts were not easily wiped out when Western psychiatry gained a foothold in Japan after the Meiji Restoration in 1868. This was not only because psychiatric treatment was a scarce commodity in its early days, but even more so because the traditional views had greater appeal to common folk [5].

The three types of mental/behavioural symptoms/complaints for which *ema* are or have been offered are childhood behaviour, moderation, and senility.

261
Hand-painted reproduction for a Japanese club of *ema* collectors called *Nihon Ema Tomo no Kai* (Friends of Japanese Ema Society). No.379. Late 20th century. W 18.3 cm. Original design from *Yōgōji* 影向寺 (Kawasaki, Kanagawa Prefecture)

Several *ema* designs are directed to moderation of addictive behaviour. This example shows a padlock (*jō*) with a sake cup (*sakazuki*), a dice (*sai*) and a playing card (*hanafuda*). It can be used for moderation in drinking (*sesshu*) or temperance in gambling (*kinshu de tobaku*) [IH2-100].

The main purpose of the *hanafuda* card game is to associate images. It can be used for gambling by assigning points for completed image combinations. The *hanafuda* card shown here is a special card for August (full moon with red sky).

262

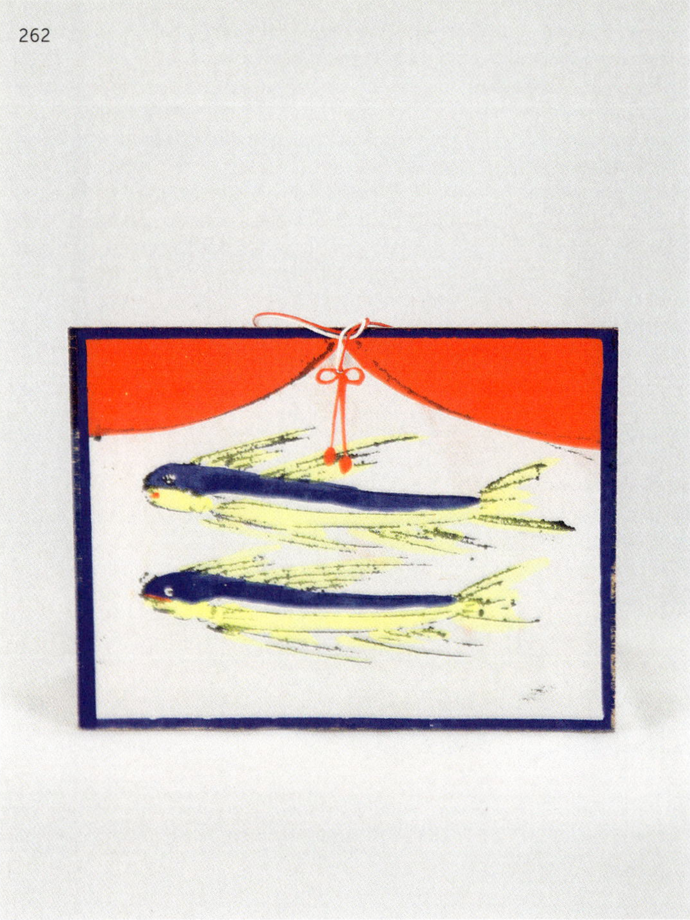

263

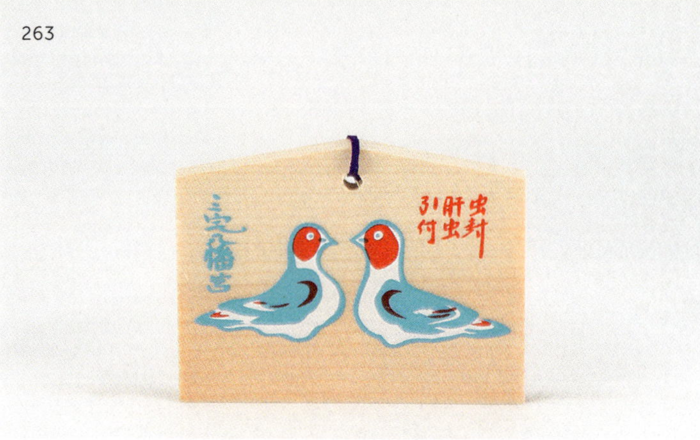

264

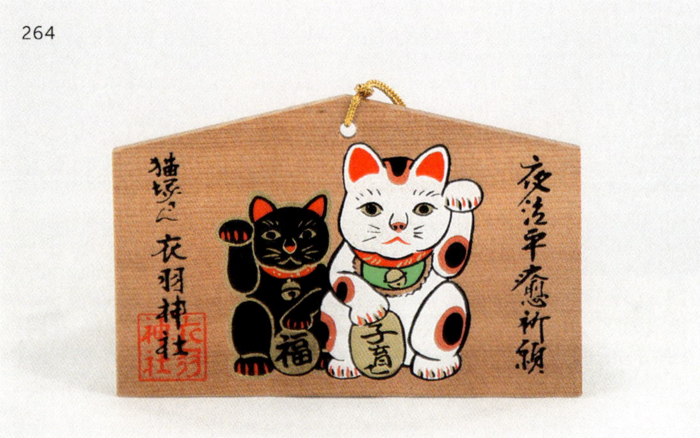

265

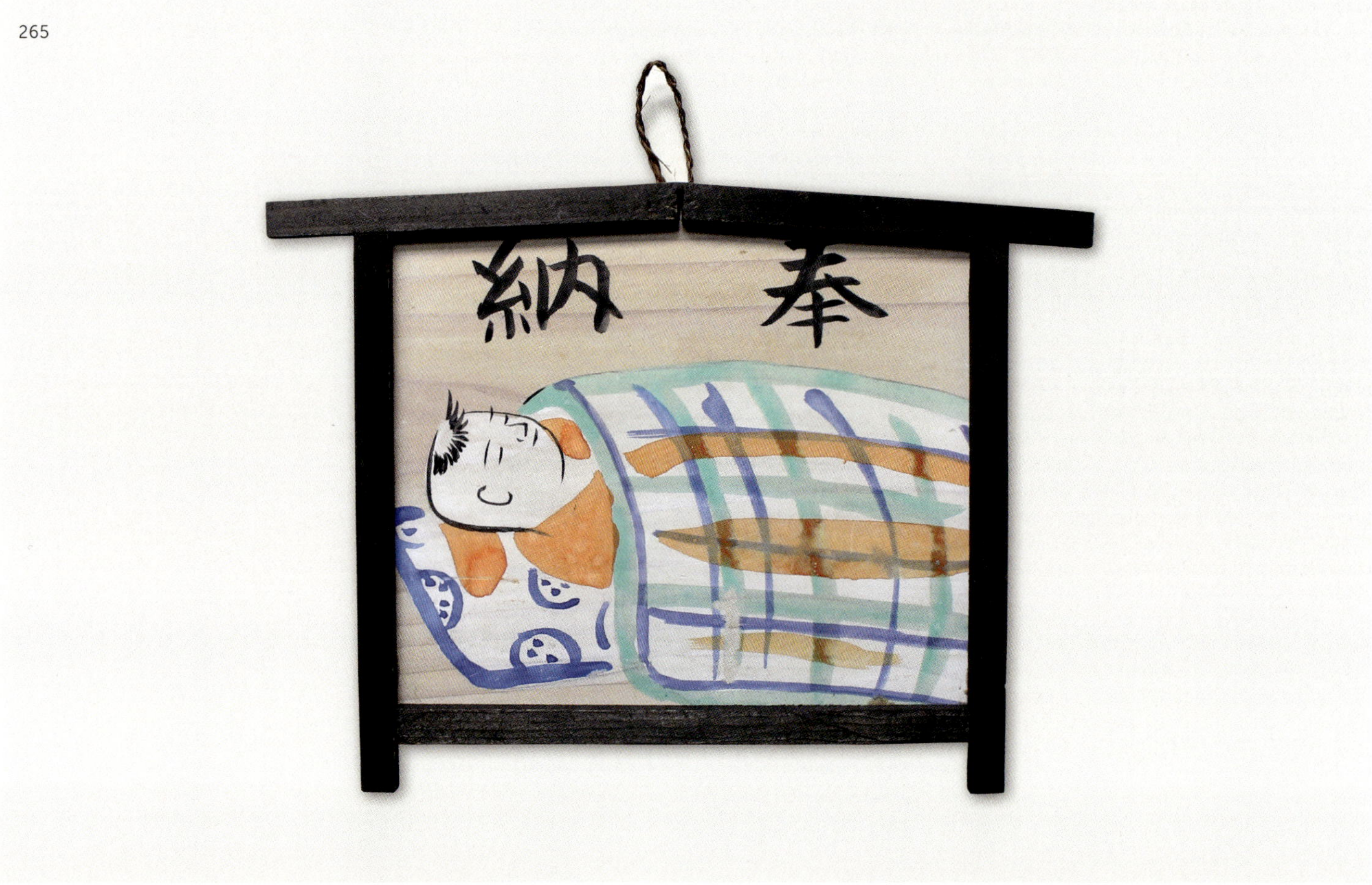

Childhood behaviour 小児期の行動 (*shōniki no kōdō*)

Background

Childhood behaviour disorders that are recognised in Japan but do not have an equivalent in biomedicine include *kannomushi* 疳の虫 (short-temperedness) and *yonaki* 夜泣き (crying of infant at night). *Kodomo no anmin* 子供の安眠 (quiet sleep of child) is also presented here. *Ema* for this purpose may have served for *yonaki* (crying at night) and *neshōben* (bedwetting). Bedwetting at night is a common disorder in Japanese children.

Kannomushi literally means the *mushi* (bug, worm) thought to cause or increase *kan* (temper, nerves). In Chinese medicine, *kan* refers to infantile neurosis characterised by crying at night and convulsions. As the Japanese belief in illness-causing worms has greatly declined, *kannomushi* nowadays stands for short-temperedness, nervousness and convulsions in children [ML-95]. It has been classified here and not in the section on nerve symptoms/complaints because the Japanese distinguished it from children's convulsions (*kyōkan*, *kyūkyō*).

Among the various Japanese shrines and temples that offer benefits to parents seeking a cure for the *kannomushi* or *dada* (tantrums) of their children are *Tsurugi Jinja* and *Miyake Hachimangū* in Kyoto and *Kannon-in* at *Nakayamadera* (Takarazuka, Hyogo Prefecture).

Yonaki (*yo* = night and *naki* = crying) is sleep-related night-time crying of infants and young children. They may experience distressed waking at night from which they do not resettle without parental intervention. *Yonaki* mostly emerges when children are 4 to 24 months of age. Although *yonaki* is a frequent complaint of parents, it is considered a benign phenomenon that disappears naturally over time. It occurs most often after midnight, when infants have been asleep for some time, whereas colic tends to peak in the late afternoon and early evening [6].

Among the Buddhist figures of worship who can be invoked for the prevention and curing of the crying of infants at night are *Yonaki Jizō* at *Mibudera* (壬生寺, Nakagyo Ward, Kyoto) and *Asahi Jizō* (Morning Sun Jizō) at *Jōkakuji* (成覚寺, Shinjuku Ward, Tokyo).

Ema designs

Flying fish 飛魚 *(tobiuo)*

262
Tsurugi Jinja 剣神社. Higashiyama Ward, Kyoto. Early 21st century. W. 17.0 cm

The shrine can be visited to cure *kannomushi* (short-temperedness), *yonaki* (crying at night) and *shinkeishō* (nervous disorders) in children. The offering of an *ema* for such purposes may be reinforced by promising to abstain from eating flying fish [TS-6].

Pigeons 鳩 *(hato)*

263
Miyake Hachimangū 三宅八幡宮. Sakyo Ward, Kyoto. Early 21st century. W. 9.1 cm
The inscriptions read:
虫封 = *mushifūji* (blocking the *mushi* = worm)
肝虫 = *kanmushi* (worm increasing *kan* = temper, nerves).
引付 = *hikitsuke* (convulsions)

The enshrined *Ōkami Hachiman* is a guardian deity who can cure children's illnesses. He is particularly capable of *kanmushi fūji*, i.e., blocking the *mushi* (bug, worm) that increases *kan* (temper, nerves). Hence he is also popularly known as *Mushi Hachiman*. The doves on the *ema* represent his messengers.

Elsewhere, *ema* with one or two pigeons are recommended for the removal of blisters from one's hands and feet, because pigeons like to eat grain (see p.185).

Beckoning cat 招き猫 *(manekineko)*

The *manekineko* (beckoning cat) is an ubiquitous Japanese charm that beckons good luck with its paw.

264
Horoha Jinja 衣羽神社 (subshrine of *Shinmei Jinja* 神明神社). Fukui, Fukui Prefecture. Early 21st century. W. 14.2 cm
The inscriptions read:
夜泣き平癒祈願 = *yonaki heiyu kigan* (prayer for recovery from *yonaki*)
猫塚さん = *Nekozuka-san* (lit. honourable cat mound)
衣羽神社 = *Horoha Jinja*

The shrine is popularly known as *Nekozuka-san*. Parents visit it to stop *yonaki* (crying at night) and for *buji seichō* (the safe growing up) of their children. [GG2-2013/04].

Quiet sleep of child 子供の安眠 *(kodomo no anmin)*

265
Ema hand-painted by *Norihito Yasuda* (Nagoya) on commission from the Naito Museum of Pharmaceutical Sciences and Industry (Kakamigahara, Gifu Prefecture). Late 20th century. Museum inv.no. Z22683. The inscription reads: 奉納 = *hōnō* (dedication, offering)

Ema design for *anmin* (quiet sleep) of *shōni* (infants) and *kodomo* (children) [NM-Z22683; TS-26]. There is another *ema* design in a similar style from *Horakuji* (Ikoma, Nara Prefecture). It shows a mother watching over her sleeping child and may have been offered for the healing of *yonaki* (crying at night) or *neshōben* (bedwetting).

Additional *ema* designs for childhood behaviour (not illustrated here) are:

- Chickens 鶏 (*niwatori*). See p.171 for an example of this design. It could be used for *yonaki* (crying at night), *fumin* (insomnia), *torime* (night blindness), *ganbyō* (eye illness), whooping cough and fire prevention. The rooster was associated with *yonaki* because it does not crow during the night [TS-22; IH2-70].
- *Jizō* 地蔵. Some *ema* with *Jizō* as their design were recommended for *kannomushi* (short-temperedness), *yonaki* (crying at night) and *neshōben* (bedwetting) [IH2-60].

266

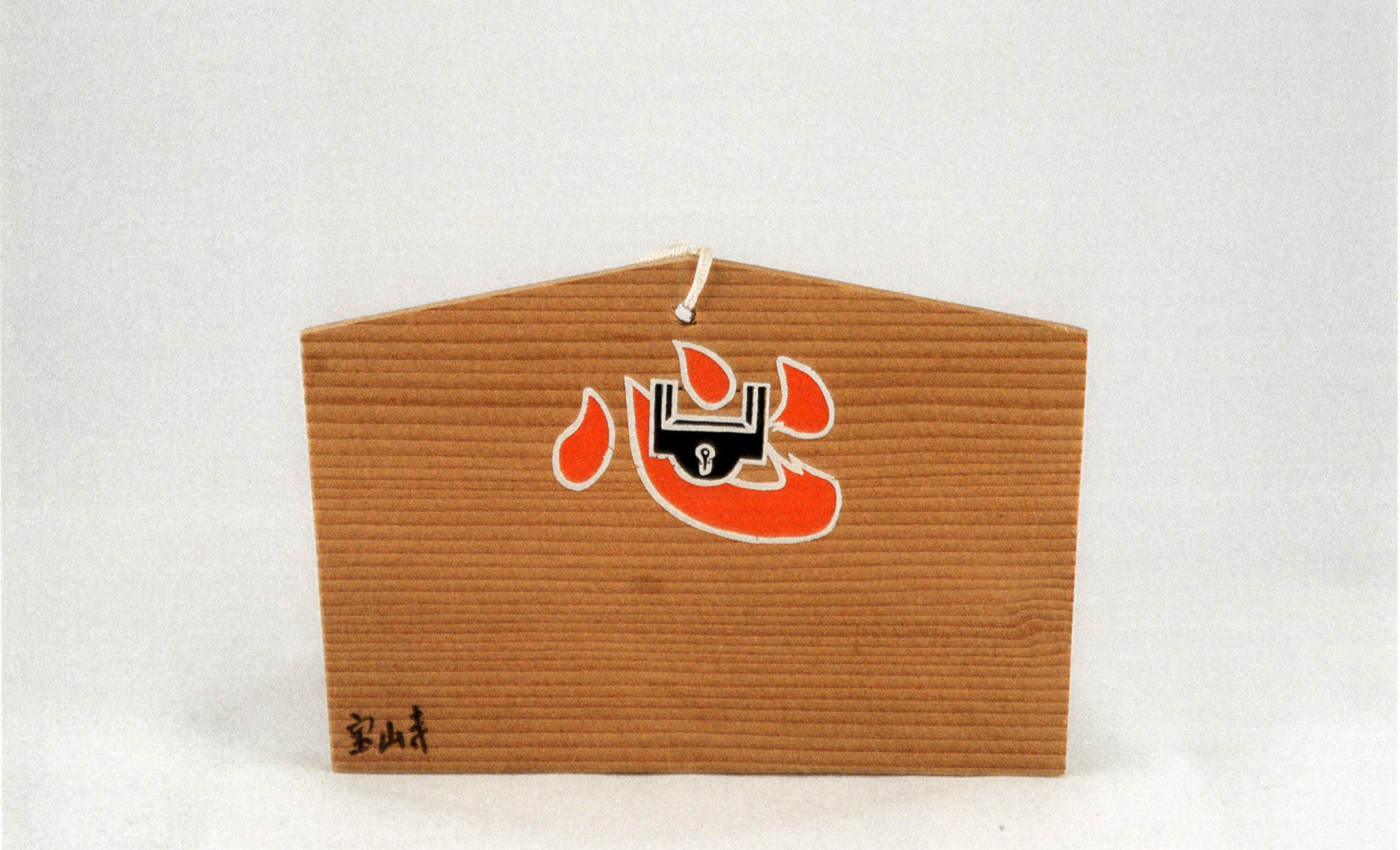

267

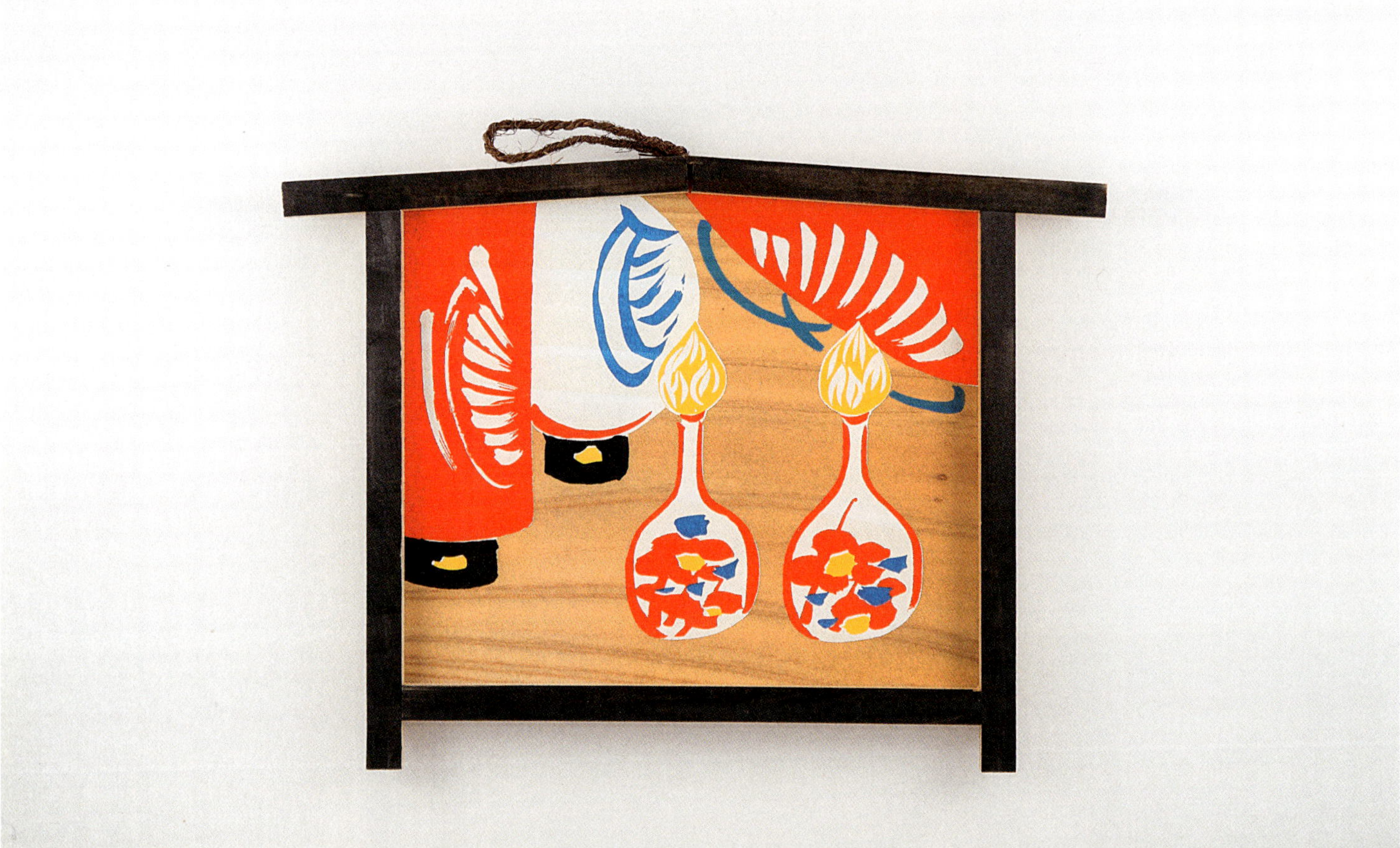

Moderation
節度
(*setsudo*)

Background

Moderation in drinking 節酒 *(sesshu)*

Until recently, alcohol consumption was not regarded as a major societal problem in Japan, and few legal measures against its production or use had been taken. Today, alcohol still fulfils an important function in social life. For instance, many employees believe that getting drunk with clients or co-workers is part of the job and a mark of company loyalty. This is not to say, however, that alcohol abuse does not exist in Japan. According to a nationwide survey among adults in 2003, 2.5% of the respondents engaged in hazardous alcohol use and almost 1% were alcohol dependent by biomedical criteria [7].

The major types of alcoholic beverages are *nihonshu*, *shōchū*, beer and whisky. *Nihonshu* (sake) is brewed from rice and contains 14-17% alcohol. Since early history, it has played a ceremonial role in Shinto shrine activities and rituals. *Shōchū* is a vodka-like liquor produced from various raw materials by distillation and contains at least 25% alcohol. The popularity of beer and whisky has substantially increased since World War II. Besides a shift in taste, alcohol consumption in Japan has undergone two other changes in the second half of the 20th century. First, its volume increased considerably in relation to further industrial development and urbanisation. Second, the alcohol drinking population diversified: while alcohol was traditionally consumed by middle-aged and older males, non-traditional drinkers (females and youths) have also become prominent [8].

Moderation in smoking 節煙 *(setsuen)*

Tobacco entered the Japanese archipelago in the 16th century, when Portuguese merchants brought it to southern Japan. From there, its cultivation and use spread to the rest of the country. At the end of the 19th century, the Meiji government claimed a governmental monopoly over tobacco. Since then, government has been directly involved in promoting tobacco sales, with the result that cigarette smoking became quite popular. According to a large survey in 1994, 50-70% of men smoked compared to 7-12% of women [9].

Temperance in gambling 禁酒で賭博 *(kinshu de tobaku)*

Ema designs for this purpose may show a padlock over *sai* (dice) and/or *hanafuda* (playing cards) [IH2-100]. Cf. the picture on p.158.

Ema designs

***Ema* for moderation in drinking (*sesshu*) were often presented by parents, wives or friends of the victim. Their design most commonly shows one or two sake containers (bottles, gourds or a cask). The cask is sometimes combined with an empty sake cup with a firmly shut lock over it (and the key thrown away). On other *ema* (not illustrated here), the cask stands next to the gravestone of *Honda Tadatomo* (at *Isshinji*, Osaka). Today, this grave is a historical tourist attraction for those wanting to stop alcohol addiction [FS-17,18; TS-11,13; IH2-98; NM-Z22689].**

Kanji character 心 *(kokoro) with padlock* 錠 *(jō)*

266
Hōzanji 宝山寺, Ikoma, Nara Prefecture.
Late 20th century. W. 15.4 cm

The padlock in front of the kanji 心 = *kokoro* (mind; heart; spirit) expresses the locking of the mind against temptation (e.g., giving up alcohol, tobacco, illicit drugs or an extramarital relationship) [RT-39].

Sake bottles 徳利 *(tokkuri)*

267
Hand-painted reproduction for a Japanese club of *ema* collectors called *Nihon Ema Tomo no Kai* (Friends of Japanese Ema Society). No.150. Late 20th century. W. 17.9 cm. Original design from Fujioka, Gunma Prefecture.

This design is for wishes to give up alcohol but also represents the sake bottles that can be offered to the gods for this purpose.

268

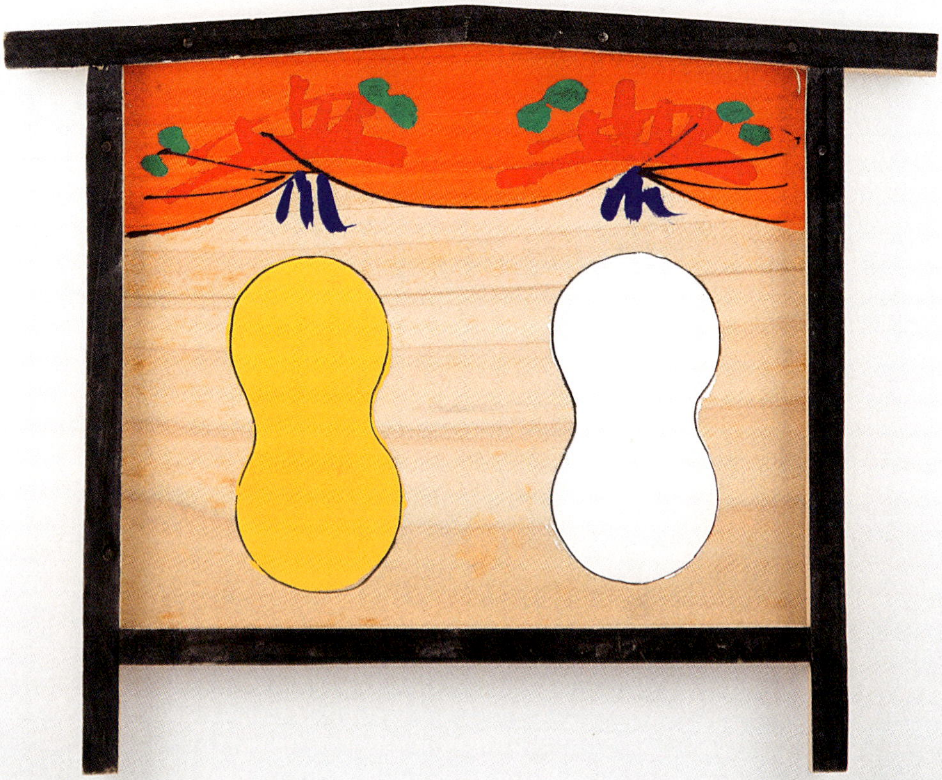

269

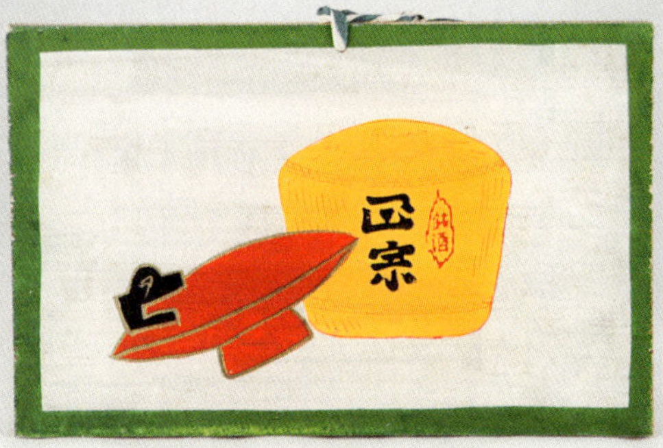

270

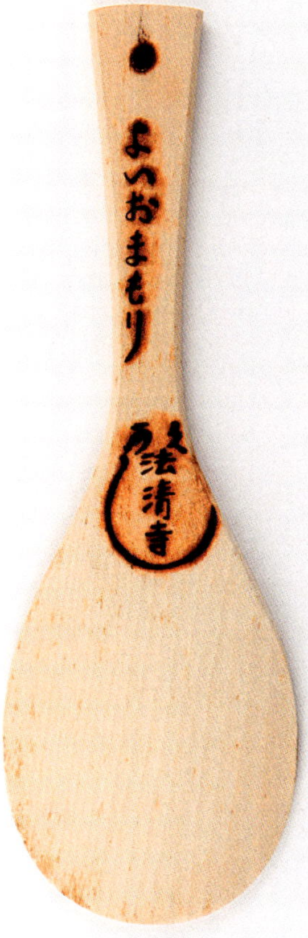

271

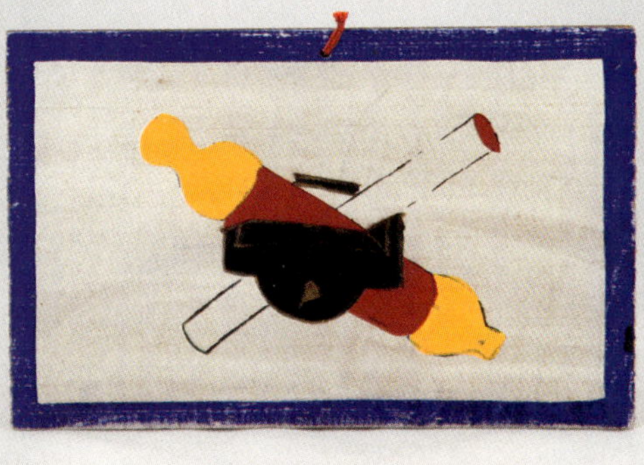

Sake gourds 酒ひょうたん (shu hyōtan)

268
Hand-painted. Middle to late 20th century. W. 18.1 cm. An annotation on the reverse reads Tokyo Asakusa.

Sake cup 杯 (sakazuki) with padlock 錠 (jō) and sake cask 酒樽 (sakadaru)

269
Hand-painted. Middle to late 20th century. W. 20.7 cm

Wooden scoop 杓文字 (shamoji)

270
Hōseiji 法清寺 Kita Ward, Osaka. Early 21st century. H. 23.5 cm
The inscriptions read:
よいおまもり= *yoi omamori* (good charm)
法清寺 = *Hōseiji*

The originating temple is located in the red light district and houses the grave of the alcoholic prostitute *Kashiku*. According to legend, she was executed after murdering her brother when he tried to stop her drinking. The temple is still visited by people who wish to ask for sobriety.

Tobacco pipe 煙管 (kiseru) and cigarette 紙巻 (kamimaki) with padlock 錠 (jō)

271
Hōzanji 宝山寺. Mount Ikoma, Nara Prefecture. Mid-20th century. W. 20.4 cm

This design is intended for moderation in smoking [TS-13; IH2-102]. It shows a tobacco pipe in an old-fashioned padlock (without the key in sight). The additional presence of a cigarette in the lock suggests that the *ema* may date from the 1960s, because cigarettes did not become popular among the Japanese until the late 1950s.

Hōzanji also offers an *ema* design of a padlocked character 心 (*kokoro* = mind; heart; spirit). This general design signifies the locking of the mind against any temptation (see p.163).

An additional *ema* design for moderation (not illustrated here) is that of the padlocked character *kokoro* for refraining from another addictive drug, namely methamphetamine (trade name Philopon) [TS-13]. Immediately after World War II, military stocks of this drug became widely available and pharmaceutical companies started to promote it for over-the-counter sales to civilians. Awareness of its dangerous effects had not yet emerged, and its abuse rapidly reached epidemic proportions. The younger generation was particularly interested in the euphoric and mood-elevating effects of the drug [10].

The consulted sources have yielded no evidence of *ema* to abandon opium use. A likely reason may well be the low rate of opium addiction in Japan in the past. The rulers in the Edo and Meiji periods were aware of the devastating effects of opium on China, and seriously punished its possession, distribution and non-medical use. In the period between 1931 and 1945, Japan continued to forbid opium for the domestic market, but at the same time manufactured large quantities of opium (and heroin) for distribution in occupied China [11].

272

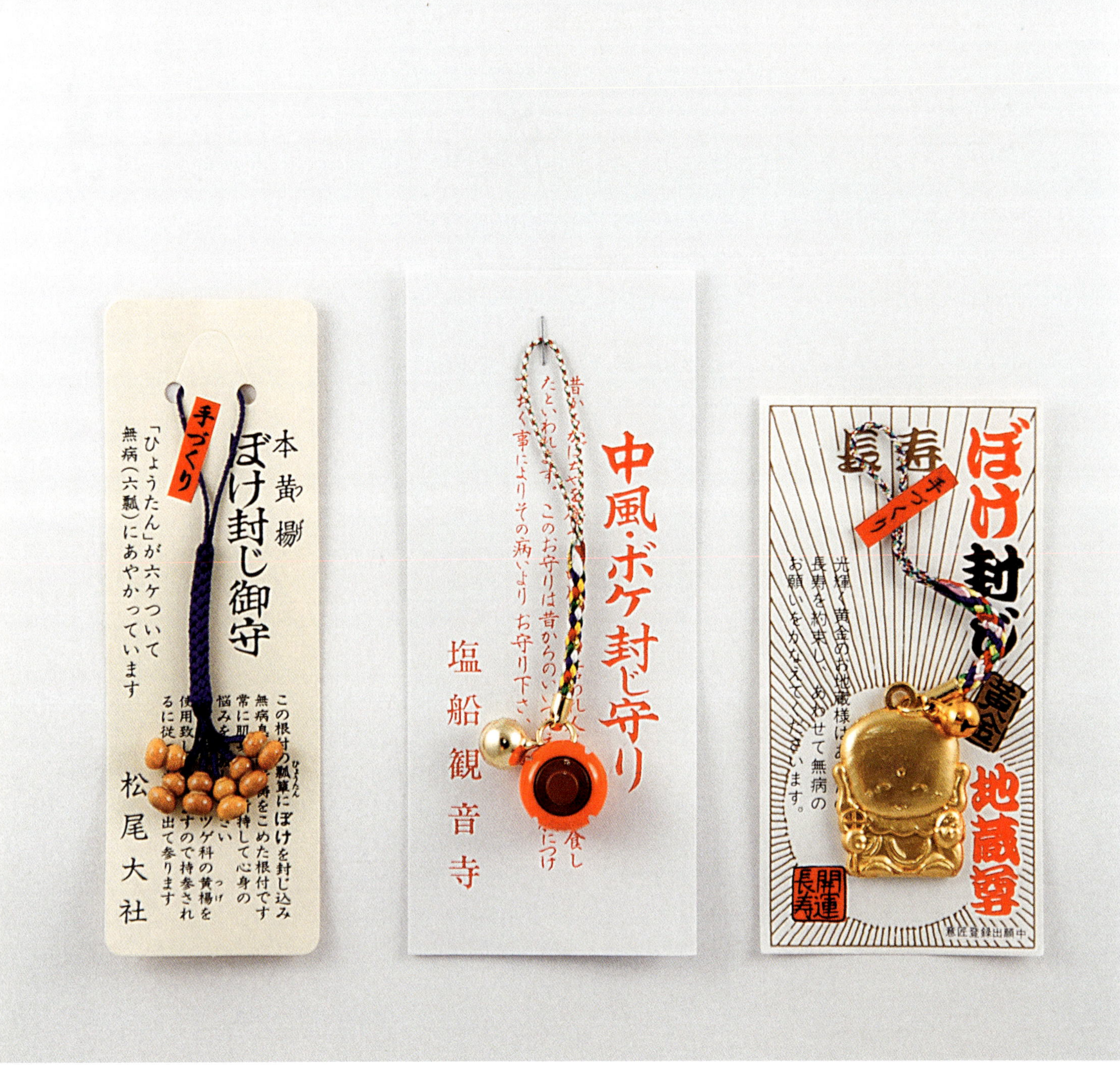

手づくり
本黄楊
ぼけ封じ御守
「ひょうたん」が六ケついて
無病（六瓢）にあやかっています
松尾大社
中風・ボケ封じ守り
塩船観音寺
ぼけ封じ
地蔵尊
長寿
手づくり
黄金
開運長寿

273

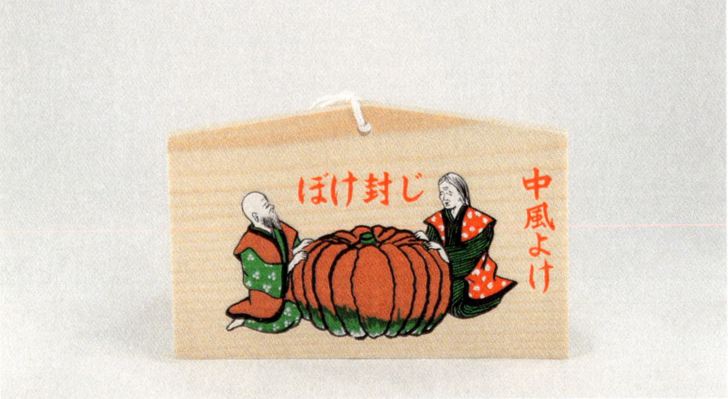

ぼけ封じ
中風よけ

274

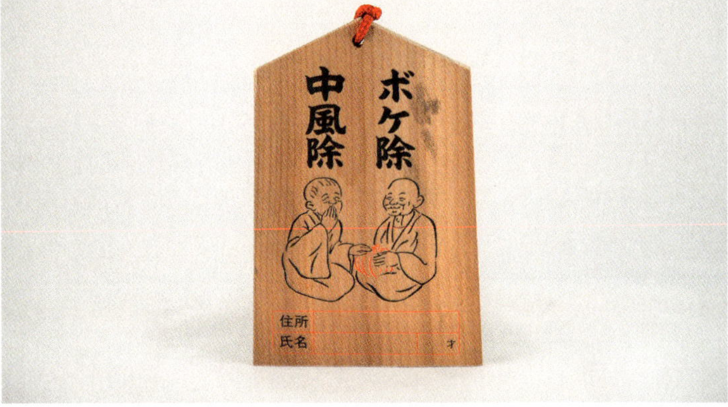

ボケ除
中風除
住所
氏名

Senility
ぼけ or ボケ
(*boke*)

Background

The translation of *boke* as senility does not do justice to the existence of three different Japanese concepts of senility from a professional perspective: *ninchishō* (dementia which was designated as *chihō* until 2004), *arutsuhaimā* (Alzheimer's disease), and *boke*. The former two conditions are biomedical diseases that lie outside one's own control. In contrast, *boke* is primarily viewed as an illness over which one may have some degree of control. By engaging in physical and mental activities within the framework of social gatherings that encourage interaction with others, one may be able to delay or even prevent its onset. The question can be raised, however, how well laymen distinguish the three concepts from each other. Many people consider being active as a way to ward off all these forms [12].

A prominent Buddhist deity for the prevention of senility is *Boke Fūji Kannon*. She became popular in the 1980s in response to concerns that the ageing of the Japanese population would substantially increase the incidence of senility. More and more elderly people started to invoke her for *pokkuri* (sudden death), that is, before succumbing to a helpless state of senility). In 1987, priests in Fukuoka Prefecture even created a new thirty-three-stage pilgrimage around *Boke Fūji Kannon*. They argued that senility was more likely to advance in anxious and inactive people and that the pilgrimage would result in more physical activity and more openness about fears of becoming dependent on others [13].

272

Charms for *boke fūji* (prevention of senility) or *boke yoke* (protection against senility).
From right to left:

- *Jizō* charm for *boke fūji*
- Charm in the shape of a pumpkin. This *kabocha* design is also encountered on *ema* for *boke fūji* (see the *ema* design of a pumpkin below)
- Charm in the shape of six gourds for *boke fūji* and *mubyōsokusai* (sound health)

Ema designs

Pumpkin 南瓜 *(kabocha)*

The same pumpkin designs that are recommended for the prevention of *boke* (senility) are also used for protection against *chūfū* (paralysis). The most common cause of paralysis in the Japanese elderly is presumably cerebrovascular diseases, which ranked 4th among all causes of death in 2012 and were outnumbered only by malignant neoplasms, heart/hypertensive diseases and pneumonia [SY15].

273

Shiofune Kannonji 塩船観音寺. Ome, Tokyo Metropolis. Early 21st century. W. 13.8 cm
The inscriptions read:
中風よけ = *chūfū yoke* = protection against paralysis
ぼけ封じ = *boke fūji* = prevention of senility

This *ema* portrays an elderly couple with a pumpkin in the middle. The originating temple enshrines *Yakushi Nyorai* (Medicine Buddha). As reflected by the inscriptions, the temple is especially visited to prevent *boke* (senility) or *chūfū* (palsy, paralysis).

274

Jōmanji 常満寺. Hidaka, Saitama Prefecture. Early 21st century. W. 10.7 cm
The inscriptions read:
ボケ除[け] = *boke yoke* = protection against senility
中風除[け] = *chūfū yoke* = protection against paralysis

This *ema* originates from a *pokkuridera* [GG1-2014/04]. This is a temple where one can pray for *pokkuri* (sudden death; see the section on incontinence on p.197). The *ema* design shows similarities to the previous *ema* and to a bronze statue by the sculptor *Mitsuo Ishida* at *Hitokotonushi Jinja* (located in the Katsuragi mountains south of Osaka).

275

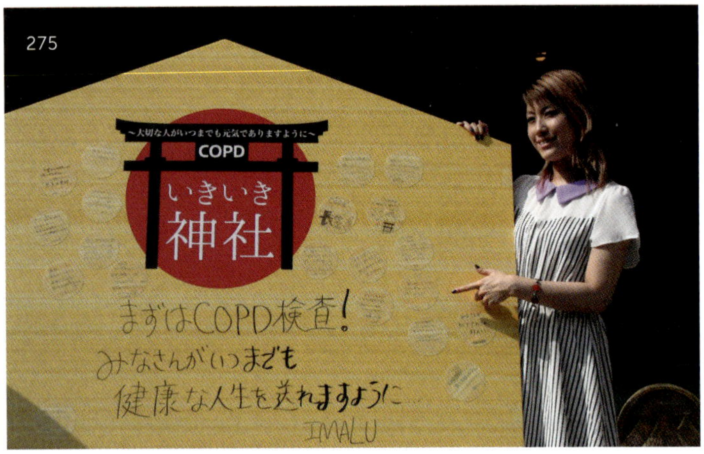

276

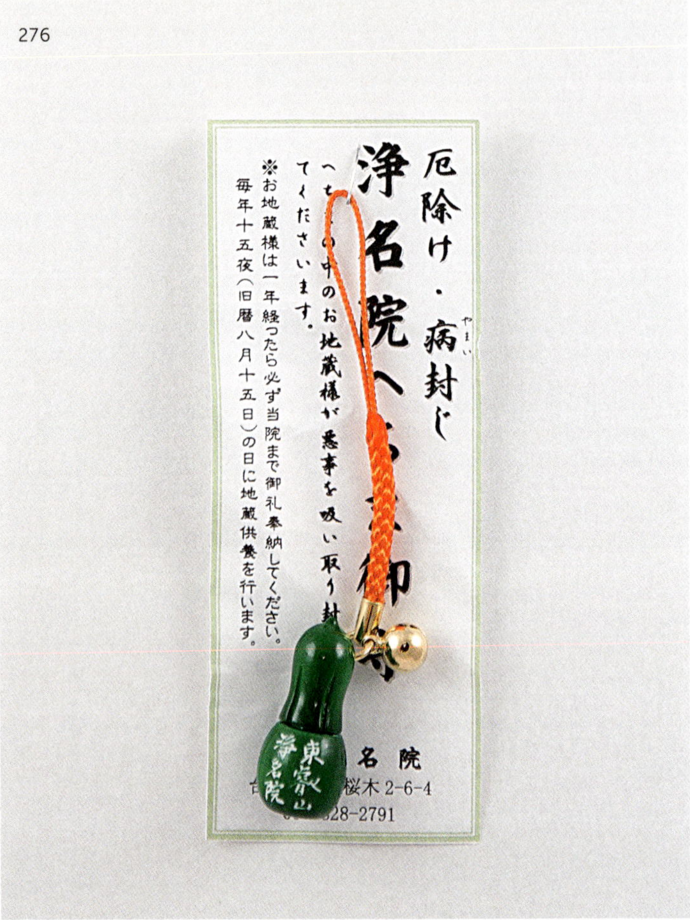

277

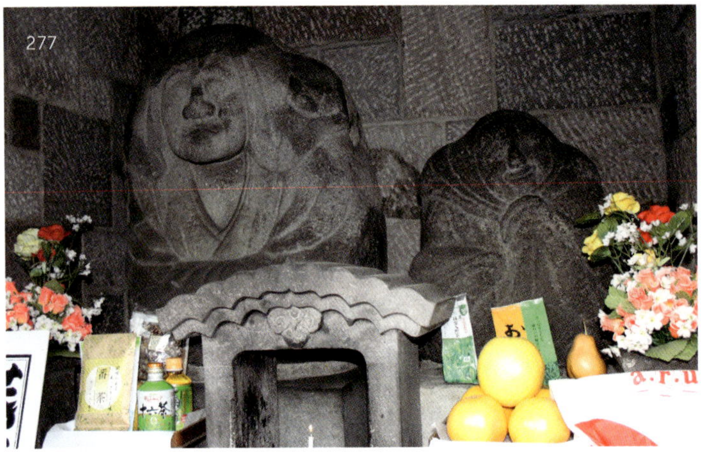

278

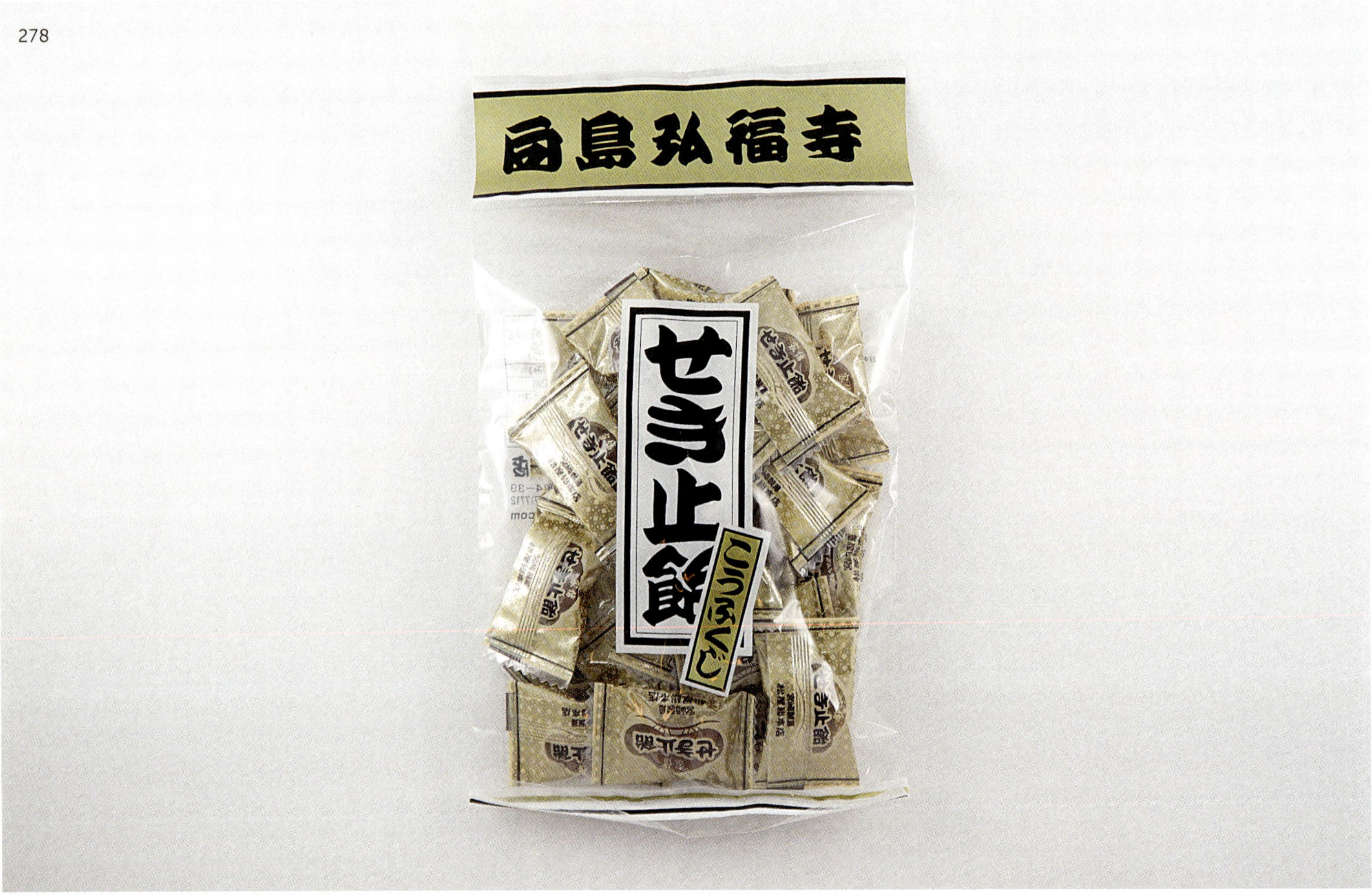

Respiratory symptoms/ complaints 呼吸器 症状／愁訴 (*kokyūki shōjō/shūso*)

Background

Common respiratory complaints in Japanese outpatients are coughing, sneezing, nasal congestion, shortness of breath, throat symptoms, sinus symptoms, and acute upper respiratory tract infections [IO; TT]. In 2012, the most common respiratory causes of death were pneumonia, trachea/bronchus/lung neoplasms, chronic obstructive pulmonary disease (COPD) and, to a lesser extent, tuberculosis and asthma [SY15]. In contrast, the respiratory burden of disease was largely determined by infectious diseases (such as tuberculosis, influenza, pneumonia and whooping cough) in the pre-war past [US-67]. This shift in respiratory causes of death is reflected in the worship of *Shiwabuki Sama* (Deity of Coughing). This deity was very popular for curing and preventing influenza but since this disease has become much better controlled, the deity is now also consulted for chronic respiratory disorders, such as *zensoku* (asthma) [EO-153].

Archaeological studies suggest that tuberculosis first reached Japan through the Korean peninsula in the Yayoi period (ca. 300 BC to AD 300) [1]. Until the late 19th century, tuberculosis remained endemic (i.e., present in the population without the need for new external sources of infection and without leading to the sharply increasing numbers of victims seen in epidemics). This changed in the 1890s, when tuberculosis started to produce epidemic mortality rates under the pressure of Japan's rapid industrialisation and urbanisation. In parallel, its name changed from *rōgai* (consuming and coughing) to *haibyō* (lung disease). The epidemic nature of tuberculosis would not level off until after the arrival of effective antibiotic therapy around 1950 [2].

Examples of shrines and temples that offer benefits for respiratory symptoms/ complaints are:

- *Jyomyōin* 浄名院 (Taito ward, Tokyo). This temple can be visited for respiratory problems, such as asthma, coughing and hay fever. Every year the temple holds a special service called *Hechima Kuyō* (Memorial Service of the *Hechima*) in the hope that this will cure respiratory illnesses. The *hechima* is a sponge gourd (also known as sponge cucumber). It is an edible vegetable to which health benefits are attributed. Cf. picture 276.
- *Fukushuin* 福聚院 (Bunkyo ward, Tokyo). This temple enshrines *Sekidome Jizō* (Cough Stopping *Jizō*) who may cure coughing or protect from coughing. He is also known as *Tōgarashi Jizō*, because he is wearing a necklace consisting of *tōgarashi* (chili peppers) [RT-249]. *Sekidome Jizō* statues are also found elsewhere in Japan, e.g., in Shinjuku ward of Tokyo and at the Shibutagawa riverside near Isehara (Kanagawa Prefecture).
- *Kōsaiji* 広済寺 (Kawagoe, Saitama Prefecture). There is a statue at this temple which is covered with ropes and cloth. It is known as *Shiwabuki Baba* (Grandmother of Coughing) and can be worshipped when seeking help for coughing.
- *Kōfukuji* 弘福寺 (Sumida ward, Tokyo). See pictures 277-278.
- *Yakurikisha* 薬力社 (Mount Inari, Kyoto). The shrine houses *Yakuriki Ōkami* (deity of medicinal power) and *Oseki Ōkami* (deity for protecting the throat). *Nodoame* (cough drops) are sold near the shrine.
- *Goō Jinja* 護王神社 (Kamigyo Ward, Kyoto). The shrine sells wine made from the fruits of local *karin* (Chinese quince) trees. It is said to be good for patients with asthma.

275
The Japanese TV celebrity *Imalu* posing besides a large *ema*-shaped board in 2013 at *Asakusa Jinja* (Taito Ward, Tokyo). She draws attention to *hai no hi* (day of the lungs) and to the large number of deaths from chronic obstructive pulmonary disease (COPD) each year. This was an initiative of Nippon Boehringer Ingelheim Co, a pharmaceutical company selling COPD drugs. This firm also created a virtual website called *Ikiiki Jinja* for an online contest in writing COPD-related texts on digital *ema*.
Photograph reproduced by courtesy of Nippon Boehringer Ingelheim Co, Tokyo

276
Charm from *Jyomyōin* in the shape of a *hechima* (sponge gourd)

277–278
Two stone sculptures at *Kōfukuji* which represent an elderly couple called *Seki No Jiji Baba Son* (Revered Grandma and Grandpa of Cough). The smaller Grandpa statue protects against a sore throat, while the taller Grandma statue protects against cough in general and whooping cough.
The temple shop sells bags of *sekidome ame* (cough-stopping sweets) [RT-249; GG1-2013/01].

279

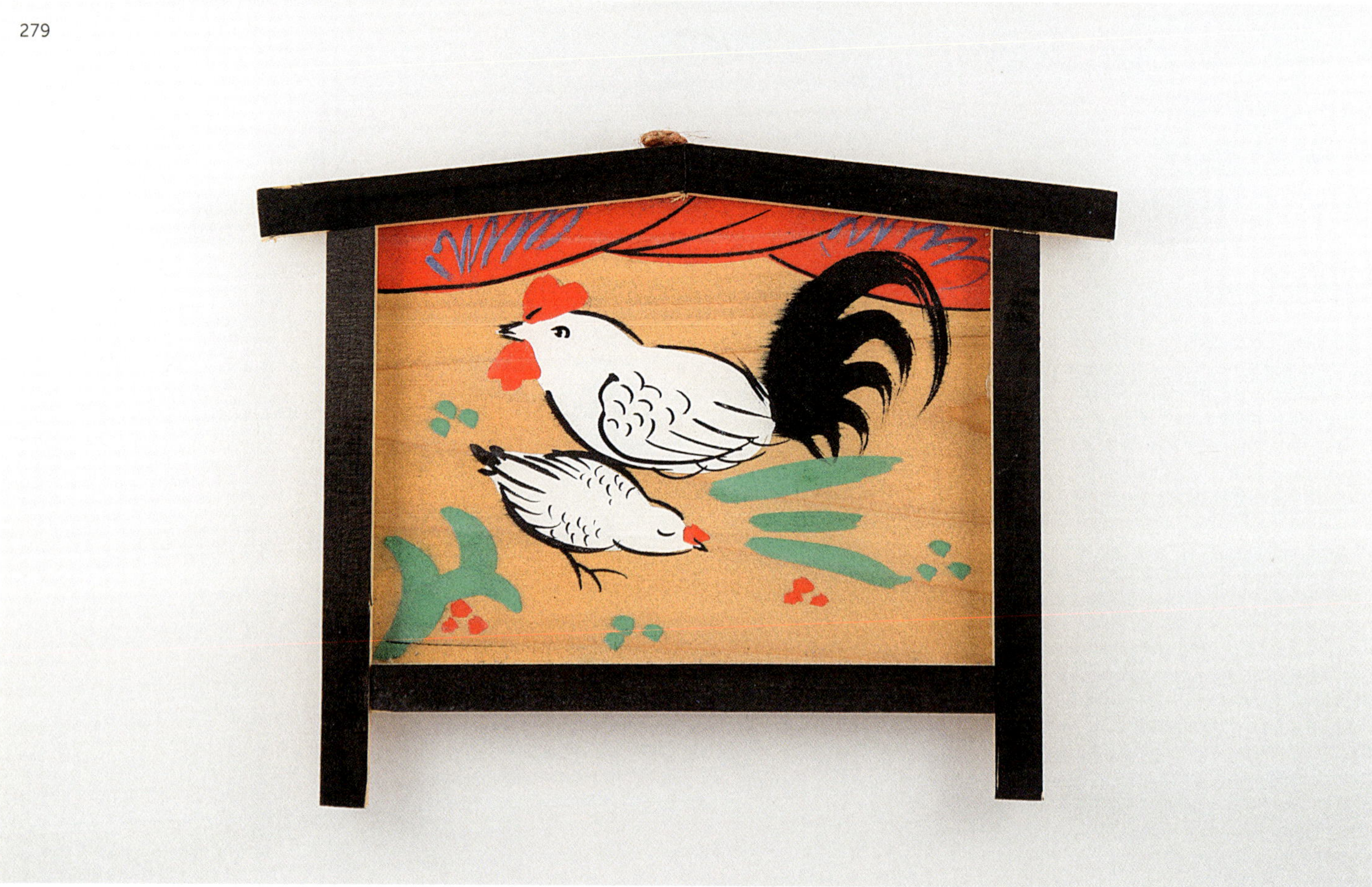

280

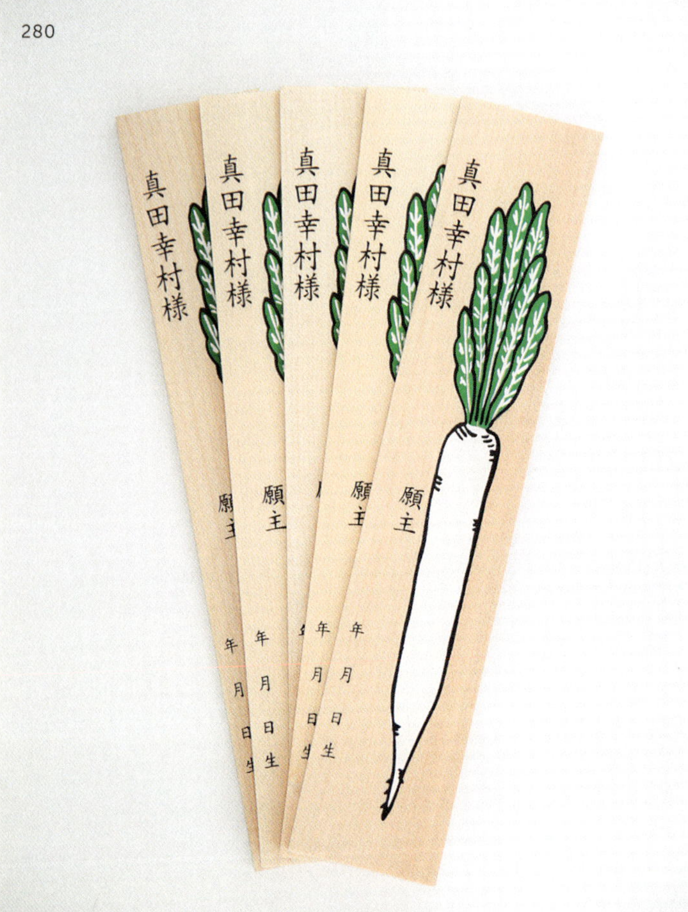

281

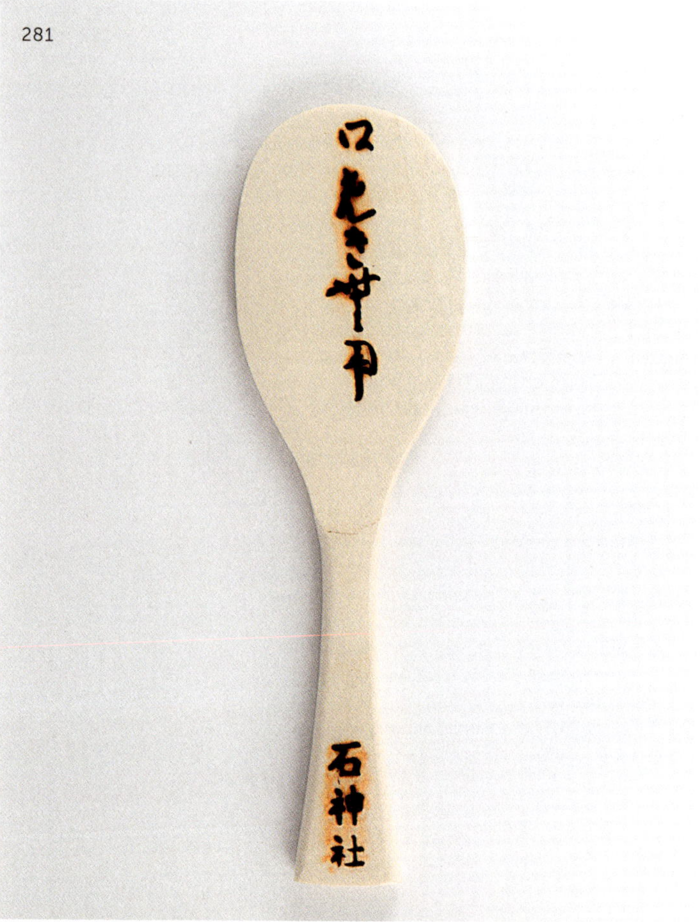

Ema designs

Chickens 鶏 (*niwatori*)

279
Hand-painted reproduction for a Japanese club of *ema* collectors called *Nihon Ema Tomo no Kai* (Friends of Japanese Ema Society). No.312. Late 20th century. W. 17.7 cm. Original design from Kanagawa Prefecture.

Ema design for *sekidome* (to stop cough) and for *yonaki* (crying of infant at night). The rooster was associated with *yonaki* because it does not crow during the night [TS-22; IH2-70].

Radish 大根 (*daikon*)

Sanada Jinja (Toyohashi, Aichi Prefecture) holds an annual *Sanada matsuri* (*Sanada* festival) in December where participants can pray for a cure for asthma. *Sanada Yukimura* (a famous samurai from the Edo Period) once appeared in the dream of a man with asthma and told him to float a *daikon* (radish) with his name on it. The man followed this advice and was cured of his asthma. Today, the participants no longer float radishes, but *ema* tablets with the picture of a radish.

280
Sanada Jinja 真田神社. Toyohashi, Aichi Prefecture. Early 21st century. W. 6.0 cm
The inscriptions read:
真田幸村様 = *Sanada Yukimura-sama*
願主 = *ganshu* (petitioner)
年月日生 = *toshi tsuki bi sei* (year month day of birth)

Rice scoop 杓文字 (*shamoji*)

281
Ishi Jinja 石神社 on the grounds of *Kotohira Jinja* 金刀比羅神社 (commonly known as *Koyasu Jinja*). Hachioji, Tokyo Metropolis. Early 21st century. H. 20.9 cm

This sanctuary enshrines *Sekidome No Kami* (deity of stopping cough). Its offers a paddle-shaped *ema* for *seki* (cough) and *zensoku* (asthma). The first character in 石神社 (the name of the shrine) is not only readable as *ishi* but also as *seki* (cough).

An additional *ema* design for respiratory symptoms/complaints (not illustrated here) is the serving of boiled rice '飯盛 (*meshimori*). Japanese sources agree that this *ema* design was used for *mune no tsukae* [IH2-84; NM-Z22673]. One source translates this concept as "obstruction in the chest" [3], while another source prefers "an upset stomach" [TS-26]. As the latter interpretation seems to be the more common one, this *ema* design has been classified and presented in the section on digestive symptoms/complaints (see pp.130-131 where an illustration of the design can also be found). However, it should be reiterated here that pulmonary tuberculosis was sometimes designated as *munen-oke* (chest trouble) in premodern Japan [WF].

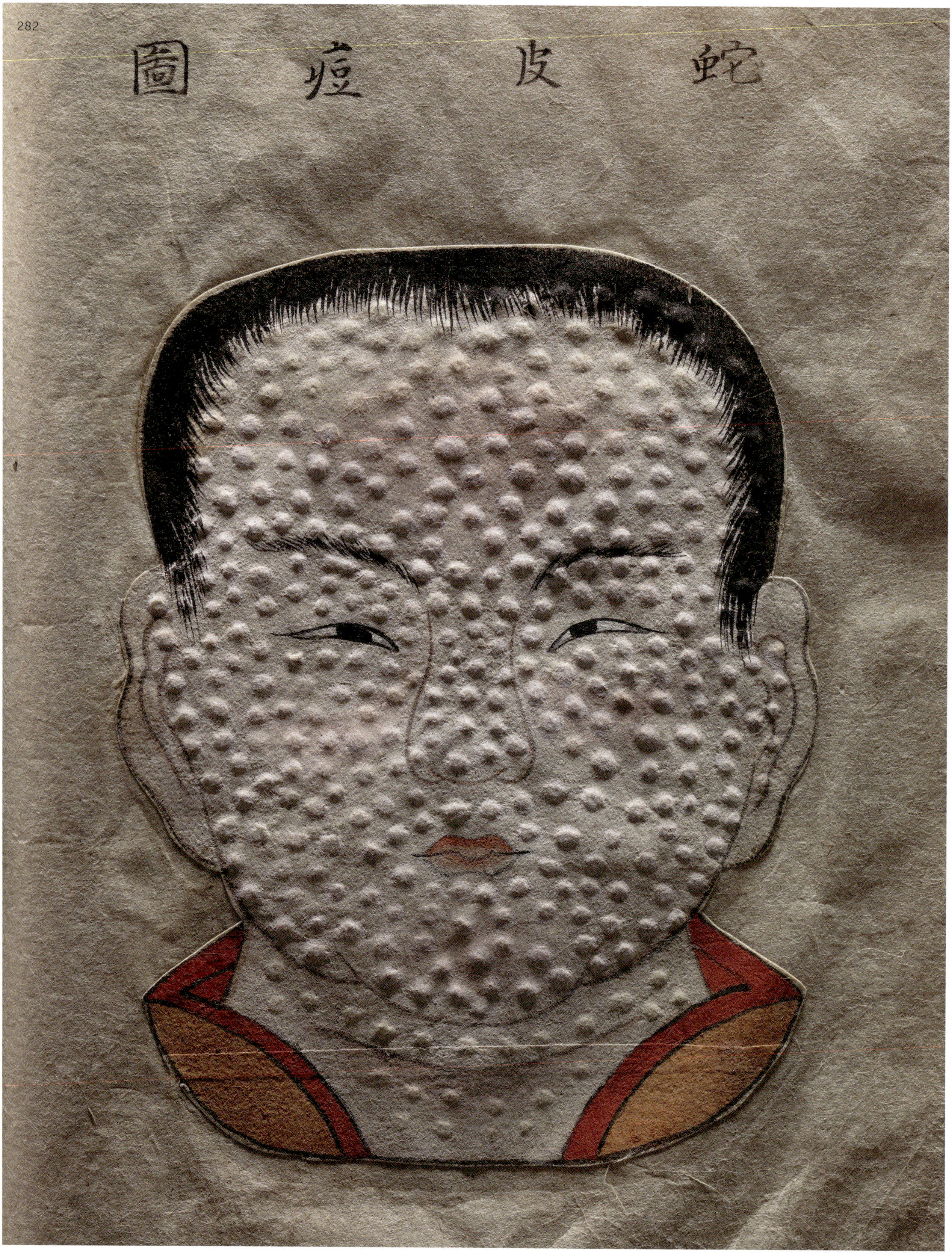
蛇皮痘圖

Skin illnesses
皮膚病 (*hifubyō*)

Background

Common skin complaints of Japanese outpatients seeking professional medical help are *kayumi* (itching), *ibo* (warts), *kessetsu* (nodule) or *shuchō* (swelling), *hosshin* (rash), *mushi kōshō/togeshō* (insect bite/sting), and *ressō* (laceration) or *sessō* (cut wound) [IO; TT].

One of the most widespread medical *goriyaku* (divine benefits) in Japan is the healing of *ibo* (warts). One website [http://hiramatu-hifuka.com/iboibo/ibozen1.html] lists more than 580 locations where one can pray for the healing or prevention of this problem. The most common figure of worship invoked for this purpose is *Ibotori Jizō* (Wart-Removing *Jizō*).

Other figures of worship and locations that offer recovery from skin illnesses include:

- Statues of *Doronuri Jizō* (Mud-Plastering *Jizō*) which are said to have the power to heal not only *ibo* (warts) but also other *hifubyō* (skin illnesses). To be cured, all one has to do is to put some mud on the part of the statue that corresponds to the affected part of one's body.
- *Ishikiri Tsurugiya Jinja* (Osaka) which has evolved into a shrine for neoplasms and for recovery from surgery but was originally known for healing various boils and growths [EO-153; RT-38].
- A pond-well near *Kongōji* (Matsue, Shimane Prefecture) which is known as the Well of Beauty. According to legend, the daughter of a 15th century warlord, who had been cursed with a disfiguring skin illness because of her father's misdeeds, was cured by bathing in this pond-well.
- A rock called *kaisen-iwa* (scabies rock) on Mount Misen (Miyajima Island, Hiroshima Prefecture). A patient with scabies may be cured by touching the rock, because the rock then takes his illness away. It is also believed, however, that an imprudent person can catch a skin illness by passing by the rock.
- A statue of *Shiokake Jizō* (Putting-Salt *Jizō*) which is located at *Taisōji* 太宗寺 (Shinjuku Ward, Tokyo) and which is said to offer *odeki chiyu* (healing of boils) [GK].

282
Textured watercolour illustration from the 18th century Japanese book *Toshin seiyo* (the essentials of smallpox) by *Kanda Gensen*. Wellcome Library, London Image L0074708.

This picture illustrates that external skin lesions can be the result of a systemic infectious disease (in this case smallpox).

283

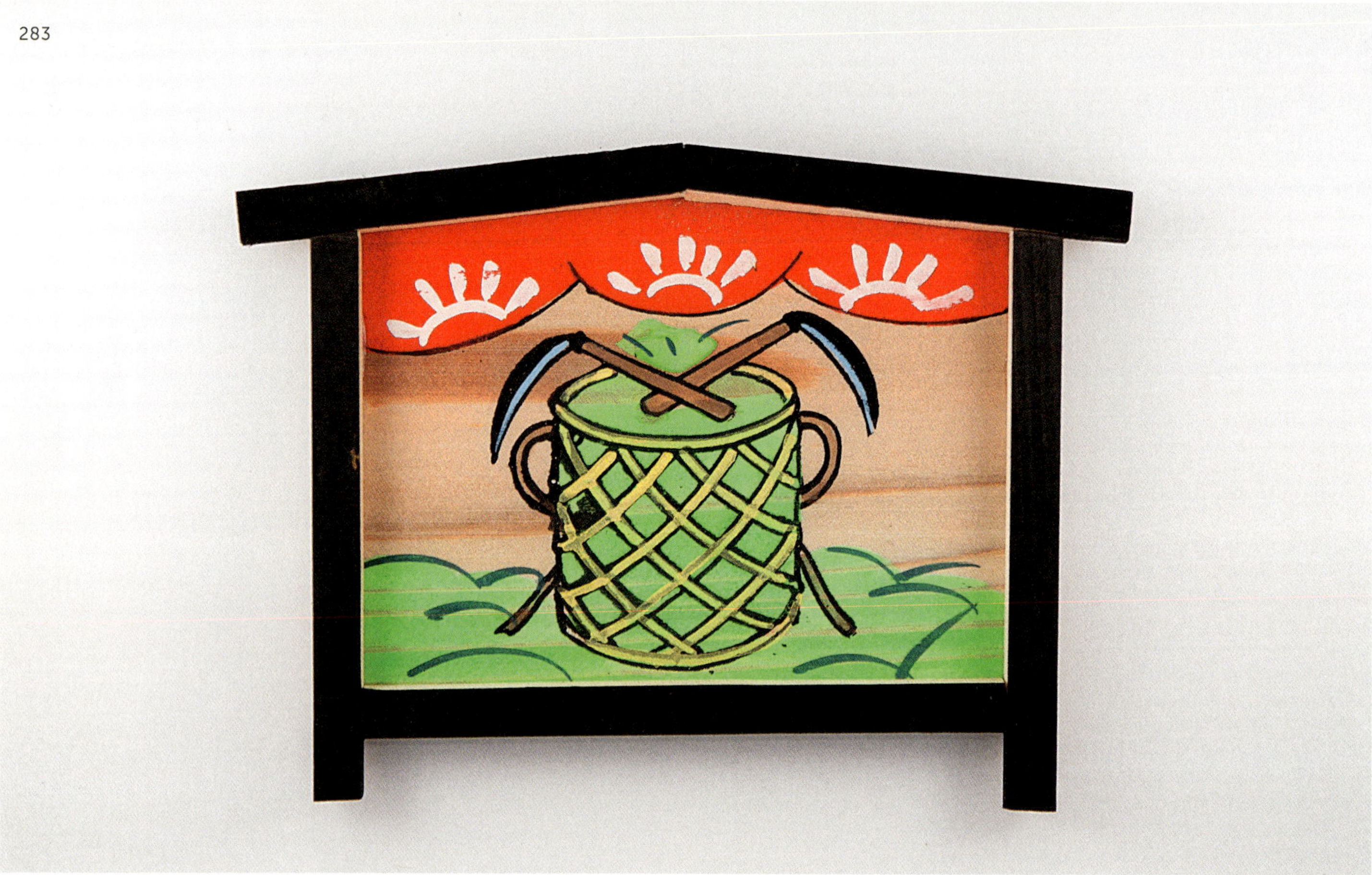

284

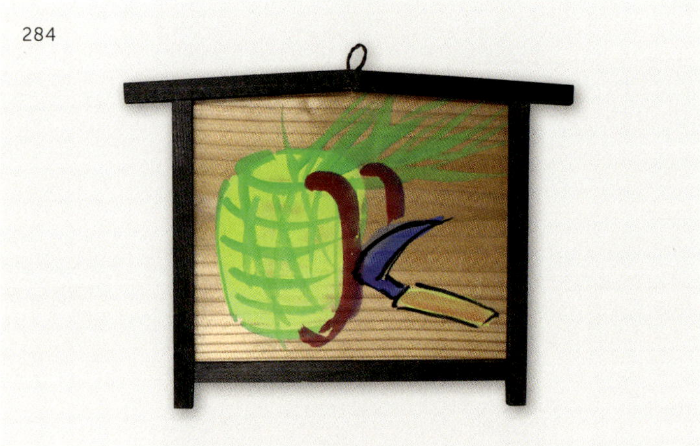

285

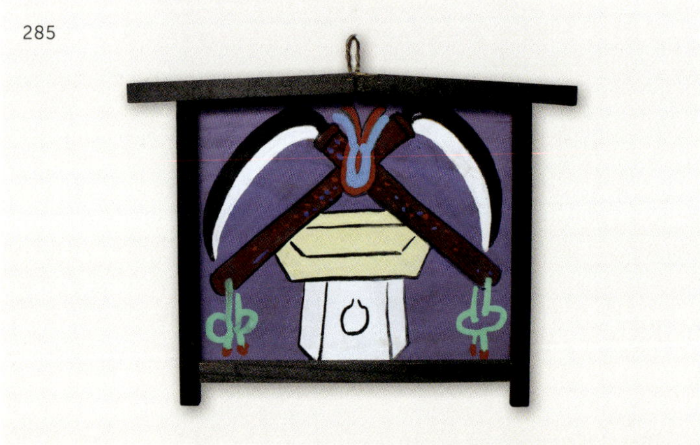

286

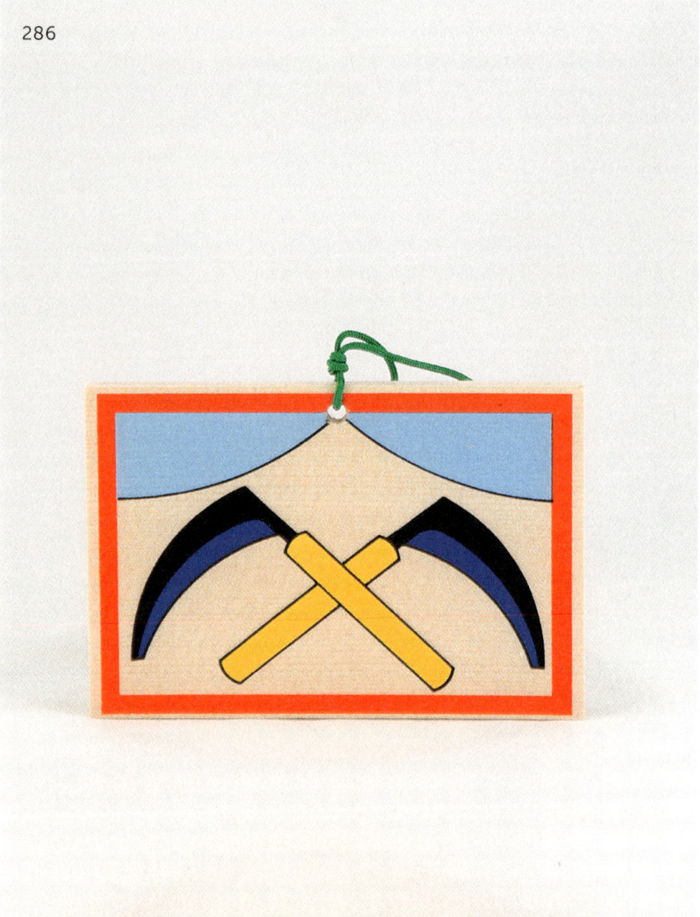

Ema designs

Grass-mowing sickle(s) and basket 草刈り鎌と篭 *(kusakari kama to kago)*

This *ema* design was primarily used for *hifubyō* (skin illnesses), such as *kusa* (eczema) and *haremono* (tumour, swelling). The underlying thought was that a sickle could cut off skin illness as cleanly as it could cut grass. Its use was associated with two different kinds of wordplay [OT; AE; TS-9; IH2-82]:

1 The Japanese terms for eczema and for grass are written differently (瘡 and 草, respectively), but they sound the same (*kusa*).

2 The kanji character for eczema (瘡) cannot only be read as *kusa* but also as *kasa* (which means boil or syphilis). Skin rash is a well-documented manifestation of secondary syphilis.

283

Hand-painted reproduction for a Japanese club of *ema* collectors called *Nihon Ema Tomo no Kai* (Friends of Japanese Ema Society). No.378. Late 20th century. W. 18.3 cm

This design was associated with *Kusakari Yakushi* (Grass-mowing *Yakushi*) in the neighbourhood of Ushigome (Shinjuku Ward, Tokyo). It was used for *kusa* (eczema) or *kasa* (syphilis) [OT; AE; TS-9].

284

Ema hand-painted by *Norihito Yasuda* (Nagoya) on commission from the Naito Museum of Pharmaceutical Sciences and Industry (Kakamigahara, Gifu Prefecture). Late 20th century. Museum inv.no. Z22686.

Used for *kusa* (eczema) or *kasa* (syphilis) [NM-Z22686].

Crossed sickles 交差鎌 *(kōsa kama)*

Just like the previous design, this *ema* design was primarily used for *hifubyō* (skin illnesses), such as *haremono* (tumour, swelling), or for the skin manifestations of *kasa* (syphilis) [TS-9; IH2-82; NM-Z22677].

285

Ema hand-painted by *Norihito Yasuda* (Nagoya) on commission from the Naito Museum of Pharmaceutical Sciences and Industry (Kakamigahara, Gifu Prefecture). Late 20th century. Museum inv.no. Z22677.

286

Kama Hachimangū 鎌八幡宮. Tennoji Ward, Osaka. Early 21st century. W. 13.5 cm

The *ema* design of crossed sickles serves other purposes at *Kama Hachimangū*, which is an *engiri* (karma cutting) shrine. If someone believes that s/he has an undesirable karmic connection with another person, s/he may go there to sever this connection. *Kama Hachimangū* has thousands of *kama* (sickles) that people have stuck in a huge old tree to escape from people they no longer want in their lives. The shrine is also believed to cure headaches, asthma, haemorrhoids, and other sicknesses, and it can help to get rid of evil spirits.

287

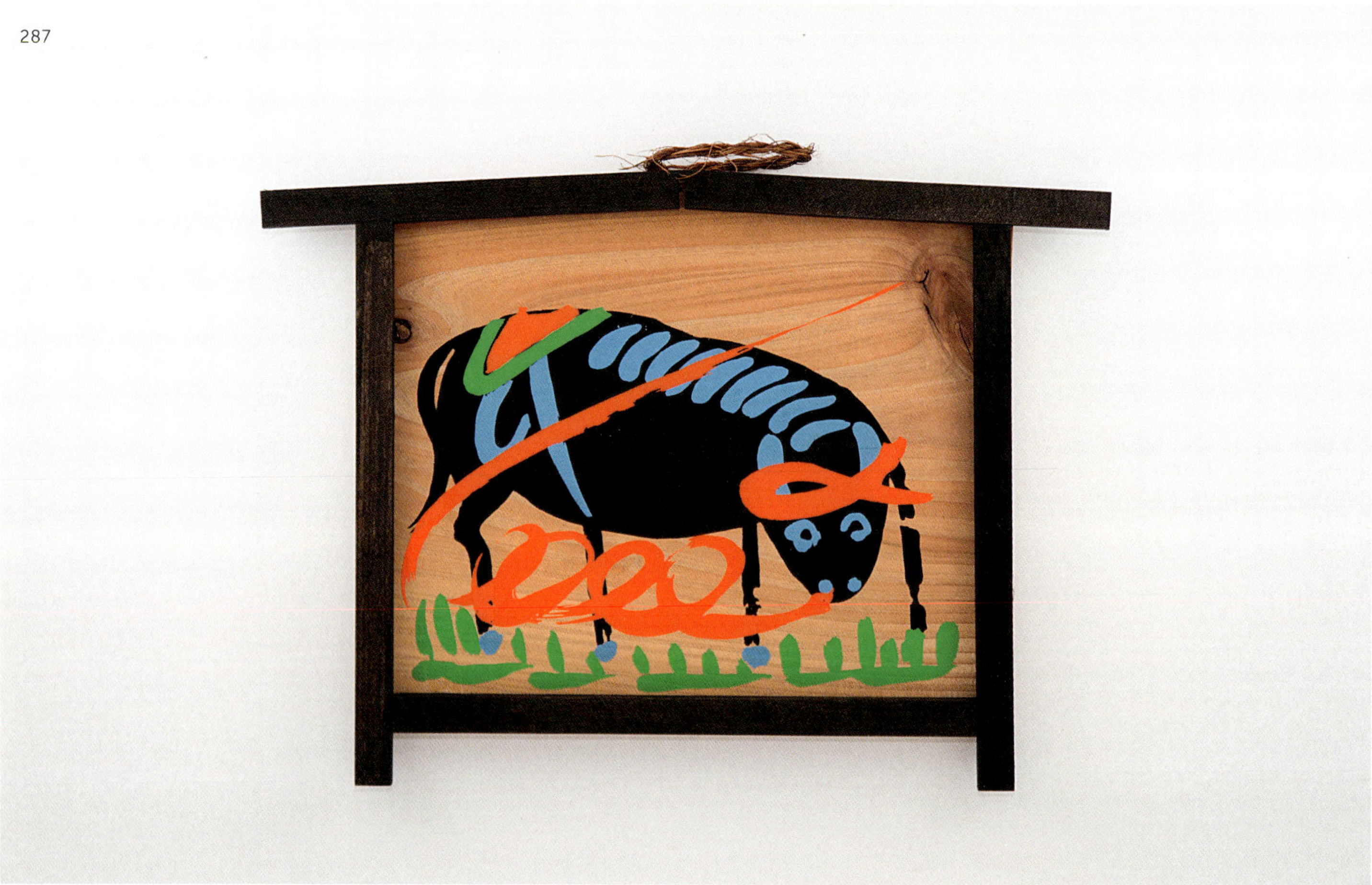

288

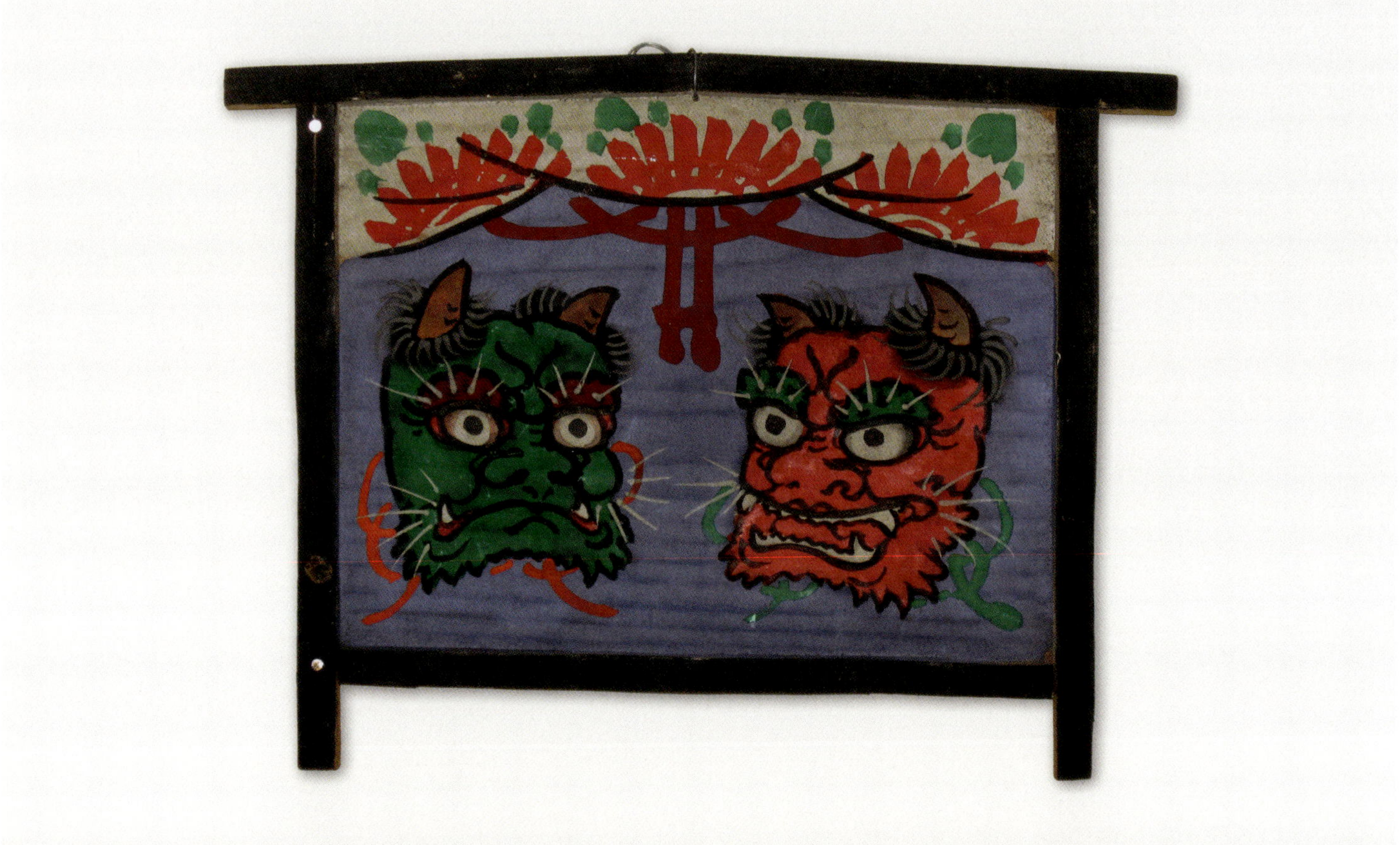

Cow/ox and grass 牛や草 (ushi ya kusa)

Ema with this design were inter alia used for *hifubyō* (skin illnesses), such as *kusa* (eczema). The underlying thought was that a cow/ox could make a skin illness disappear in the same way as it can make grass go away when grazing. The underpinning wordplay was that the Japanese words for eczema and for grass sound the same (*kusa*), even though they are written differently (瘡 and 草, respectively) [FS-21; TS-30; IH2-68; NM-Z22676]. Cf. the entry on grass-mowing sickle(s) and basket on p.175.

287
Hand-painted reproduction for a Japanese club of *ema* collectors called *Nihon Ema Tomo no Kai* (Friends of Japanese Ema Society). No.14. Late 20th century. W. 17.9 cm

Fierce gods 鬼神 (onigami)

Ema with *onigami* (fierce gods) were used in many areas for protection against *haremono* (boils, tumours) [TS-19].

288
Origin unclear; possibly from Adachi Ward, Tokyo. Early or mid-20th century. W. 25.7 cm. Tenri University Sankokan Museum (Tenri, Nara Prefecture). Museum inv.no.18193E966

289

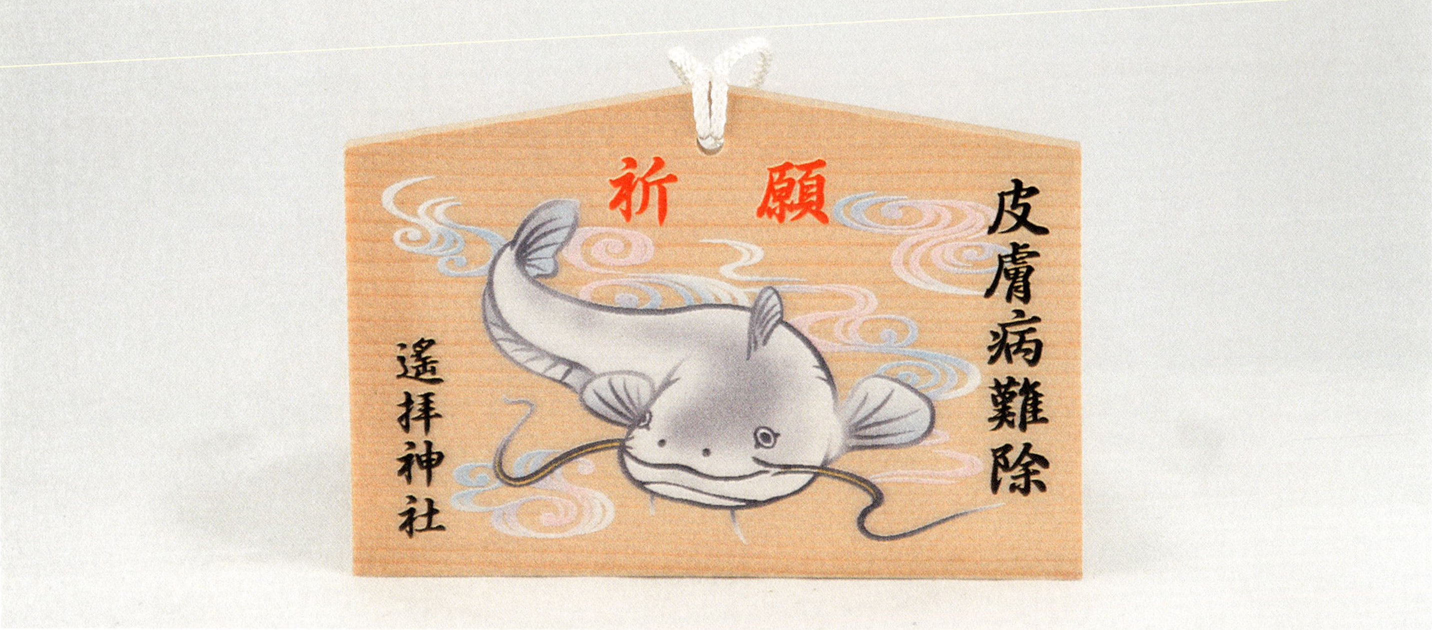

290

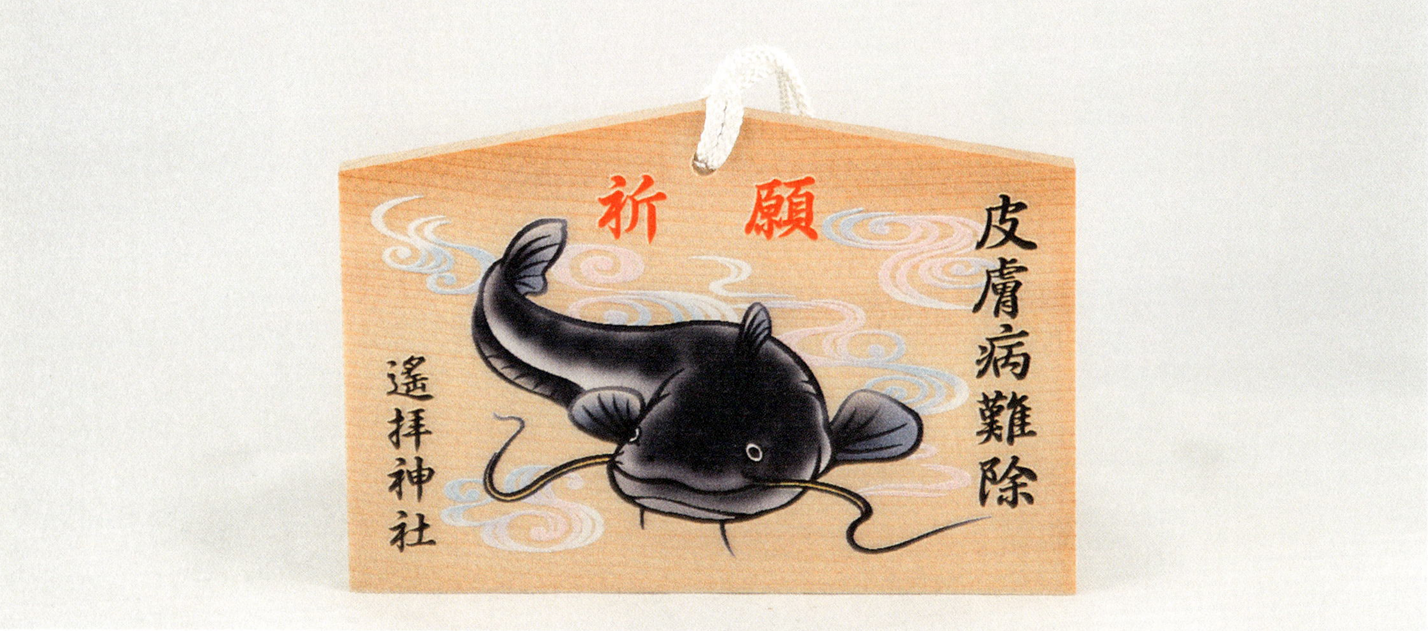

291

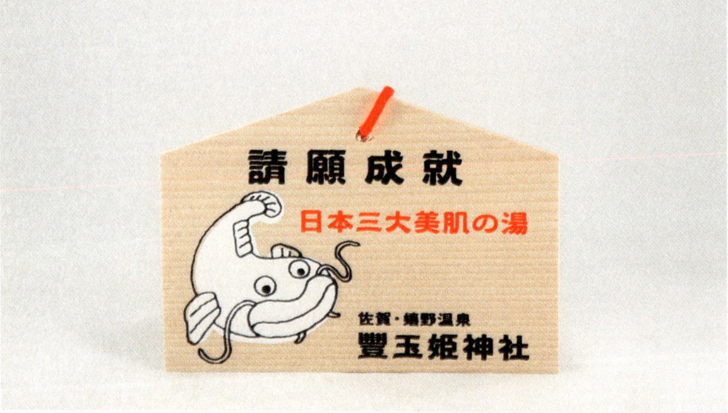

292

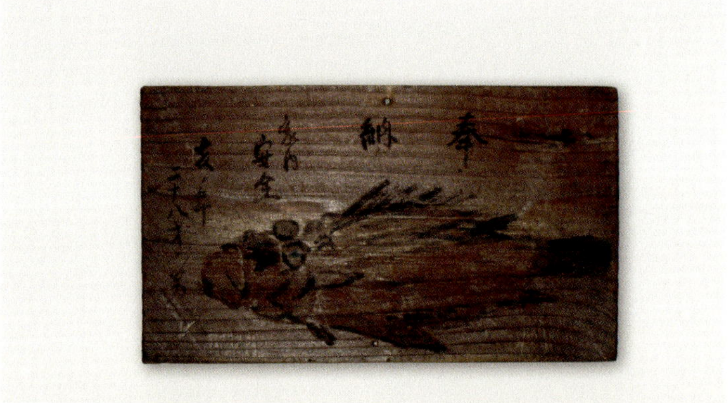

Catfish 鯰 *(namazu)*

The *ema* design of a *namazu* (catfish) is inter alia used for *bihada* (beautiful skin) and *hifubyō* (skin illnesses). In the past, it was particularly valued for a skin order called leukoderma, which is characterised by local skin depigmentation. The underlying reason was that one of the Japanese terms for leukoderma (*shironamazu*) sounds the same as white catfish (*shironamazu*) [FS-21; AE; TS-6; IH2-83; GG1-2012/06; NM-Z22692,Z22712] Leukoderma can be a manifestation of secondary syphilis that appears several months after the initial rash [1].

Among the other reported uses of catfish *ema* are toothache (see p.127); easy delivery or happy marriage [TS-6]; and protection from earthquakes. According to mythology, earthquakes were caused by a giant catfish living under the Japanese islands that was normally restrained by the deity *Kashima* by means of a large rock. Sometimes, however, the catfish was able to escape from this restraint and when it did so the vibrations that occurred as a result were the cause of the earthquakes that afflicted Japan. In 1855, when an enormous earthquake claimed thousands of victims among the inhabitants of Edo (now Tokyo), woodblock prints depicting the responsible catfish (*namazu-e*) rapidly became popular among the survivors. In addition to providing humour and social commentary, many prints were claimed to offer protection from future earthquakes [2].

289–290
Yōhai Jinja 遥拝神社. Yatsushiro, Kumamoto Prefecture. Early 21st century. W. 13.6 cm
The inscriptions read:
皮膚病難除 = *hifubyō nan yoke*
(warding off the problem of skin illnesses)
祈願 = *kigan* (prayer)
遥拝神社 = *Yōhai Jinja*

291
Toyotama-hime Jinja 豊玉姫神社. Ureshino, Saga Prefecture. Early 21st century. W. 15.2 cm
The inscriptions read:
請願成就 = *seigan jōju* (fulfilment of all vows/requests)
日本三大美肌の湯 = *nihon sandai bihada no yu* (Japan's big three hot springs for a beautiful skin)
佐賀・嬉野温泉 = Saga Ureshino *onsen* (hot springs)
豊玉姫神社 = *Toyotama-hime Jinja*

The *onsen* (hot spring) in Ureshino is reputed to be one of Japan's three best *onsen* for the skin. One can also make one's skin more beautiful there by visiting the shrine of *Toyotama-hime* (princess *Toyotama*). She was a daughter of the god of the sea and was famous for her beautiful white skin. On the grounds of her shrine there is a sanctuary for *shironamuzu* (white catfish) . According to legend, there once was an outbreak of skin illness in the village where the princess lived. All the villagers became healthy again by touching the statue of the white catfish [GG1-2012/06].

Stonefish 虎魚 *(okoze)*

This *ema* design is still found at *Kasayama Jinja* 笠山神社 (Koka, Shiga Prefecture). The name of this shrine is also written as 瘡山神社 and its enshrined deity is 瘡神 (= *Kasakami*). The first character (瘡) can be read as *kasa* (boil, pustule, or syphilis) and as *kusa* (eczema) [3]. Elsewhere, the design of a stonefish has been offered for *byōki heiyu* (recovery from illness), for protection from harmful *mushi* (worms), and for large catches of fish [TS-5; IH2-93].

292
Sarutahiko Jinja 猿田彦神社 Kobe, Hyogo Prefecture. Early or mid-20th century. W. 22.2 cm
The main inscription reads:
奉納 = *hōnō* (dedication, offering)

Tenri University Sankokan Museum (Tenri, Nara Prefecture). Museum inv.no.16808E71 [acquired in 1942]

This particular *ema* was employed for *mushiyoke* (protection against *mushi*) and for success in fishery.

293

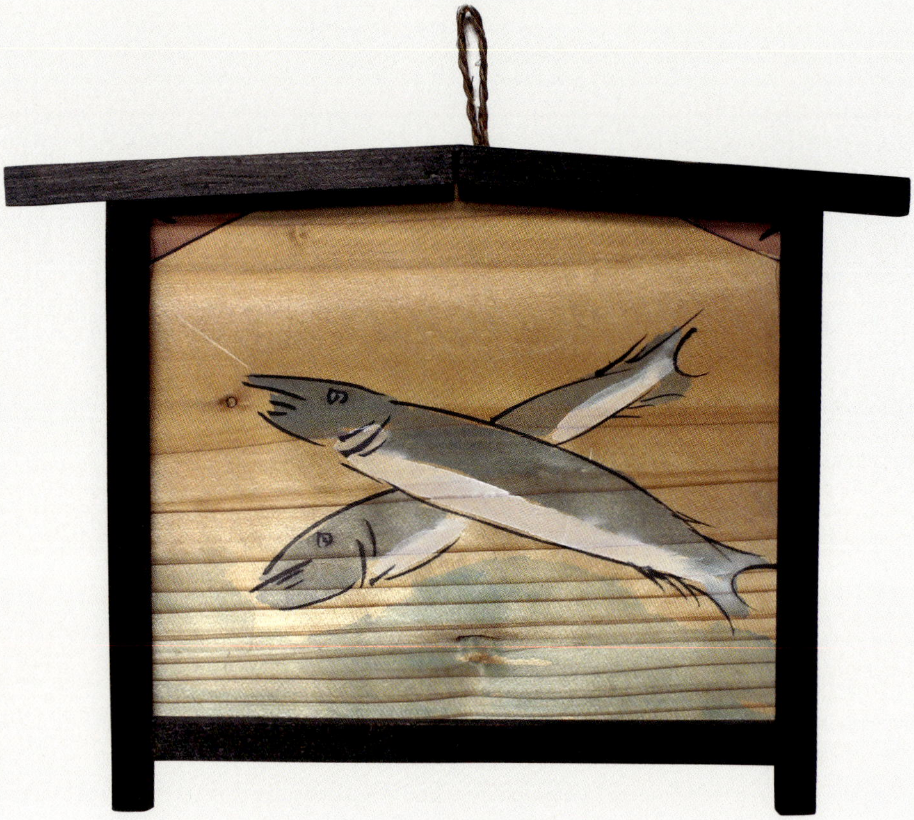

294

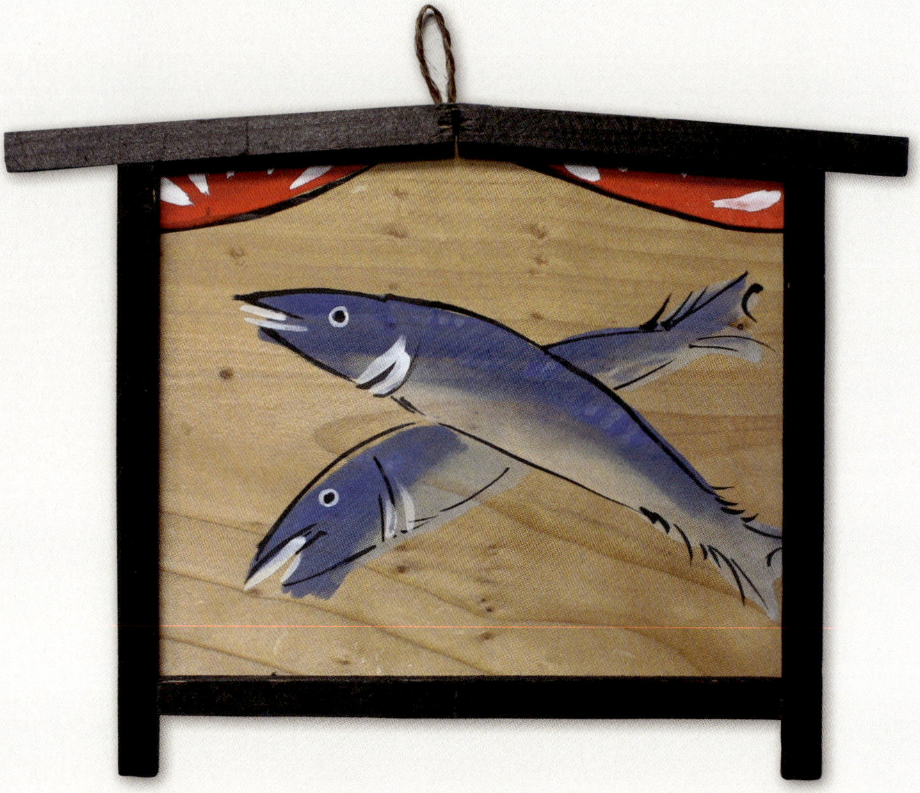

Sardines 鰯 (iwashi)

The consulted sources attribute different functions to the *ema* design of *iwashi* (sardines) [IH2-74]. The example illustrated here was used for *jinmashin* (urticaria) and *seibyō* (venereal diseases) [NM-Z22639]. At *Bannaji* (Ashikaga, Tochigi Prefecture), the design served to ask or thank for *anzan* (easy delivery) and this could be accompanied by a vow to refrain from eating *iwashi* [FS-13]. Another source associates the design with *ganbyō* (eye illnesses) and points to the similarity between *iwashi* (sardines) and *iyashi* (healing) [4].

293
Ema hand-painted by *Norihito Yasuda* (Nagoya) on commission from the Naito Museum of Pharmaceutical Sciences and Industry (Kakamigahara, Gifu Prefecture). Museum inv.no. Z22639. Late 20th century.

Mackerel 鯖 (saba)

This *ema* design was meant for *jinmashin* (urticaria) and for *shitsū* (toothache – cf. p.127 in the section on tooth and mouth symptoms/complaints) [TS-6; IH2-74; NM-Z22659].

294
Ema hand-painted by *Norihito Yasuda* (Nagoya) on commission from the Naito Museum of Pharmaceutical Sciences and Industry (Kakamigahara, Gifu Prefecture). Museum inv.no. Z22659. Late 20th century.

295

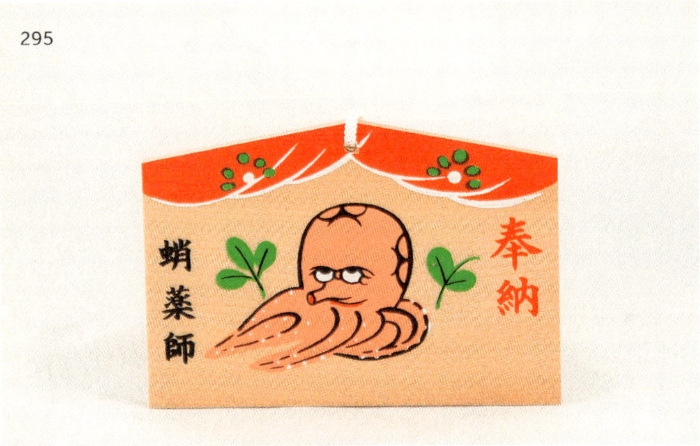

296

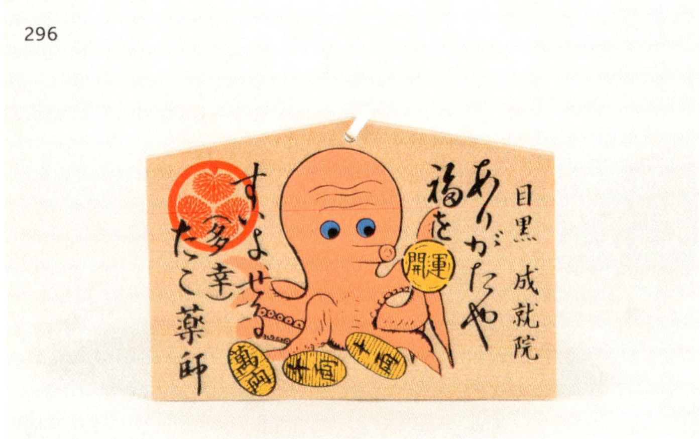

297

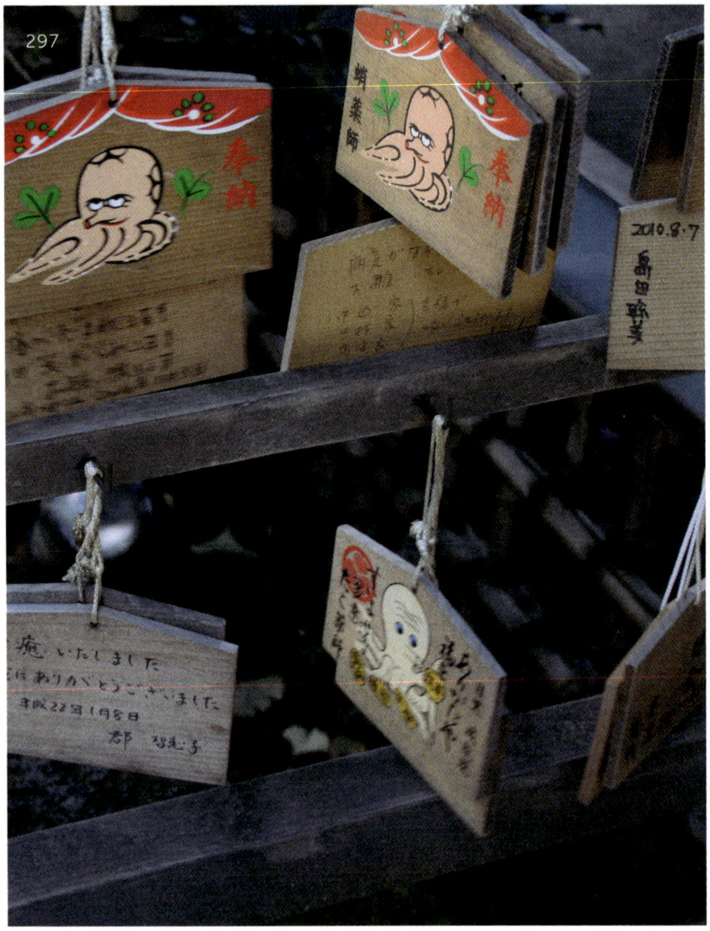

298

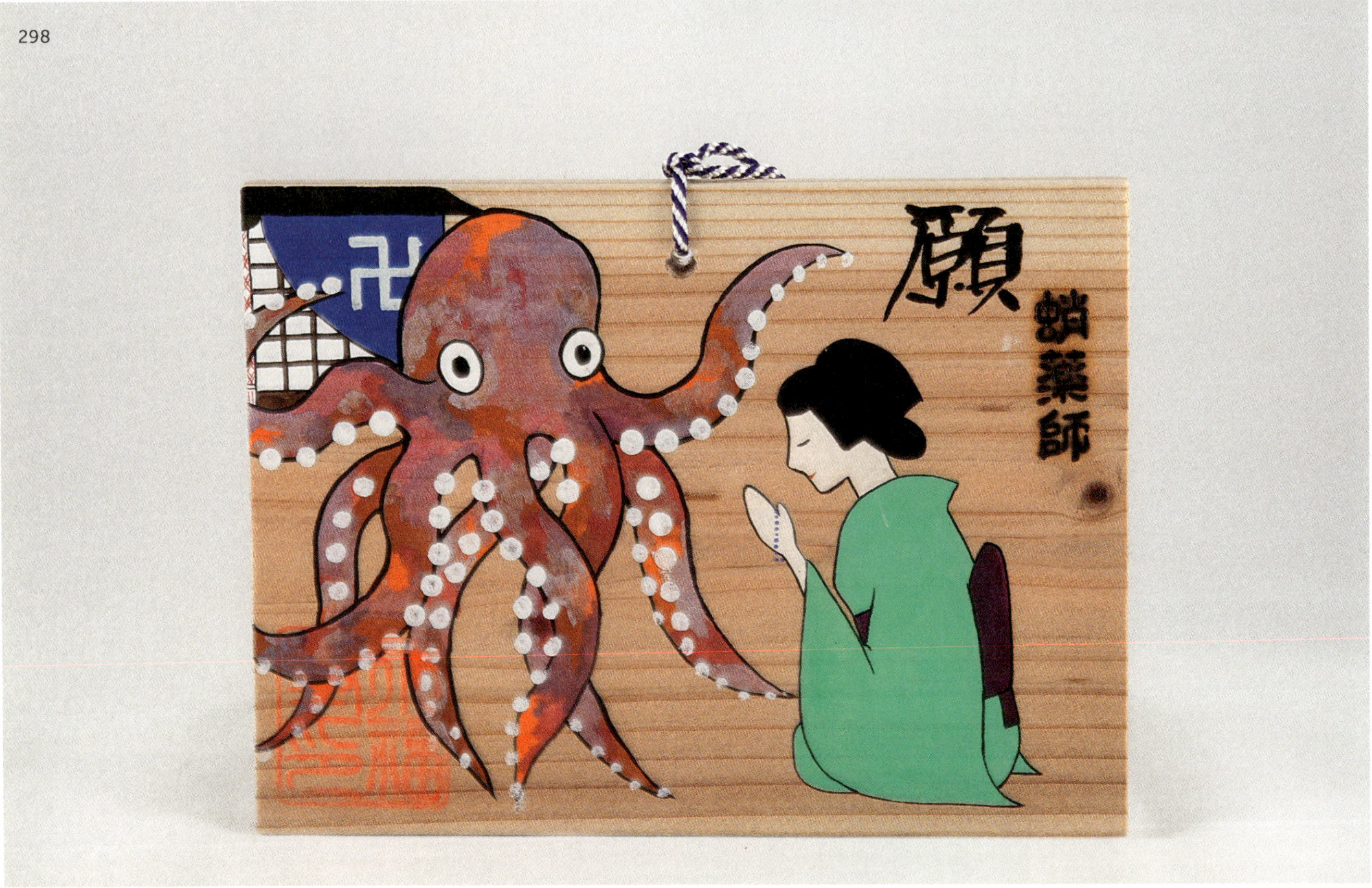

Octopus 蛸 *(tako)*

Tako is the Japanese word for octopus, but when written with different ideograms, it can also refer to callus or corn (胼胝) [RT-249]. Based on this similarity of sounds, *ema* depicting *tako* are recommended for *mame* (blister; corn), *tako* (callus;corn), *keigan* (corn), and *ibo* (warts). *Ema* with an octopus design have also been used for *haremono* (swellings, tumours), papules, rashes, coughing, *fujinbyō* (women's illnesses), *shōnibyō* (childhood illnesses) and *ganbyō* (eye illnesses) [TS-7,17; IH2-90; NM-Z22766]. See p.131 for the *ema* design of an octopus for *dacchō* (abdominal hernia).

295
Takoyakushi Jōjūin 蛸薬師 成就院. Meguro Ward, Tokyo. Early 21st century. W. 13.0 cm.
The inscriptions read:
奉納 = *hōnō* (dedication, offering)
蛸薬師 = *Takoyakushi*

296
Takoyakushi Jōjūin 蛸薬師 成就院. Meguro Ward, Tokyo. Early 21st century. W. 12.9 cm.
The inscriptions read:
目黒 = *Meguro*
成就院 = *Jōjūin*
ありがたや福をすいよせるたこ薬師 = *arigataya fuku wo suiyoseru Takoyakushi* (*Takoyakushi* attracts luck for those with unwavering faith)
開運 = *kaiun* (opening up good luck)
十両 = *jūryō* (ten *ryō* = old golden coin)
千両 = *senryō* (thousand *ryō* = old golden coin)
萬両 = *manryō* (ten thousand *ryō* = old golden coin)
多幸 = *takō* (great happiness) – note the wordplay with *tako* (octopus)

297
Ema rack at *Takoyakushi Jōjūin* (Meguro Ward, Tokyo).

The temple enshrines a statue of three octopuses carrying *Yaskushi Nyorai* (Medicine Buddha). This represents the legend of a figurine that went overboard during a storm, was brought safely to shore by an octopus, which carried it on its head, and was then carved into the form of *Yakushi*. As *Takoyakushi* has the protruding shape of an octopus's head, he is specifically a healer of illnesses related to protruding things, such as corns, warts and haemorrhoids [RT-249].

298
Takoyakushidō 蛸薬師堂 at *Eifukuji* 永福寺 Nakagyo Ward, Kyoto. Early 21st century. W. 18.1 cm
The inscriptions read:
願 = *gan* (wish)
蛸薬師 = *Takoyakushi*
Takoyakushidō can be visited for *odeki* (boils), *gan heiyu* (recovery from cancer) and *byōki heiyu* (recovery from illness) [GK].

According to legend, it happened in the 13th century that the mother of a monk who was living in the temple fell ill. When she did not recover, she asked him if he could bring her some *tako* (octopus) to eat. As a Buddhist monk, however, he was not allowed to buy a living creature for food. Yet his mother's wish prevailed. He bought an octopus in the market and took it back in a wooden box. Some people became suspicious that he had broken the rules and pressed him to reveal the contents of his box. The monk asked *Yakushi* to help him out. When he opened the box, the octopus had been transformed into a set of sutra scrolls. At the temple, these scriptures turned again into an octopus which jumped into the pond in front of the temple. There he changed into *Yakushi* and immediately healed the monk's mother. From then on, people visiting the temple for relief from illness were immediately healed and women praying for children were blessed with offspring [5].

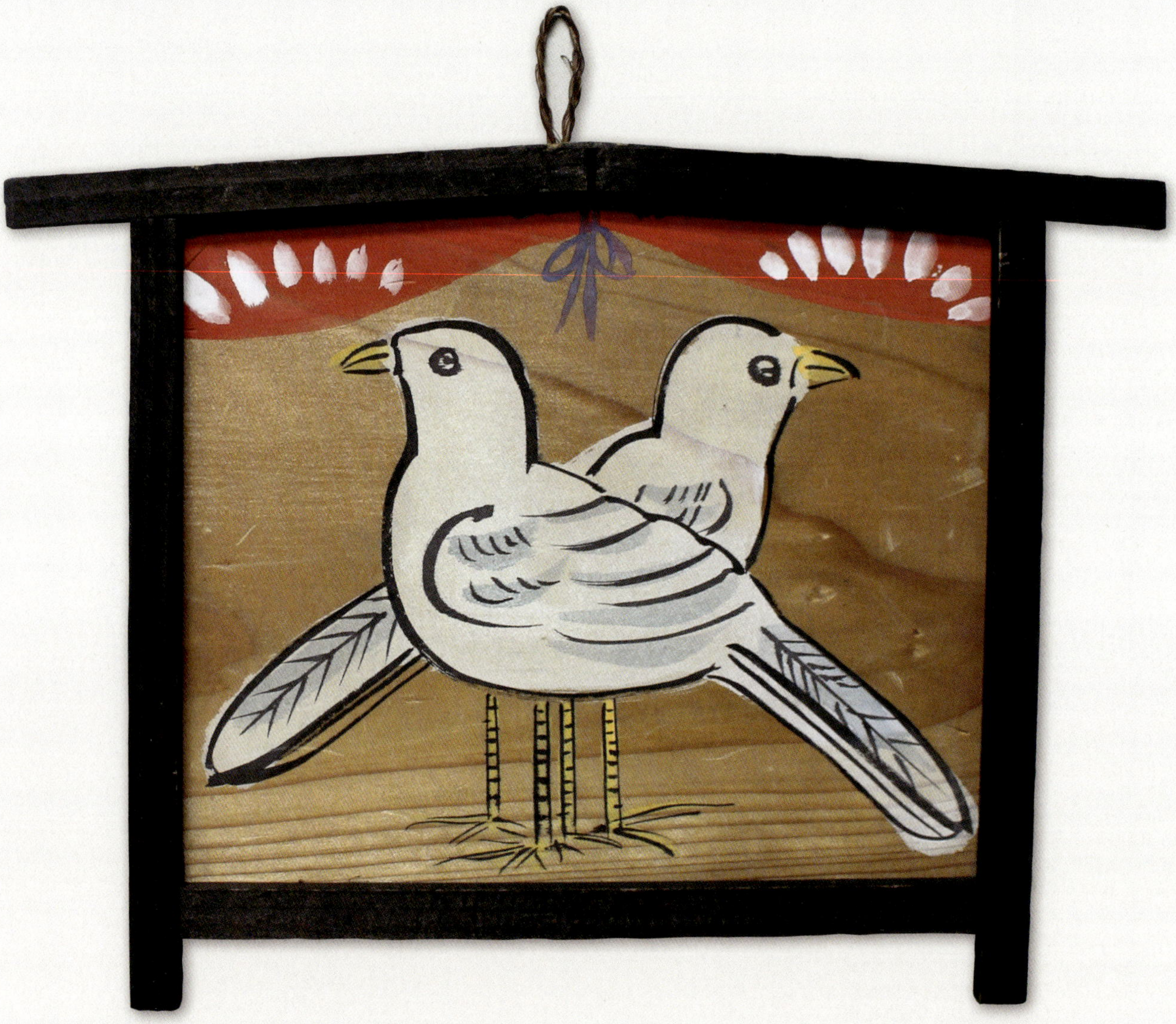

Pigeons 鳩 *(hato)*
As the pigeon is a messenger of *Hachiman* (God of War), images of this bird can be especially encountered at *Hachimangū*. *Ema* designs with two pigeons can be recommended for various purposes, such as *mame* (blisters, corns), *kannomushi* (short-temperedness; see p.161), love and marriage, and *kosodate* (raising children) [TS-22; IH2-80; NM-Z22767].

299
Ema hand-painted by *Norihito Yasuda* (Nagoya) on commission from the Naito Museum of Pharmaceutical Sciences and Industry (Kakamigahara, Gifu Prefecture). Museum inv.no. Z22767. Late 20th century.

Used for *mame* (blisters, corns) on the hands and feet, because pigeons like to pick grains. Its probable origin is a *Hachimangū* (*Hachiman* Shrine).

Nutritional and metabolic symptoms/ complaints 栄養と代謝の症状／愁訴 *(eiyō to taisha no shōjō/shūso)*

Beriberi 脚気 *(kakke)*

Background

Between 1900 and 1940, beriberi was the most devastating nutritional disorder in Japan. At its peak in 1923, its annual death rate was 46 per 100,000 inhabitants; 43% of these fatalities consisted of cases of infantile beriberi. After World War II, the incidence of beriberi steadily declined and resurgence became exceptional [US-67,137; 1].

Beriberi results from thiamine (vitamin B1) deficiency due to an unbalanced diet.
In Western society, it can be seen in chronic alcoholism, but the principal cause in Japan was heavy reliance on white rice as a staple food. The dehusking of rice extends its shelf life, but also removes thiamine. The two main types of beriberi in adults are:

- dry beriberi: gradual degeneration of the long nerves (first of the legs and then of the arms); death occurs due to paralysis;
- wet beriberi: oedema due to heart failure. These types constitute the same disease and a mixture of the two is common. The onset of beriberi is insidious, but acute heart failure leading to rapid death without nervous system symptoms may also occur. This acute fulminant form is known as *shōshin* beriberi. Beriberi can also emerge in breast-fed infants of thiamine-deficient mothers. This infantile beriberi is characterised by progressive heart failure [2].

In the 17th century the eating of dehusked white rice without many side dishes became fashionable among the richest classes of Japan, which produced an increase in the incidence of beriberi in the major cities. The rural population was not equally affected, because peasants were generally too poor to afford white rice as a staple food. In the Meiji Period, however, the custom of eating dehusked rice became more widespread and this particularly took a high toll among the military serving in the Japanese army and navy [3].

Examples of sanctuaries that were visited in the past to pray for the healing or prevention of beriberi are:

- *Shōtsurugi Jinja* 勝剣神社 (Hirosaki, Aomori Prefecture). The walls of the *haiden* (hall of worship) are covered with *ema* with a *tsurugi no kumi* (pair of swords) design.
- *Mikawashima Inari Jinja* 三河島稲荷神社 (Arakawa Ward, Tokyo). When the prayer was answered it was customary to offer *waraji* (straw sandals) [GK].
- *Konoshima Jinja* 木嶋神社 (also known as *Kaiko no Yashiro*), Ukyo Ward, Kyoto. There was a spring at this shrine; wetting one's hands and feet in its water in summertime was believed to protect from chilblains and beriberi [GK].
- *Nichikadō* 日荷堂 (*Mutsūrasan Enjūji*), Taito Ward, Tokyo The shrine still sells *ema* for leg/foot difficulties (see the entry on *Nichika* on p.151).
- *Hattori Tenjingū* 服部天神宮 (Toyonaka, Osaka Prefecture) The shrine still sells *ema* for leg/foot difficulties (see the entry on sandals = *zōri* on p.151).

Ema designs

Straw sandals 草鞋 *waraji and sandals* 草履 *zōri* (illustrated on p.150).

The earliest sign of beriberi may be a sensory loss in the foot and calf so that the patient is not aware that he is walking barefoot when his sandal has slipped off [4]. In pre-war days, *ema* with *zōri* (sandals) or *waraji* (straw sandals) attached to them were offered in connection with beriberi [HD; TS-4]. Such ema can still be seen at *Nichikadō* (Taito Ward, Tokyo).

Diabetes mellitus 糖尿病 *(tōnyōbyō)*

Background

In the course of the 20th century, diabetes mellitus became a significant cause of mortality in Japan. In recent years its prevalence has grown further, making Japan one of the nations most affected by the global diabetes epidemic. As the prevalence of type 1 diabetes is very low, type 2 diabetes accounts for the vast majority of diabetic patients in Japan. In 2002, 13.5% of the population (equivalent to 8.8 million) suffered from either type 2 diabetes or its pre-stage (impaired glucose tolerance) [SY15; 5].

There are some sanctuaries that offer benefits to patients with diabetes:

- *Rakuyaji* 櫟野寺 (Koka, Shiga Prefecture) houses a wooden statue of *Jūichimen Kannon* (Eleven Faces *Kannon*), which dates from the Late Heian Period and is 312 cm high. It is imputed with the power to prevent and cure diabetes. According to a story from the Meiji Period, a man was cured of diabetes by praying to the statue and drinking a tea made by boiling its wooden chips. On 3 November of each year, the statue is publicly displayed. People offer their prayers, drink tea made from the wood of oak trees (*ichii*), and purchase charms for the prevention of diabetes [RT-166; GK].
- *Jōrakuji* 常楽寺 (Tokushima, Tokushima Prefecture) enshrines *Miroku Bosatsu* as main deity. It is said that one can be cured of diabetes, if one prays at the temple and also drinks the boiled leaves from the yew tree beside the main hall.
- *Ōtori Jinja* 大鳥神社 (Meguro Ward, Tokyo). Among the diseases, for which this shrine offers benefits are *tōnyōbyō* (diabetes mellitus) and *seikatsushūkanbyō* (lifestyle diseases) [GK].

Ema designs

Shrines or temples that offer an *ema* for diabetes have not been found.

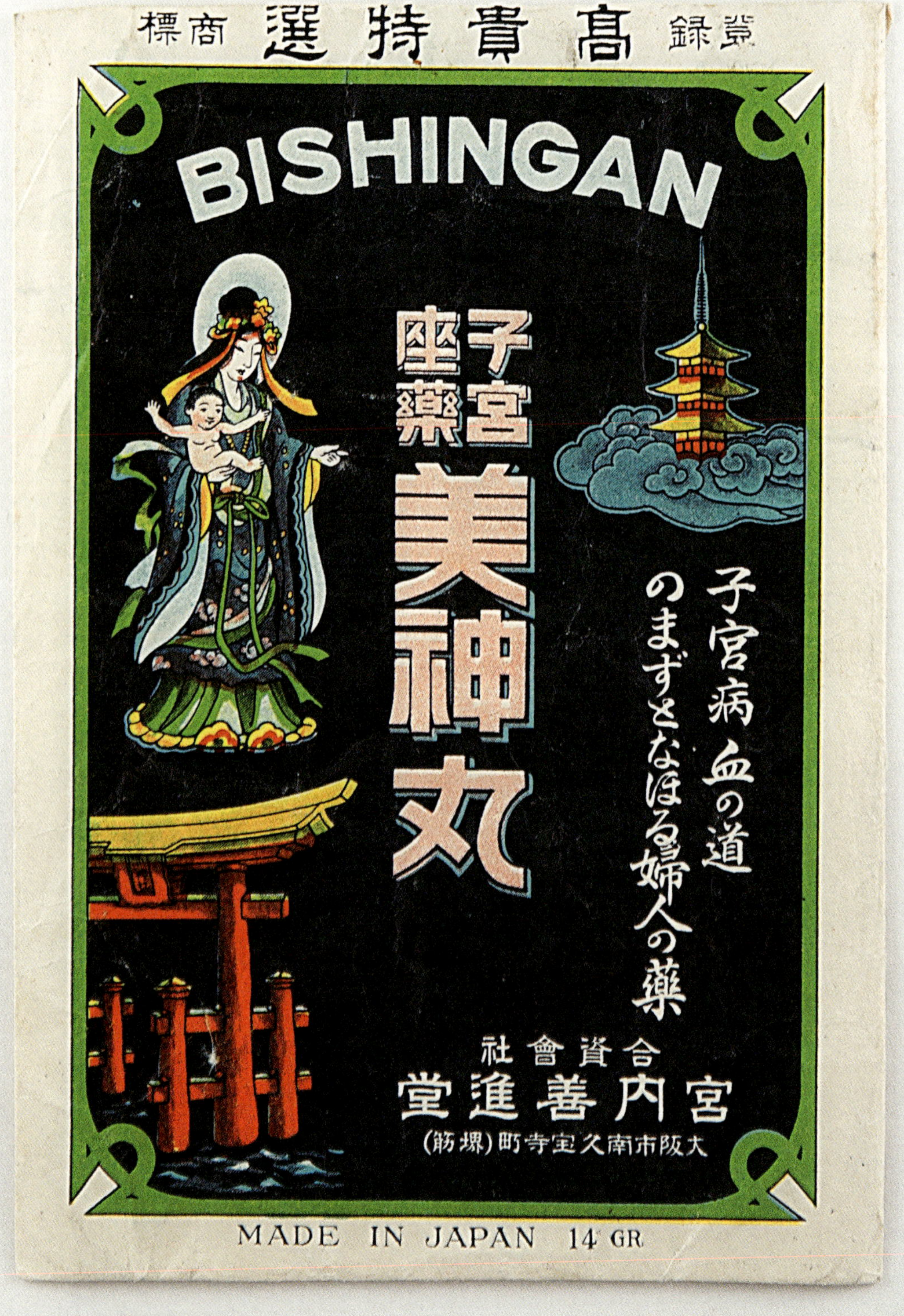
登錄 高貴特選 商標
BISHINGAN
子宮座藥
美神丸
子宮病血の道
のまずとなほる婦人の藥
合資會社
宮内善進堂
大阪市南久宝寺町(堺筋)
MADE IN JAPAN 14 GR

Women's illnesses
婦人病 (*fujinbyō*)

Background

Ema for fertility, safe childbirth and breast-feeding have already been presented in part three on human life issues (p.67). Here the focus is on *ema* for *fujinbyō* (women's illnesses). These illnesses not only included specific female complaints, such as problems of the *shikyū* (uterus) or *chichi* (breasts), but also referred to *seibyō* (venereal diseases) or *karyūbyō* (sexually transmitted diseases = STDs), as if only females were to blame for the spread of STDs.

It is generally assumed that bacterial STDs (such as syphilis and gonorrhoea) were common in Edo and Meiji Japan. Among the suggested causes are lenience towards having multiple sexual partners during one's lifetime and the existence of many licensed red-light quarters. According to surveys conducted in the late 19th century, most prostitutes were infected with an STD. There is evidence from archaeological bone remains that syphilis was already rampant in the Edo period. The first Japanese epidemic of syphilis probably took place in the early 16th century, i.e., after the discovery of the New World in 1492, but before the first arrival of Westerners in Japan. Evidence that gonorrhoea was also widespread in Edo Japan is more circumstantial, because this disease does not cause characteristic bone lesions and because the differentiation of STDs was still difficult in those days [WF; AJ; 1].

In the immediate period after the Second World War, STDs were more prevalent in the military Defence Forces than in the civilian population. Between 1947 and 1956, the official rates of STD cases started to decline (especially for syphilis). It remains unknown, however, how many prostitutes escaped inspection, both before and after the Prohibition of Prostitution Act was promulgated in 1958 [2].

300
Package of vaginal suppositories
美神丸 = *Bishingan* (lit. beauty just like a deity)
Early to mid-20th century

As the package illustrates, the deity concerned is *Kannon*. The suppositories were used for *fujinbyō* (women's illnesses), such as *koshike* (a mucous discharge from the female private parts called leucorrhoea).

301

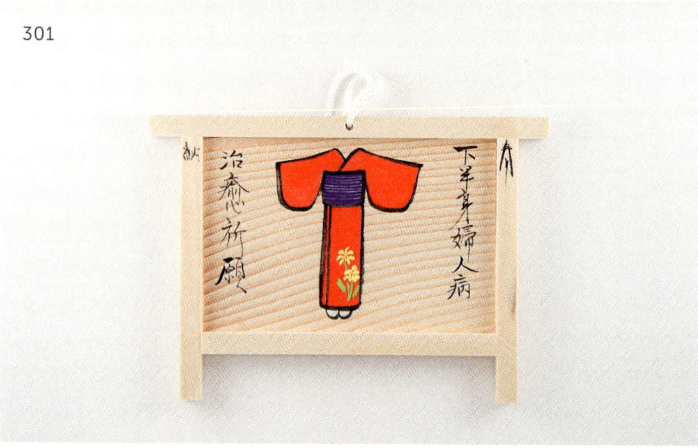

302

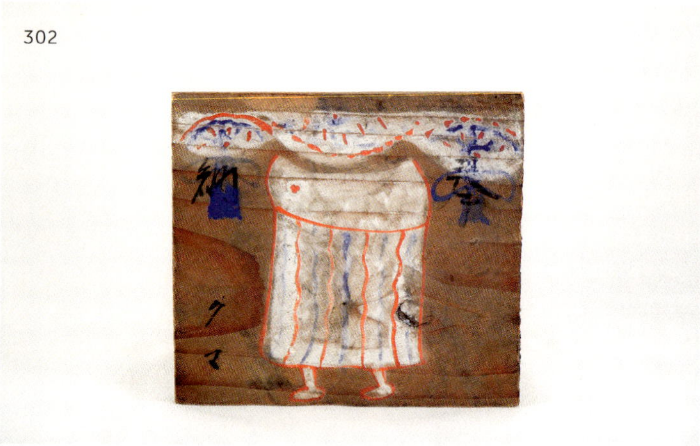

304

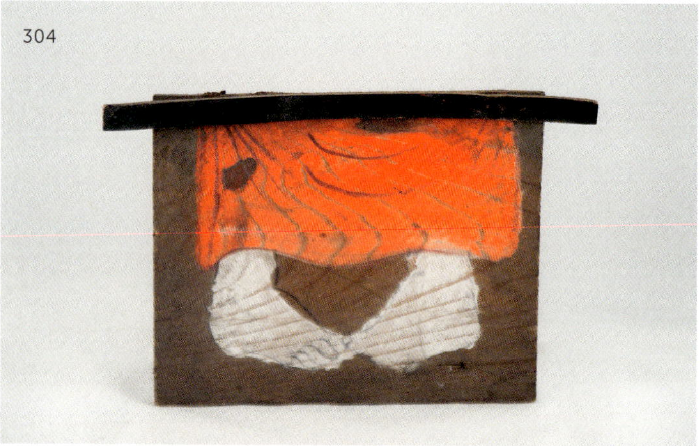

305

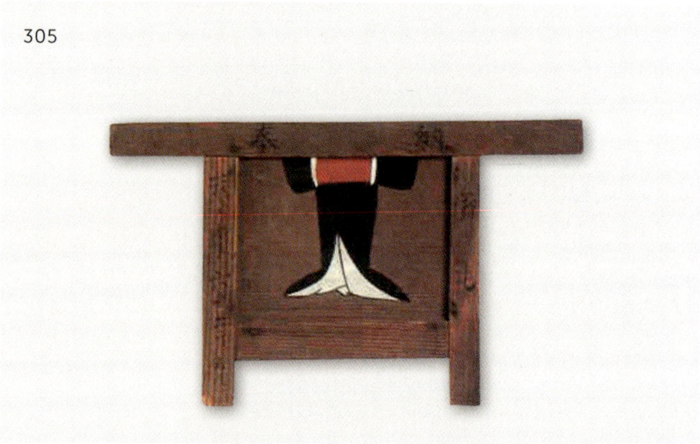

303

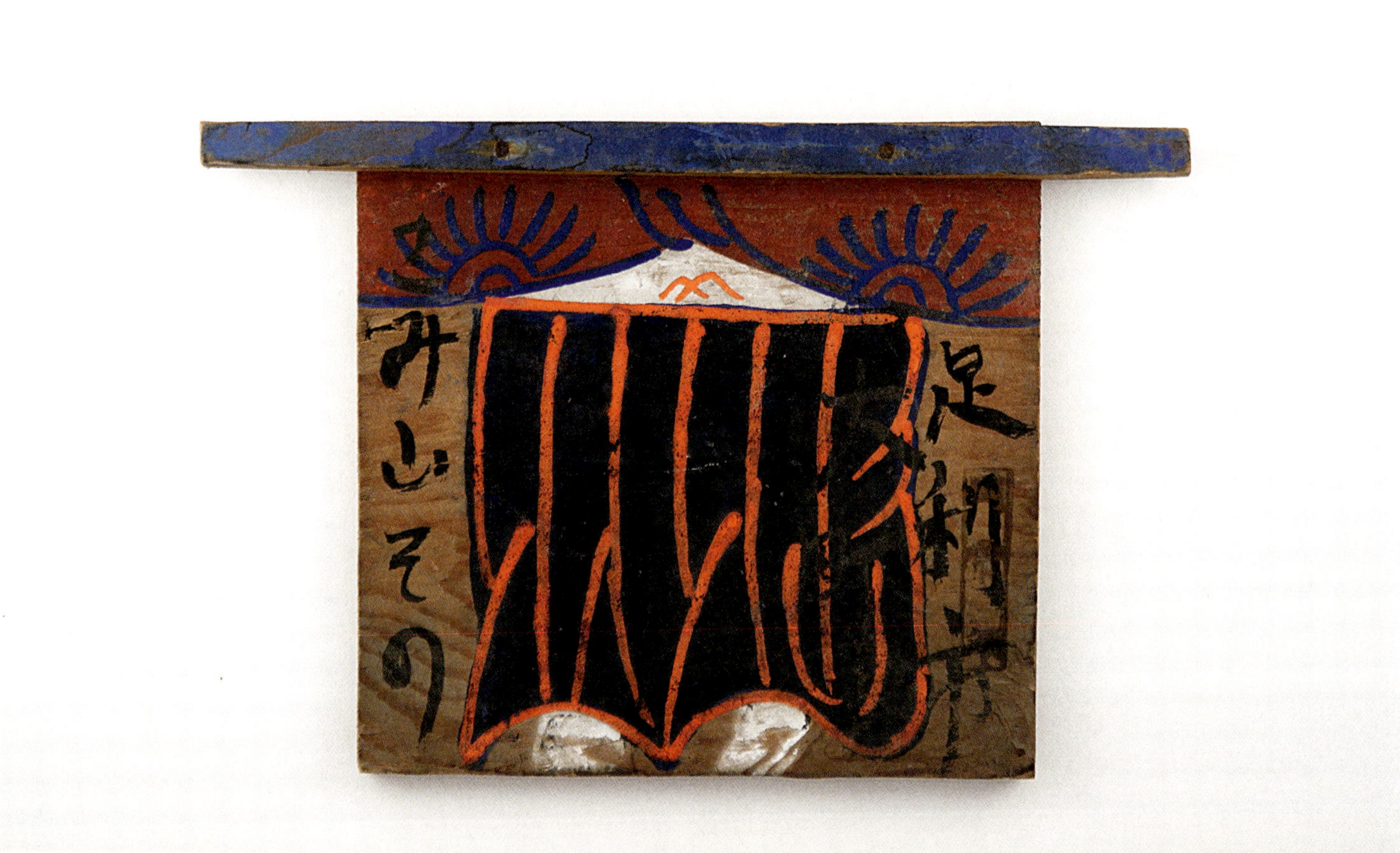

Lower half of the body 下半身 *(kahanshin)*

Kahanshin (lower half of the body) of a female worshipper or *koshi kara shita* (from the waist down) are older terms for *ema* designs that were used for the healing or prevention of female illnesses or "illnesses from the waist down" (more particularly venereal diseases) [FS-13; OT; TS-10; IH2-86; NM-Z22658]. An early source on *ema* designs distinguishes [AE]:

- *Fujin no ashi*: bare feet of a female wearing a red waist cloth; offered at *Mizushi Jinja*, Ashikaga, Tochigi Prefecture.
- *Kokue no kahanshin*: lower half of the body wearing black cloth; offered at *Kushida Jinja*, Fukuoka, Fukuoka Prefecture.

301
Akachichi Jinja 赤乳神社 (near *Kasuga Taisha* 春日大社). Nara, Nara Prefecture. Early 21st century. W. 15.9 cm
The inscriptions read:
下半身婦人病 = *kahanshin fujinbyō* (women's illnesses of the lower half of the body)
治癒祈願 = *chiyu kigan* (prayer for recovery)

The red colour of the kimono on the *ema* echoes the colour mentioned in the name of the shrine (*aka* = red). The nearby *Shirochichi Jinja* (*shiro* = white) offers a corresponding *ema* for the upper part of the body (see p.191).

302
Mizushi Jinja 水使神社 Ashikaga, Tochigi Prefecture [KM-26; IH2-86]. Early to mid-20th century. W. 15.1 cm

---

303
Mizushi Jinja 水使神社 Ashikaga, Tochigi Prefecture [KM-26; IH2-86]. Early to mid-20th century. W. 14.6 cm

---

304
Mizushi Jinja 水使神社 Ashikaga, Tochigi Prefecture [KM-26; IH2-86]. Early to mid-20th century. W. 17.1 cm

---

305
Awashima Jinja 淡島神社 in precincts of *Sumiyoshi Jinja* 住吉神社. Reproduced with permission of the publisher from Iwai H. *Ema ni negai o*. Tokyo: Nigensha, 2007:87

306

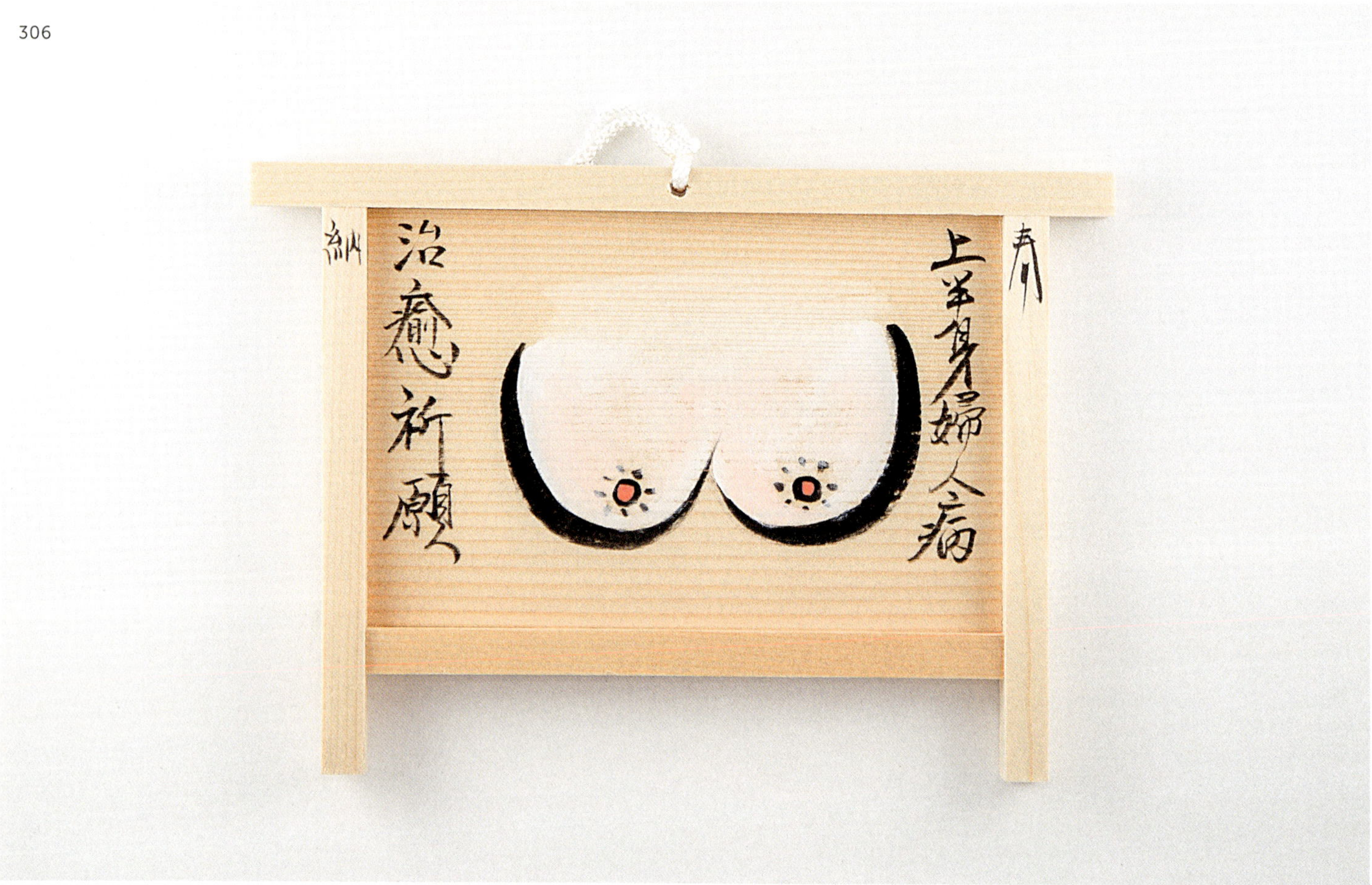

307

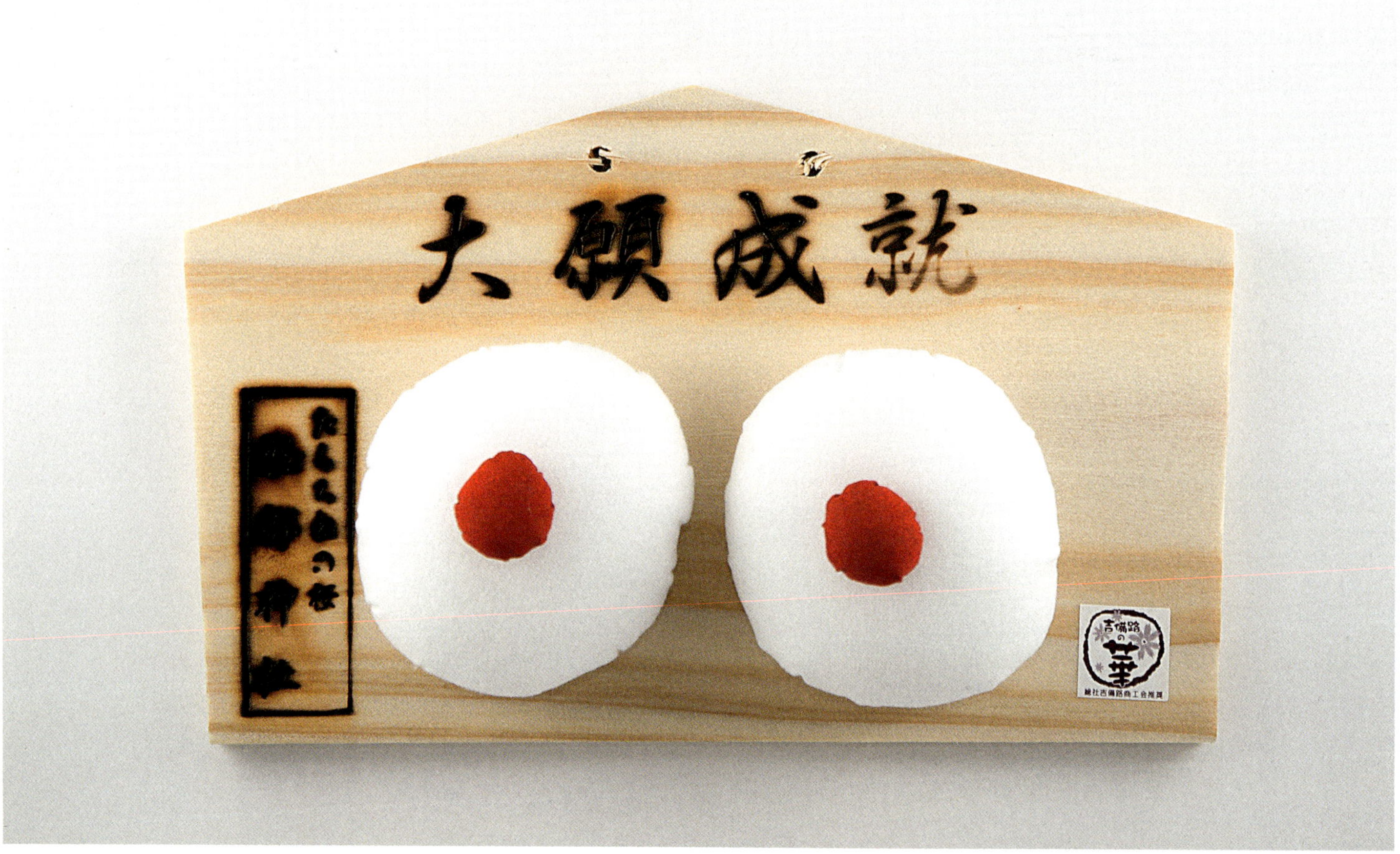

Upper half of the body 上半身 *jōhanshin*

306
Shirochichi Jinja 白乳神社 (near *Kasuga Taisha* 春日大社). Nara, Nara Prefecture. Early 21st century. W. 15.9 cm
The inscriptions read:
上半身婦人病 = *jōhanshin fujinbyō* (women's illnesses of the upper half of the body)
治癒祈願 = *chiyu kigan* (prayer for recovery)

The white colour of the breasts on the *ema* echoes the colour that is mentioned in the name of the shrine (*shiro* = white). The nearby *Akachichi Jinja* (*aka* = red) offers a corresponding *ema* for the lower part of the body (see the entry on *kahanshin* on p.189).

Breasts 乳 *chichi*

307
Karube Jinja 軽部神社. Soja, Okayama Prefecture. Early 21st century. W. 23.6 cm
The inscriptions read:
大願成就 = *daiganjōju* (realisation of a great ambition)
たらちねの桜 = *tarachine no sakura* (mother cherry tree)
軽部神社 = *Karube Jinja*

Karube Jinja was originally a fertility shrine dedicated to *Chichigamisama* 乳神様 (Goddess of Breasts). Nowadays women come there not only to pray for a safe child birth, abundant lactation, or simply for large breasts, but also for the healing of *nyūgan* (breast cancer). The breast imagery may have developed from a cherry tree that apparently had some feature reminiscent of breasts. Two stumps are all that is left of that tree.

308

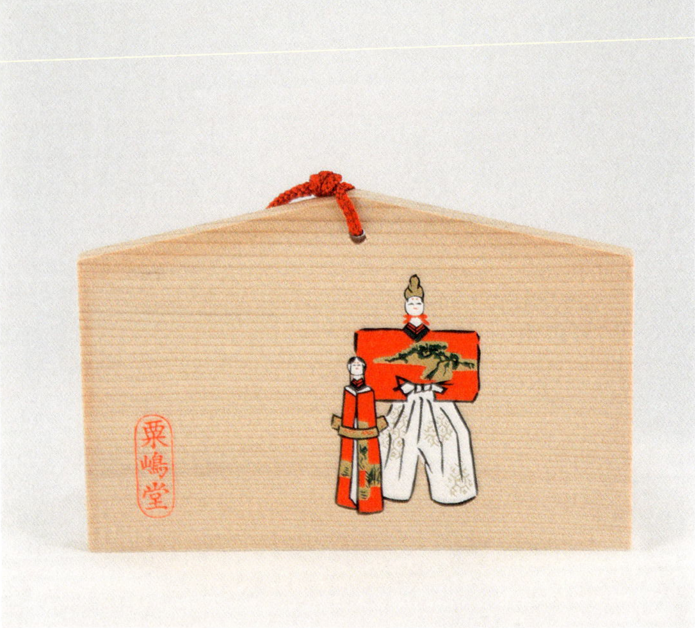

309

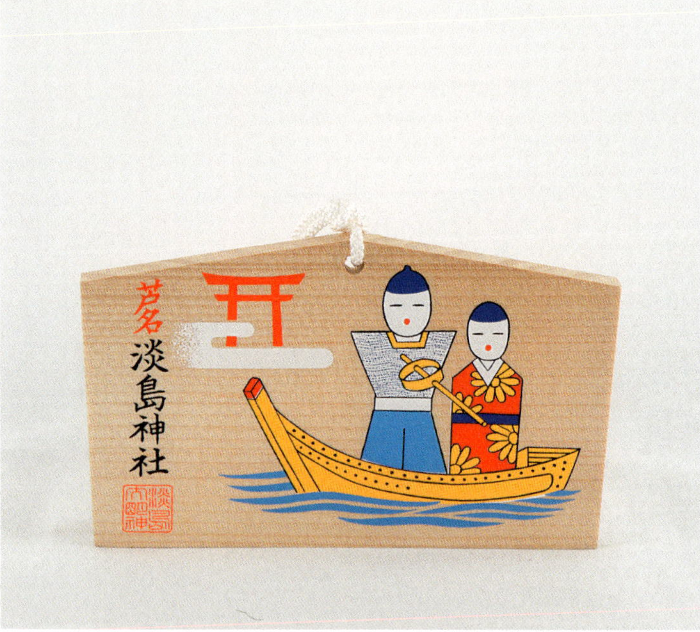

310

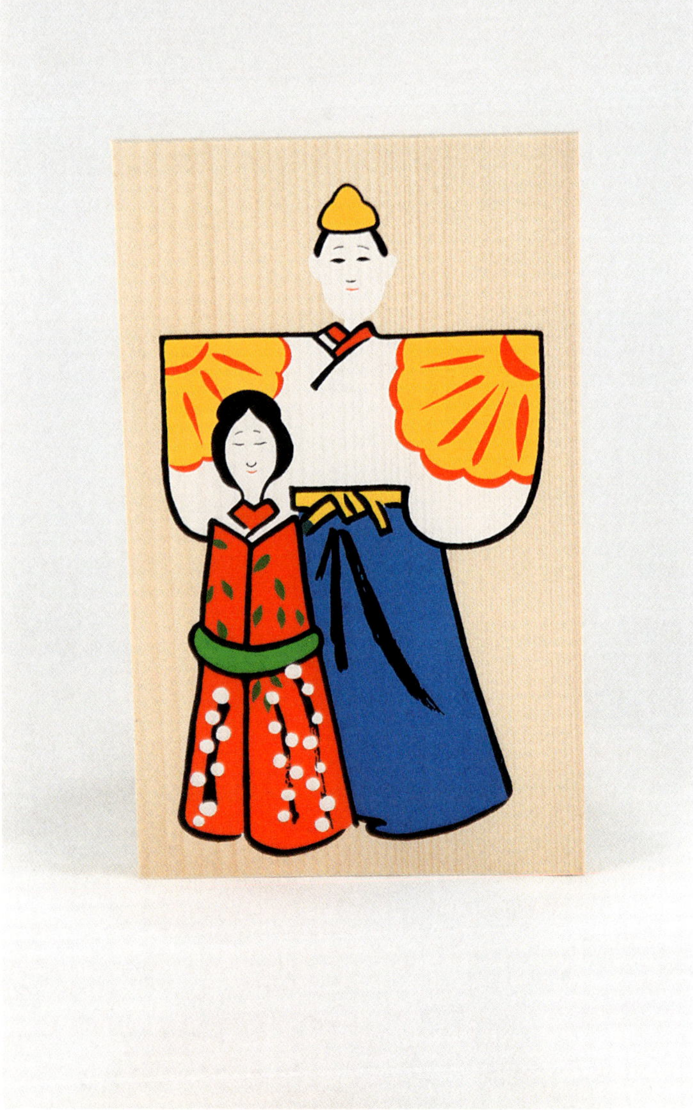

311

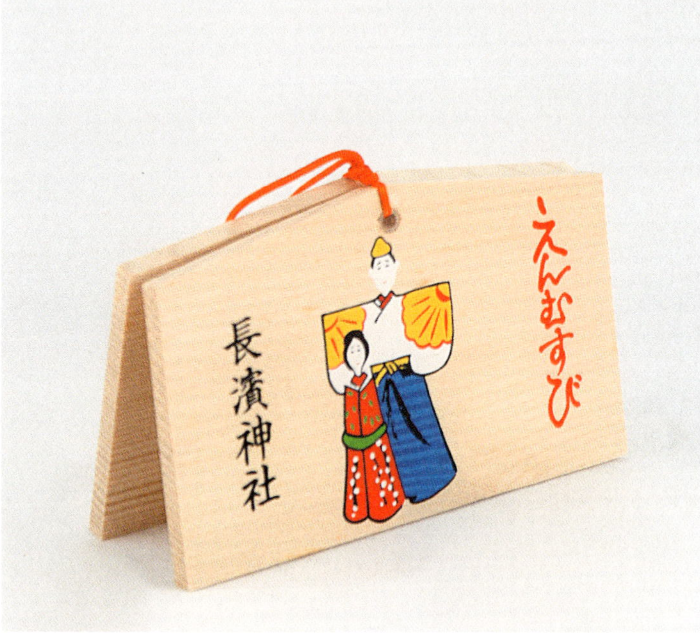

312

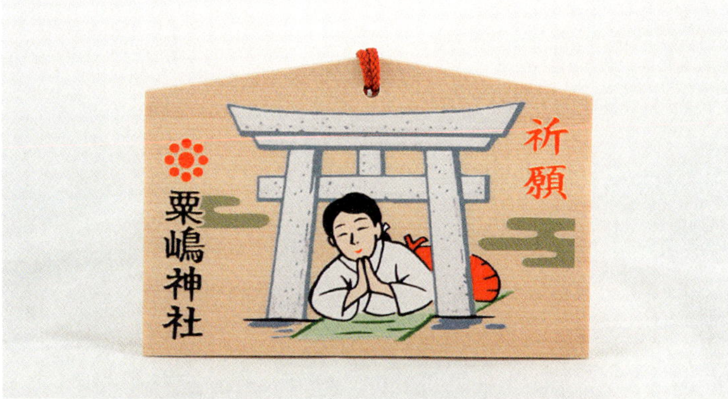

Dolls 雛 *hina*

Awashima shrines and temple halls are prominent among the sanctuaries that offer *ema* with *hina* (dolls) designs for recovery from or prevention of *fujinbyō* (women's illnesses). According to legend, the goddess *Awashima* was the divine consort of *Sumiyoshi Myōjin*, who sent her out to sea after she had become afflicted with *koshike* (a mucous discharge from the female private parts called leucorrhoea). After she had washed up back on shore, she became known as *Awashima Myōjin* and people started to worship her for *fujinbyō* (women's illnesses), *anzan* (easy childbirth) and *kodakara* (the treasure that is children) [AE; KU].

In the early Edo period, the belief in her healing powers was popularised by *gannin bōzu* (wandering monks) who would carry around small shrines and perform prayers for the sake of other people [3].

308
Awashima-dō 粟嶋堂 at *Sōtokuji* 宗徳寺. Shimogyo Ward, Kyoto. Early 21st century. W. 17.5 cm

309
Awashima Jinja 淡島神社. Ashina, Yokosuka, Kanagawa Prefecture. 神奈川県. Early 21st century. W. 16.7 cm
The inscription reads:
芦名淡島神社 = *Ashina Awashima Jinja*

Awashima Jinja in Ashina is a branch shrine of *Awashima Jinja* in Kada, Wakayama Prefecture. Every year on 3 March, the shrine organises a *Hina Matsuri* (Doll Festival): pairs of paper dolls are placed in small boats and floated out to sea. In this *ema* design, one of the dolls holds a *sokonuke hishaku* (bottomless ladle) in remembrance of that part of *Awashima*'s legend where she managed to keep her boat afloat by scooping out inflowing water with a bottomless ladle.

310–311
Ōita Nagahama Jinja 大分長浜神社. Oita, Oita Prefecture. Early 21st century.
310 W. 11.3 cm. 311 W. 13.0 cm.
The inscriptions in 311 read:
えんむすび = *enmusubi* (joining two people together in love/marriage)
大分長浜神社 = *Ōita Nagahama Jinja*

Although this *ema* design of *hina* (dolls) does not come from an *Awashima* shrine, the *ema* in 310 was used for the healing of *fujinbyō* (women's illnesses) in the past [IJ-126; TS-11]. However, as better medical treatments became available, the purpose of the *ema* shifted to *enmusubi* (joining two people together in love/marriage). The shrine currently also offers a special *awase ema* = conjoined *ema* for this latter purpose (see 311).

Mini Shinto shrine archway ミニ鳥居 *mini torii*

312
Awashima Jinja 粟嶋神社. Uto, Kumamoto Prefecture. Early 21st century
The inscriptions read:
祈願 = *kigan* (prayer)
粟嶋神社 = *Awashima Jinja*

This *ema* design shows a *miko* (shrine maiden) crawling under a *mini torii* of only 30 cm high. This act wards off evil and illnesses (especially women's illnesses) and grants *anzan* (easy childbirth) [GG2-2014/02].

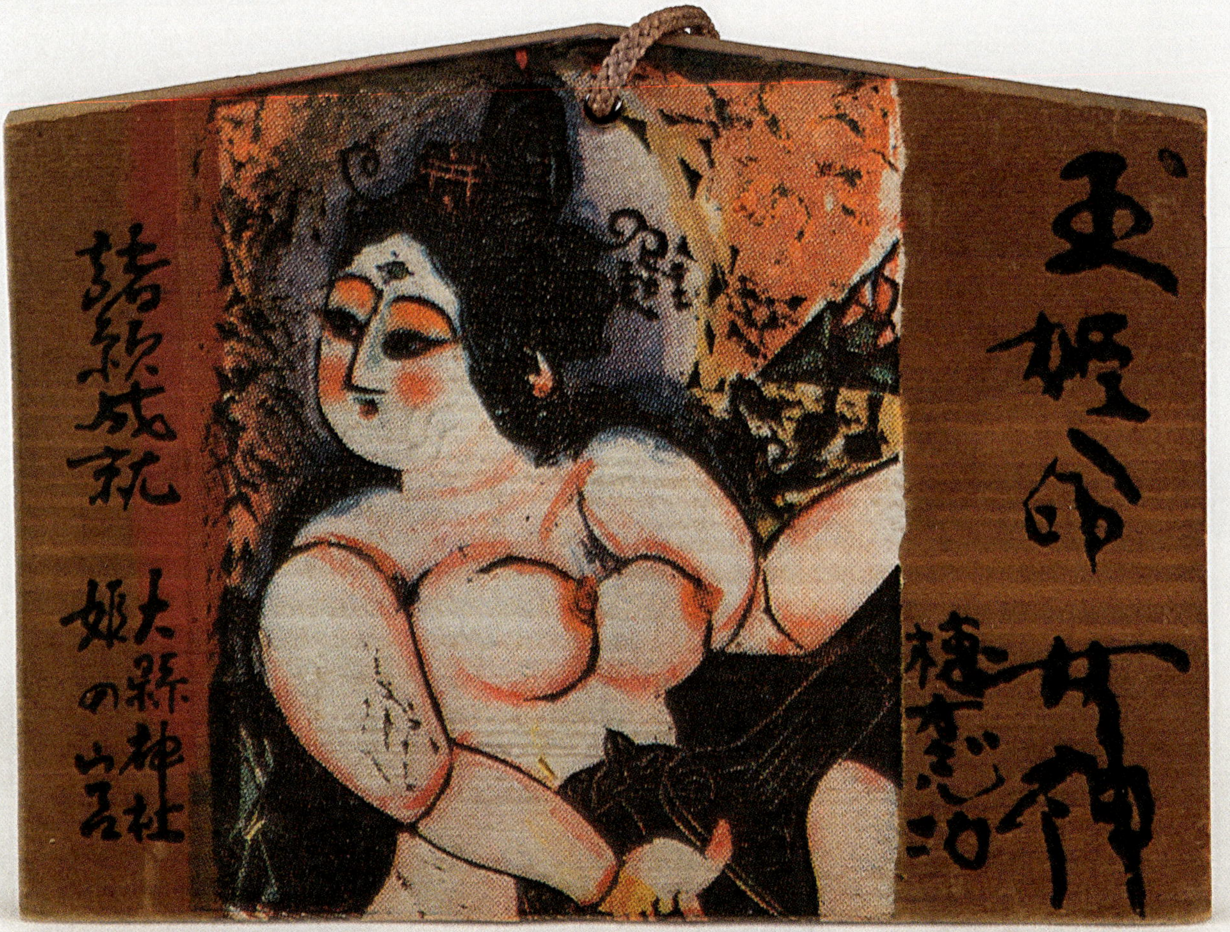
玉姫命
諸願成就
大縣神社
姫の宮

Tamahime-no-mikoto 玉姫命

Ōagata Jinja is known for its female fertility symbols. The main object of worship is a stone in the shape of female private parts. The shrine is paired with the nearby *Tagata Jinja* which is devoted to male fertility. In the *Hime no miya* subshrine of *Ōagata Jinja*, the daughter of *Ōagata* (known as *Tamahime-no-mikoto*) is worshipped as guardian goddess of women. She can be invoked for female illnesses, fertility and easy delivery. Her image on the *ema* was especially created for the shrine by the famous woodblock artist *Munakata Shiko*.

313
Ōagata Jinja 大県神社. Inuyama, Aichi Prefecture. Late 20th century. H. 12.5 cm
The main inscriptions read:
玉姫命女神 = *Tamahimeinochi megami* (goddess)
大県神社 = *Ōagata Jinja*

Additional *ema* designs for women's illnesses (not illustrated here) are:

- **Woman 婦人 (*fujin*). Among the *ema* designs that were hand-painted by *Norihito Yasuda* (Nagoya) in the late 20th century on commission from the Naito Museum of Pharmaceutical Sciences and Industry (Kakamigahara, Gifu Prefecture) is an *ema* design of a *fujin* (woman) for *fujinbyō* (women's illnessess) [NM-Z22669].**
- **Facing foxes 向い狐 (*mukai kitsune*). Among the *ema* designs that were hand-painted by *Norihito Yasuda* (Nagoya) in the late 20th century on commission from the Naito Museum of Pharmaceutical Sciences and Industry (Kakamigahara, Gifu Prefecture) is an *ema* design of foxes facing each other that was inter alia used for *fujinbyō* (women's illnessess) [NM-Z22665].**

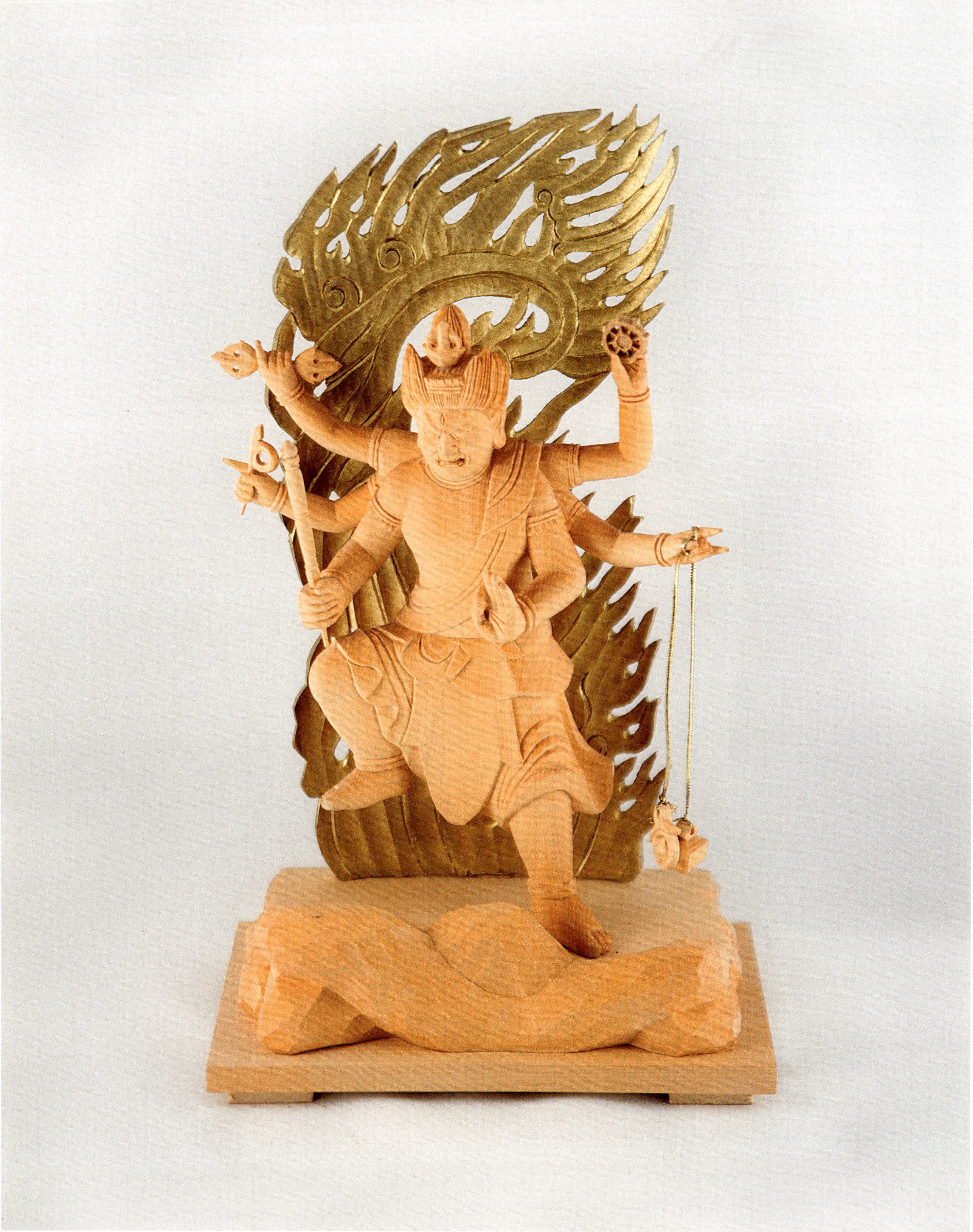

Incontinence
失禁 (*shikkin*)

Background

Japan has not escaped the worldwide trend that the risks of urinary incontinence (*nyōshikkin*) and faecal incontinence (*benshikkin*) increase with advancing age.

314
Wooden statue of *Ususama Myo-ō*. Late 20th or early 21st century. H. 30 cm

This figure of worship can be found at *pokkuridera* (temples for sudden death) where elderly people can pray for an abrupt end to life, when they fear that they will fall chronically ill and will thereby become reliant on the care of their descendants for years.

Ususama is known for his power to purify the unclean. In Japanese Zen and Shingon Buddhism, he is the protective deity of the toilet, which makes him an important deity for those who fear or suffer from incontinence [1].

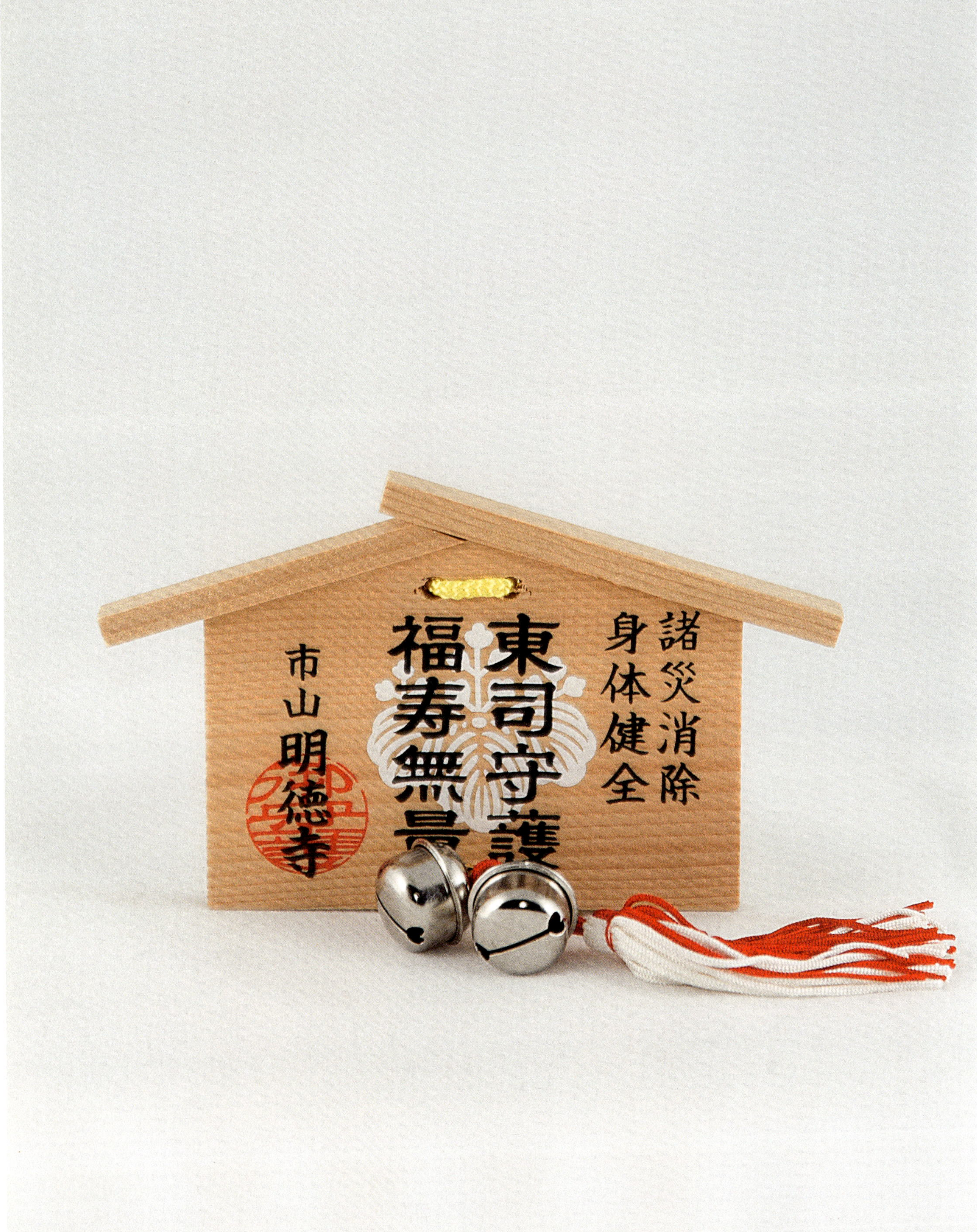
諸災消除
身体健全
東司守護
福寿無量
市山
明徳寺

315
Myōtokuji 明徳寺. Izu, Shizuoka Prefecture.
Late 20th century. W. 10.3 cm
The inscriptions read:
諸災消除 = s*ho sai shōjo* (eradication of various disasters)
身体健全 = s*hintai kenzen* (healthy body)
東司守護 = *tōsu shugo* (protection/protector of the toilet)
福寿無量 = *fukuju muryō* = immeasurable long life and happiness
市山明徳寺 = *Ichiyama Myōtokuji*

Myōtokuji is a major *pokkuridera* (temple of sudden death). Its guardian deity *Ususama Myō-ō* originally offered health and strength for male family members and the prevention of abdominal illnesses, but now elderly people come and pray for protection against genital illnesses and against becoming incontinent. This special prayer is called *omatagi*. *Ususama* is accommodated in a temple building called *tōsu* (toilet in a Zen monastery). Although the elderly pray to ask for good health for as long as possible, their prayer often implies that they want to die without suffering from long-term illness so that their family members will not have to help them to the toilet and to change their nappies (cf. the *ema* for the prevention of senility on p.167) [2].

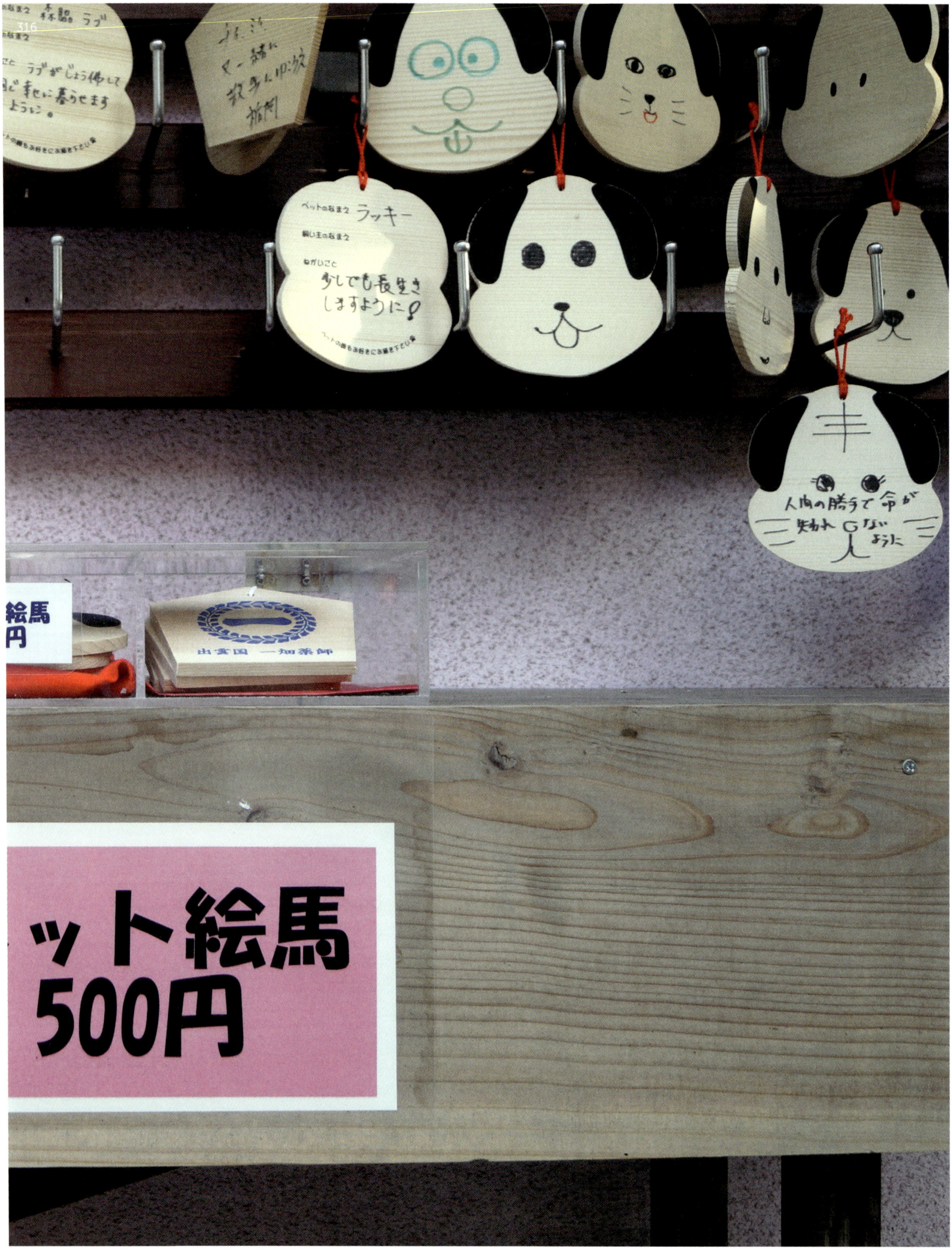
ラッキー
少しでも長生きしますように!
出雲国 一畑薬師
ット絵馬
500円

5 Animal health 動物の健康 (*Dōbutsu no kenkō*)

316
Ema at *Ichibata Yakushi* in Izumo (Shimane Prefecture)

The temple is known for healing human eye problems. According to its foundation legend, the blind mother of a fisherman regained her eyesight after her son had prayed piously to a miraculous statue of *Yakushi* (Medicine Buddha) that he had found in the sea [RT-20]. The temple has a *dōbutsu reien* (pet cemetery) and offers *ema* for pets with the design of a blank dog's head in which the petitioner has to fill in the eyes, nose and mouth.

Domesticated animals serve various purposes in present-day Japan. Dogs and cats have become important as companion animals. Horses are mainly kept for racing and only to a minor degree for recreational horseback riding. Cattle, pigs and poultry are bred for the production of meat, milk and eggs. In the late 20th century, livestock production was the fastest-growing sector in Japanese agriculture. This is in sharp contrast to the situation in ancient times. After the introduction of Buddhism in the 6th century AD, imperial edicts frequently forbade the consumption of meat from cattle, horses, dogs and poultry. Horses were used primarily for military purposes, while cattle were employed to carry weights and to haul vehicles and equipment [1].

317

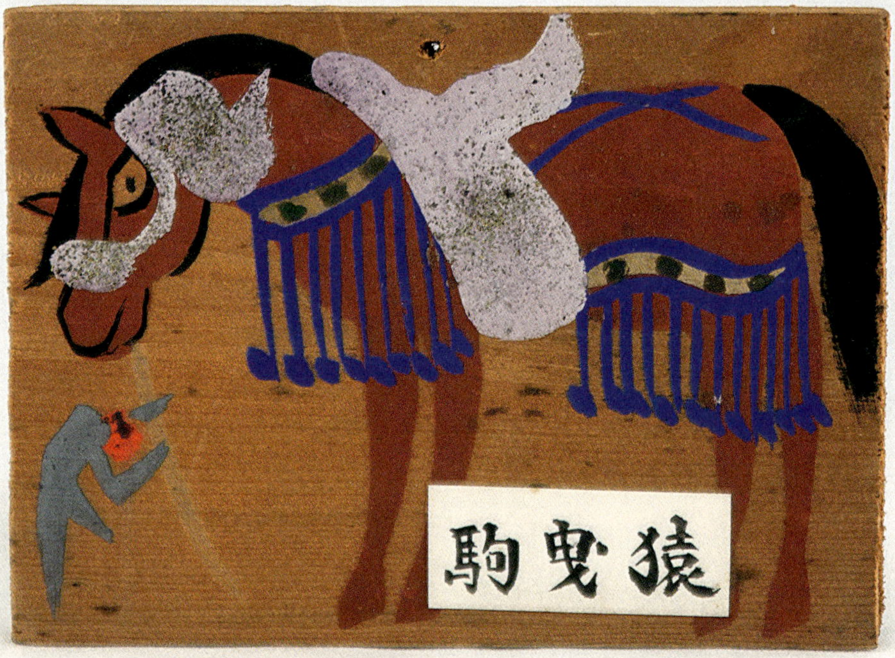

318

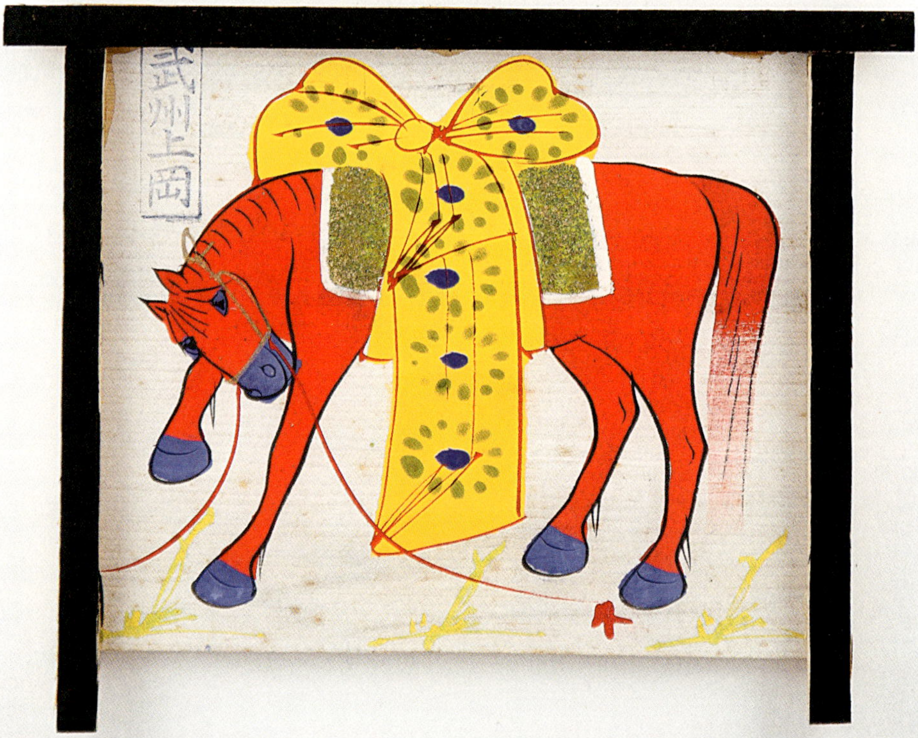

Horses and cows/oxen
馬や牛 (*uma ya ushi*)

Background

Traditional Japanese figures of worship have played a similar role in veterinary folk medicine as they have done in human healthcare. An important guardian figure for horses whose statues are found in many places in Japan is the Buddhist goddess *Batō Kannon* (Horsehead *Kannon*). She has the head of a horse in her headdress, and farmers would pray to her for the safety of their horses and cattle. She not only protects working animals in this life, but may also appease their spirits thereafter. Another Buddhist figure who can act as a guardian for cattle is *Dainichi Nyorai*. He serves as the main figure of worship for Japanese esoteric Buddhist sects (such as Shingon Buddhism), but can also be invoked for the health of cattle by offering him a pair of straw sandals (which were once widely used in Japan to protect the hooves of cattle) [MS; 2].

The Shinto deity for horses is called *Umagami* (lit. Horse Deity). At *Umagami Jinja* (in the precincts of *Nagara Jinja*, Otsu, Shiga Prefecture), *umagake* (horse coverings) would be presented to ward off the god *Daiba*, who could possess or strike horses, especially when they were outside the shelter of their stables. The equivalent deity for cattle is known as *Ushigami* (lit. Cow/Ox Deity). He was venerated as protector of the land and would receive small straw figures of *ushi* (cows, oxen) in festivals that were held in his honour. In some districts of Kyushu (southeast Japan), glittering abalone shells were hung in the entrances to stables or cattle sheds as a charm to protect horses and cattle [3].

The monkey was considered as an important guardian of horses, with the power to maintain their health and cure their illnesses. This is reflected in a large number of *ema* from various historical periods and regions of Japan with the design of *sarukomahiki* (monkey leading a horse) [4].

A noteworthy recent observation is the offering of *ema* at *Sōma Kodaka Jinja* (Minamisoma, Fukushima Prefecture) after the Fukushima Daiichi nuclear disaster. Since local livestock had to be killed because of contamination with radioactivity, *ema* with livestock designs were presented at the shrine to offer condolences to the dead animals.

317
Ema portraying *sarukomahiki* (monkey leading a horse). Mid-20th century. W. 14.0 cm

This design goes back to the second half of the 8th century and is among the oldest *ema* designs that have been discovered so far [5]. An *ema* with the *sarukomahiki* design is still offered for sale by *Sunosaki Jinja* (Nagoya, Aichi Prefecture). An early source claims that the design embodied lust and was therefore probably used at *Sunosaki Jinja* to resist the temptations of the flesh [FS-17].

Ema designs

Horse 馬 *(uma)*

The horse often appears on *ema* as a zodiac animal. However, certain *ema* with this design served to pray for the health of horses.

318
Myōanji 妙安寺. Higashimatsuyama, Saitama Prefecture. Late 20th century. W. 18.0 cm
The inscription reads:
武州上岡 = *Bushū Kamioka*

Myōanji is one of the three great *Batō Kannon* temples in the Kanto region of Honshu Island. It is situated at a location formerly known as *Bushū Kamioka*. The enshrined deity is called *Kamioka no Batō Kannon* (Horsehead *Kannon*). In the past, *ema* and *sasa* (bamboo grass) would be presented to her on a special festive day in February to protect horses and cattle against the evil god *Daiba*. Horse owners could dedicate an *ema* to the temple to pray for the health of their horses and could nail the bamboo grass at the entrance to the stable or give it to a sick horse. On 19 February of every year, the temple still organises an annual *ema ichi* (*ema* market) where *Bushū Kamioka no ema* (votive boards of *Bushū Kamioka*) are sold to anyone with a special interest in horses [TS-29,33; GG1-2011/08; 6].

319

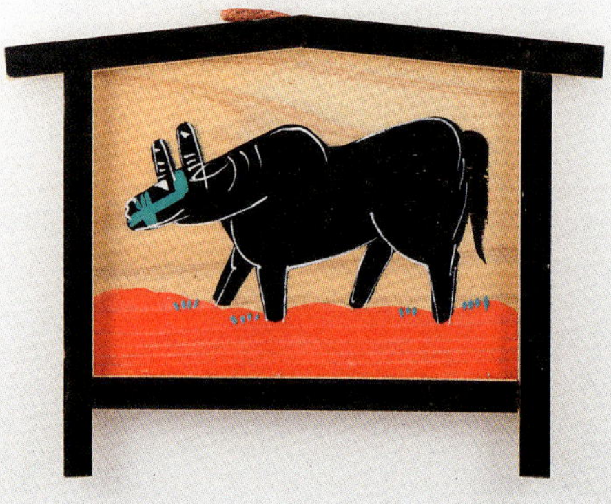

321

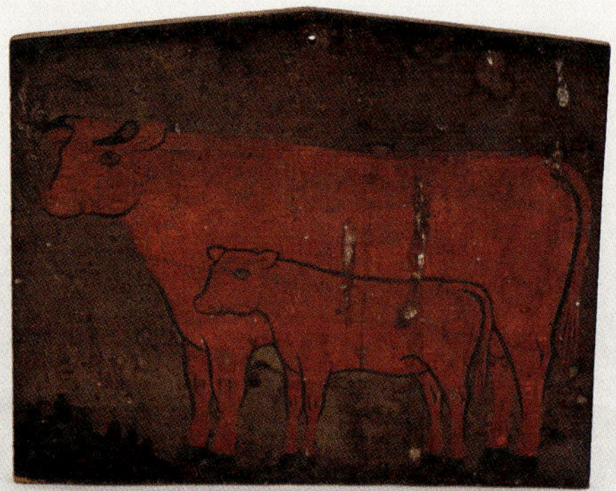

320

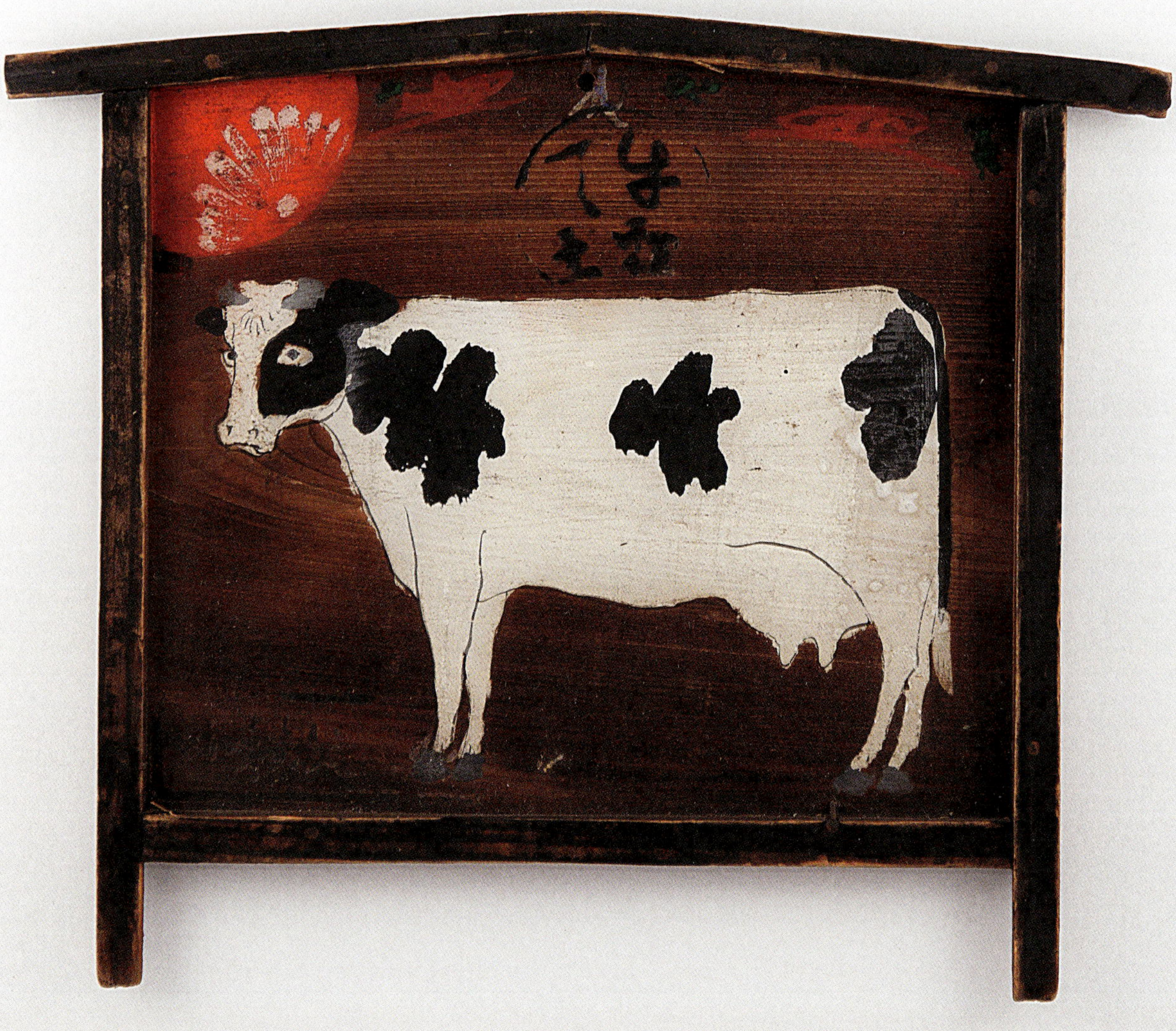

Cow/ox 牛 *(ushi)*

Ushi (cows/oxen) often appear on present-day *ema* as a zodiac animal. In the past, when cattle were still an important means of transport, this design was also used to pray for the health and safety of cattle [TS-30].

319

Hand-painted reproduction for a Japanese club of *ema* collectors called *Nihon Ema Tomo no Kai* (Friends of Japanese Ema Society). No.322. Late 20th century. W. 17.7cm. Associated with *Oku Fudōson* (Fukui, Fukui Prefecture)

According to the accompanying description, farmers regarded cattle as manifestations of local deities. The *ema* was used for human illnesses and for the prevention and eradication of *gyūeki* (cattle epidemics such as rinderpest). Rinderpest was known as *tachi* in Japan. The first two documented outbreaks there occurred in the 17th century and each cost the lives of hundreds of thousands of cattle [7].

320

Origin unclear. Early to mid-20th century. W. 17.9 cm

This *ema* design may have served to ask for protection of cattle, because in another example (not illustrated here) the inscription above the back of the animal can be read as 牛頭天王 (*Gozu Tennō* = literally Ox-Headed Heavenly King). This combinatory Shinto/Buddhist deity has been identified with the Shinto deity *Susanoo* who features in the legend of *Somin Shōrai* (see the entry on p.65). *Gozu Tennō* is inter alia worshipped at *Yasaka Jinja* (Kyoto) where he is connected to the annual *Gion* festival [KU]. This ritual was organised for the first time in the 9th or 10th century A.D. to appease *Gozu Tennō*, because a severe outbreak of pestilence was attributed to his anger (see the entry on p.53). In popular belief, *Gozu Tennō* transformed from an epidemic-causing deity into a tutelary protector with the power to ward off evil spirits and epidemics (see the entry on *Tsushima Jinja* on p.27).

Cow and calf 牛と子牛 *(ushi to koushi)*

Sanctuaries that still offer *ema* with a cow and calf design (not illustrated here) include:

- *Kasumi Jinja* 霞神社 (Takaharu, Miyazaki Prefecture). This shrine also offers *ema* for other types of farm animals, such as horses and poultry.
- *Batō Kannondō Hachimangaoka* 八幡ヶ丘馬頭観音堂 at *Kōsenji* (Ebino, Miyazaki Prefecture). On 8 May, the sanctuary organises *Batō Kannon Matsuri* (*Batō Kannon* Festival) where livestock farmers can pray for the prosperity of their cattle, pigs or chickens. Since cars have replaced farm animals as major means of transport, one can nowadays also ask for traffic safety.

321

From the locality of Hashinocho Kamaishi (Iwate Prefecture). Early to mid-20th century. W. 18.7 cm

Breeders of *tankakugyū* (short-horned cattle) in the locality of Hashinocho Kamaishi (Iwate Prefecture) hung this *ema* design in their stables for good health of the cows and for easy delivery and healthy growth of the calves. The custom fell into disuse in the late 1960s [8].

322

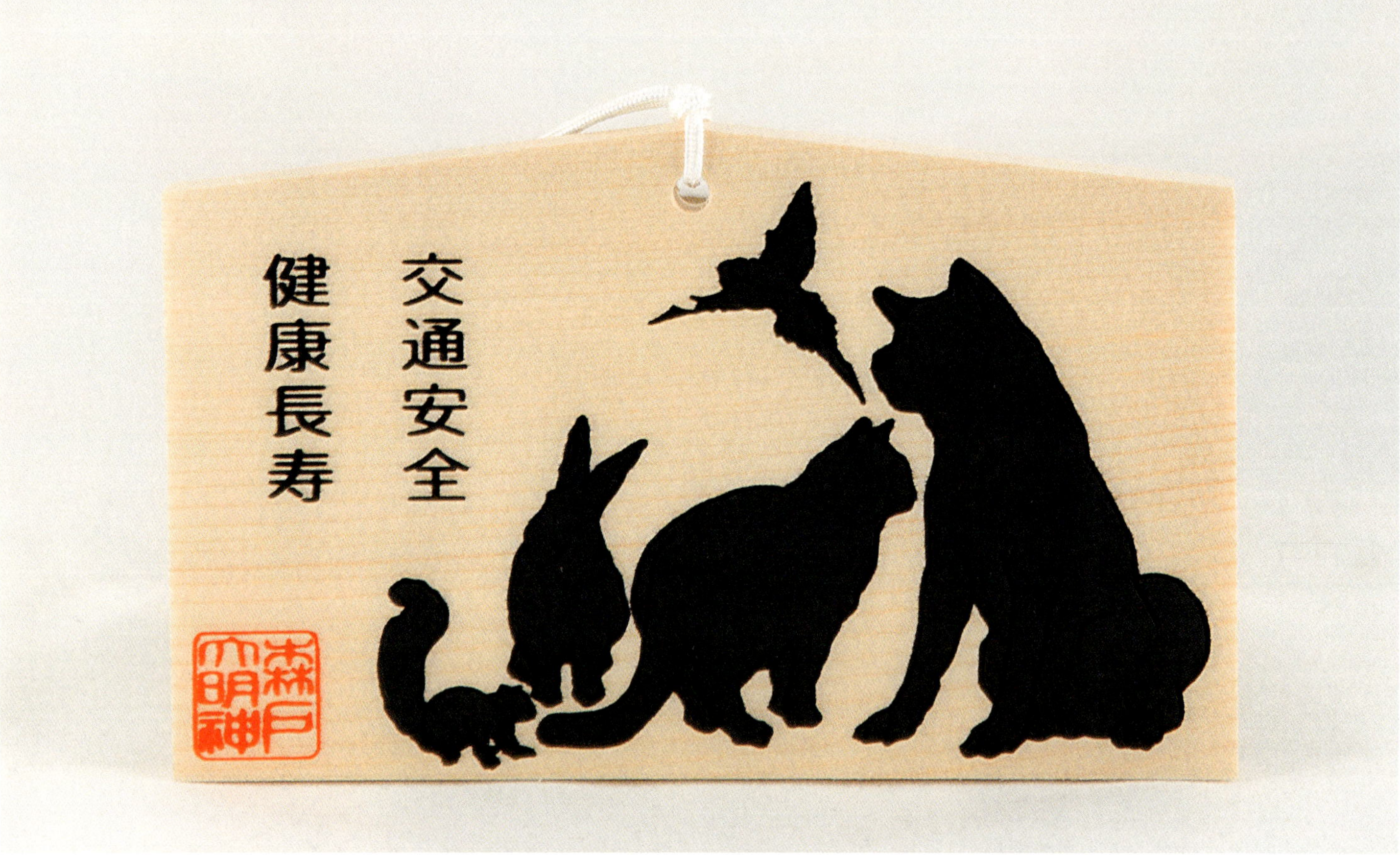

323

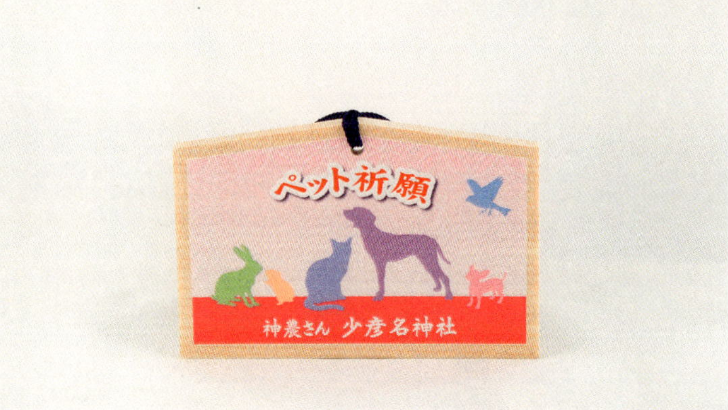

324

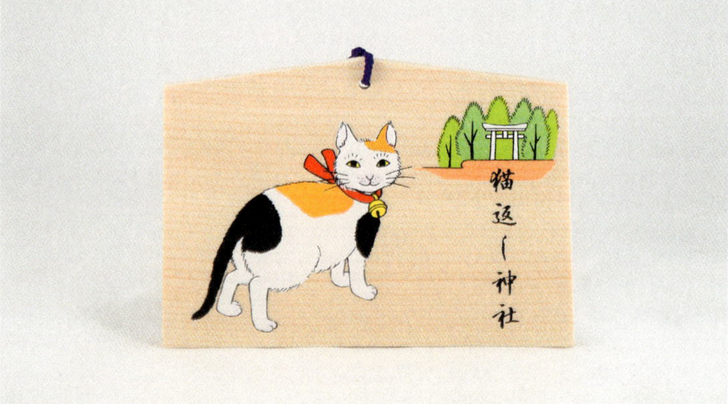

325

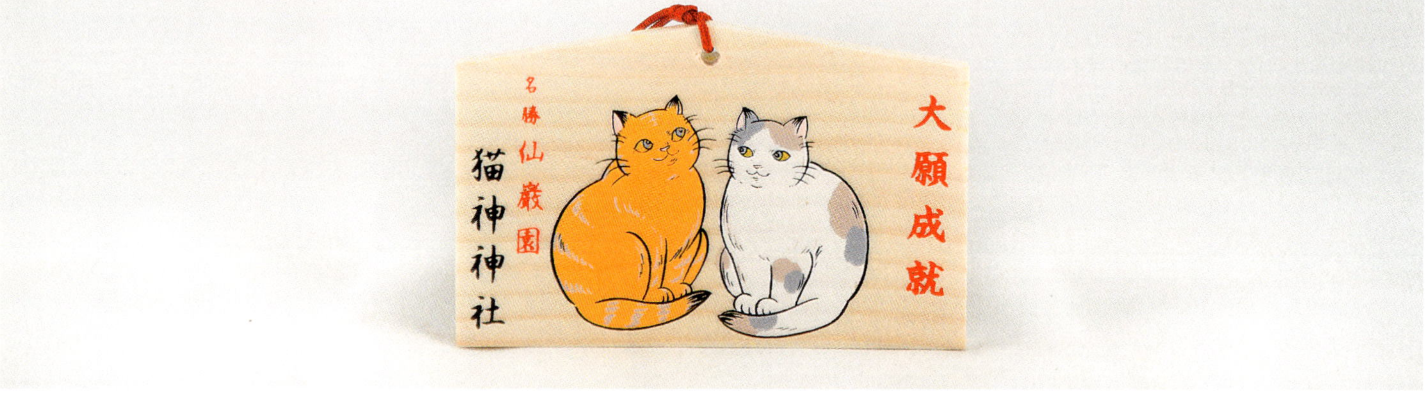

Pet animals
ペット (*petto*)

Background

In the past, dogs and cats were mostly considered to be community residents. In the late 20th century, however, Japan saw a marked increase in individual pet ownership. It is estimated that there are now more pets in Japan than children under the age of fifteen. As part of this development, a new manifestation of the goddess *Kannon* gained importance: *Dōbutsu Kannon*, who is devoted to the care of suffering animals and acts as a patron of dead pets.

Her name reflects a change from fear for *chikushō* (beasts), which could become malevolent spirits in the afterlife, to love for *dōbutsu* (animals), which become benevolent spiritual protectors after death. Special cemeteries and *petto kuyō* (memorial services for pets that may be abridged versions of rituals for humans) have become a profitable industry in Japan, in which *Dōbutsu Kannon* offers comfort to the grieving pet owners. A source from 2006 counted over 900 pet cemeteries in Japan, about 120 of which were operated by Buddhist temples [MS; 9].

Ema designs

Pets ペット *(petto)*

Pet-related *ema* may be presented as prayers for the health of a living pet. At a pet cemetery, they may also be used to ask the spirit of one's deceased pet for a kind of protection that one would expect from human ancestors. Pet spirits rank below human ancestors, however, in a position that is somewhat comparable to that of an aborted foetus (which can also be addressed through *ema*). Aborted foetuses are marginal members of the household, because they are deceased family members (hence ancestors) but have never lived as humans. A difference between pets and aborted foetuses is that the former usually have no reason for resentment which makes them good candidates to become protective spirits [10].

322
Morito Jinja 森戸神社. Hayama, Kanagawa Prefecture. Early 21st century. W. 14.3 cm
The inscriptions read:
交通安全 = *kōtsū anzen* (traffic safety)
健康長寿 = *kenkō chōju* (health and longevity)

Although the two inscriptions refer to well-being in general, this is an *ema* for *petto* (pet animals) that is associated with *petto no shugojin* (guardian deity of pet animals).

323
Sukunahikona Jinja 少彦名神社. Chuo Ward, Osaka. Early 21st century. W. 13.7 cm
The inscriptions read:
ペット祈願 = *petto kigan* (prayer for pet)
神農さん = *Shinnō-san*
少彦名神社 = *Sukunahikona Jinja*

Shinnō is the Japanese name of *Shennong*, the Chinese god of medicine. He is enshrined at *Sukunahikona Jinja*. Cf. the entry on *Sukunahikona* on p.43.

324
Nekogaeshi Jinja 猫返し神社 (in precincts of *Kokage Jinja* 蚕影神社). Tachikawa, Tokyo Metropolis. Early 21st century. W. 15.8 cm
The inscription reads:
猫返し神社 = *Nekogaeshi Jinja*

The name of the shrine is composed of the words *neko* (cat) and *kaeshi* (return). The shrine can be visited to pray for the safe return and health of a missing cat.

325
Nekogami Jinja 猫神神社. Kagoshima, Kagoshima Prefecture. Early 21st century. W. 13.1 cm
The inscriptions read:
大願成就 = *daiganjōju* (fulfilment of all wishes)
名勝仙巌園 = *meishō Senganen* (place of scenic beauty: Senganen = park in Kagoshima)
猫神神社 = *Nekogami Jinja*

The name of the shrine is composed of the words for cat (*neko*) and for Shinto deity (*kami*).

The cats on this *ema* and two ceramic cats in the centre of the shrine refer to its *engi* (foundation legend). At the end of the 16th century, a Japanese lord went to Korea on a military mission. He took seven cats with him, only two of which would survive the long journey. He used the cats as clocks by looking at their pupils (which changed with the sun) to determine the time of day [GG2-2013/04].

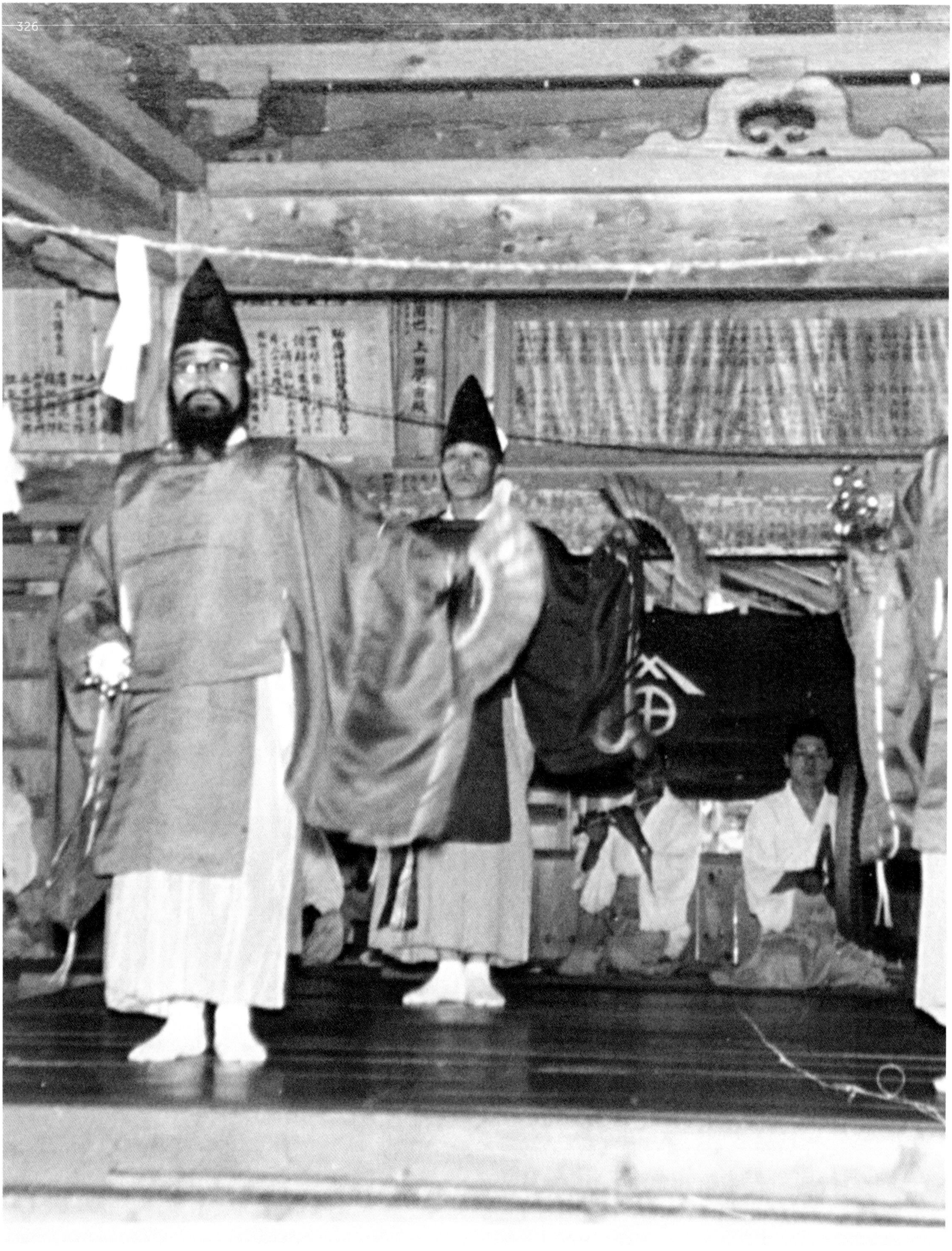

6 Commentary 解説 (*Kaisetsu*)

326
Shrines and temples in Japan do not only offer options for self-care but also perform professional healing services for a fee. According to an annotation on the reverse, this photograph represents a ritual dance for *byōki heiyu* (recovery from illness) that was associated with the ancient Shinto deity *Sai no Kami* and took place somewhere in Nagasaki Prefecture.

The offering of *ema* at Japanese shrines and temples to ask or to thank deities for *goriyaku* (divine favours) has remained a tradition up to this very day. Among the most prominent purposes are health-related *hito no isshō* (human life issues) and *byōki heiyu* (recovery from illness) or *byōki no yobō* (prevention of illness). These benefits are not restricted to humans but extend to *kachiku* (domestic animals). People may even go so far as to apologise to the animal for having it killed or to pray for its *boke fūji* (prevention of senility), *enmei* (prolonging life) and *pokkuri* (sudden death).

HITO NO ISSHŌ (HUMAN LIFE ISSUES)	
Purpose of health-related *ema*	**Possible association(s) with biomedical morbidity and mortality patterns**
Kodakara (the treasure that is children)	Infertility from sexually transmitted disease
Anzan (easy childbirth)	Maternal death from bleeding or infection after childbirth
Kosodate (child rearing)	High risk of newborn and infant death

Table 8 Potential associations between the purposes of health-related *ema* and biomedical disease patterns [1]

BYŌKI HEIYU (RECOVERY FROM ILLNESS/DISEASE)	
Purpose of health-related *ema*	**Possible association(s) with biomedical morbidity and mortality patterns**
Eye illnesses	Blindness from infectious disease (trachoma, gonorrhoea, smallpox)
Sakamatsuge (ingrown eyelashes)	Trachoma
Feet/leg illnesses	Beriberi Syphilis
Zutsū (headache) Symptoms of *hara* (abdomen/stomach) *Katakori* (neck/shoulder pain)	Depression (Japanese depressed patients in primary care mention headaches, abdominal distress and neck/shoulder pain more often than their US counterparts) (see p.159)
Palsy	Cerebrovascular disease (stroke)
Respiratory illnesses	Infectious lung disease (tuberculosis, influenza, pneumonia, whooping cough)
Skin illnesses	Can be a symptom of a systemic infectious disease (such as smallpox, syphilis, tuberculosis)
Localised loss of skin pigmentation (leukoderma)	Secondary syphilis

As indicated by some inscriptions on the *ema*, their presentation is known as *hōnō* (dedication), and *hōnōgaku* is an alternative term for these votive tablets. *Hōnō* goes back to ancient times, just like practices that include praying, visiting a sanctuary to thank the enshrined deity for answering one's prayer (*reimairi*), observing dietary abstinence after praying for a divine favour (*tachimono*), and purification by cold water prior to prayer (*mizugori*) [KU].

The health-related purposes of *ema* are the focus of this commentary. When one regards such *ema*, one has to distinguish between the direct meaning of their design (who or what is being represented on the front of the *ema*) and their ultimate purpose (for what benefit or thanks-giving is the *ema* presented to the sanctuary). This is important, because the same *ema* design may vary over time and may relate to different benefits in different locations (and even in the same location). For instance, the *ema* design of a *tako* (octopus) has served, at one time and place or another, for large catches and for such medical purposes as *kodomo no hōsōyoke* (protection of children from smallpox), *fujinbyō* (women's illnesses), *shōnibyō* (childhood illnesses), *ganbyō* (eye illnesses), *dacchō* (abdominal hernias), *haremono* (tumours, swellings), *ibo* (warts), papules and rashes, and cough (cf. the sections on digestive illnesses and on skin illnesses) [IH1-155; TS-7; IH2-90; GK]. It is also possible for an individual worshipper to write a message on the reverse that is unrelated to the purpose of the design on the front.

Continuity and change

The previous parts have made clear that contemporary Japanese *ema* cover a fairly wide range of health-related issues. Many of these designs and purposes were already well-established in the first half of the 20th century and have undergone little or no development since then [FS; HD; AE; IH1; KJ].

Besides this continuity, it is also evident that certain new health-related *ema* were developed in the course of the 20th century for modern medical and social concerns, such as protection from *eizu* (AIDS), *mizuko* (apology to a water child = aborted child), *pokkuri* (prayer for sudden death), and *petto no kenkō* (pet health). Furthermore, some sanctuaries shifted their attention from old to new medical problems in conformity with changing disease patterns [EO-153; RT-57]. For instance, the annual *Yasurai* festival in Kyoto was once organised to exorcise epidemic-spreading *ekijin* (evil spirits) but is nowadays profiled as an opportunity to pray for good health in general.

Biomedical perspective

A striking property of health-related *ema* is that they are often aimed at a symptomatic complaint (e.g., palsy, headache, cough) or broad class of complaints (e.g., stomach illnesses, eye illnesses, female illnesses) rather than at one or more biomedical diagnoses. When such complaints are

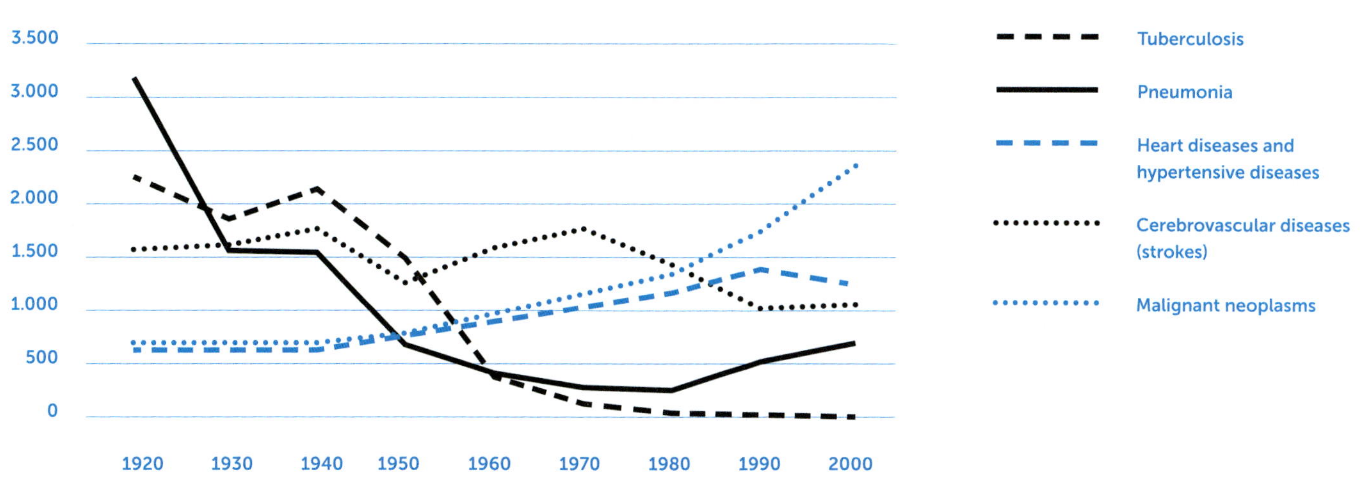

Figure 2 Changes in annual death rates (per million inhabitants) from major causes of death in Japan in the period between 1920 and 2000.
Some caution is required when comparing different years directly due to potential revisions in the classifications of causes of death.

Based on: Japan's experiences in public health and medical systems: towards improving public health and medical systems in developing countries. Tokyo, Japan International Cooperation Agency, 2005: Chapter 1 and Appendix
Available at: https://www.jica.go.jp/jica-ri/IFIC_and_JBICI-Studies/english/publications/reports/study/topical/health/index.html [accessed 27 May 2016]

compared to pre-war mortality patterns in Japan, however, it is possible to suggest several possible associations between the former and the latter (Table 8).

Differences with epidemiological patterns

What stands out most from a biomedical point of view is not so much what is present in the range of health-related *ema* designs but what is infrequent or even missing. In the 20th century, mortality patterns in Japan shifted significantly from communicable causes to non-communicable diseases (see Figure 2 for examples). This shift is only partially reflected in the *ema* designs that are currently available. The number of designs for cancer (*gan*) is not particularly abundant for such a high-ranking category of diseases. Internet searches have not yielded *ema* designs specifically aimed at heart diseases (*kokoro shikkan*), hypertensive diseases (*kōketsuatsusei shikkan*) or cerebrovascular diseases (*nōkekkan shikkan*). One type of *ema* design (*kabocha* = pumpkin) is used, inter alia, for protection against palsy (*chūfū*) and can thus be indirectly associated with cerebrovascular diseases (see p.167). Another *ema* design (*Niō* statues) comes from a temple where visitors may crawl between the legs of a *Niō* statue to prevent of stroke (*nōsocchū*), subarachnoid haemorrhage (*kumomakukashukketsu*) and paralysis (*mahi*). It cannot be inferred, however, that this *ema* is used only or specifically for cerebrovascular afflictions, as an inscription on the *ema* refers to the much broader concept of bodily health (*shintai kenzen*) (see p.143).

Chronic condition	Availability of corresponding *ema*
Hearing loss	As *ema* for *mimi byōki* (ear illnesses)
Heart failure	No
Hypertension	No
Coronary artery disease	No
Atrial fibrillation	No
Osteoarthritis	Not as such but as *ema* for musculoskeletal illnesses
Osteoporosis	No
Stroke	Not as such but as *ema* for *chūfū* (palsy)
Dementia	As *ema* for *boke* (senility)
Depression	No (but *ema* are available for certain somatic complaints of Japanese depressed patients: abdominal distress, headache and neck/shoulder pain) [5]
Chronic obstructive pulmonary disease	Not as such (*ema* are available for cough and asthma, but not for COPD-related dyspnoea with cough)
Pressure ulcers	No
Diabetes mellitus	No (but *ema* for eye illnesses could be used for the late eye complications of diabetes)
Urinary incontinence	As *ema* for *shimo no sewa ni naranai* (to go to the lavatory by oneself in old age)
Chronic renal failure	No

Table 9 Availability of *ema* for fifteen chronic conditions selected for their effects on health and functioning in ageing populations [4]

A similar picture emerges when the highest-ranking Japanese causes of disability-adjusted life years (DALYs) are considered [2]. The number one cause (lower back pain) corresponds directly to an *ema* purpose (*yōtsū*), the second cause (cerebrovascular disease) only indirectly (see above), and the third one (ischemic heart disease) not at all [3]. Links with biomedical patterns are also partial, when the purposes of health-related *ema* are juxtaposed to chronic conditions of major concern in ageing societies, such as diabetes mellitus (Table 9).

Reasons for divergence

Why do the health benefits of *ema* not correspond one-to-one to current epidemiological patterns? A number of possible reasons may have contributed to this phenomenon:

1 Health-related benefits are not biomedical concepts

As pointed out above, health-related benefits tend to focus on complaints in lay terms and not on biomedical diagnostic labels. These lay terms are often imprecise and it can be difficult to find an equivalent biomedical term (Table 10). This also applies to terms that are used for illness patterns in traditional Japanese medicine (*kanpōyaku* or *kanpō* in short). The same patient with watery diarrhoea may be diagnosed as *kakuran* by a *kanpō* doctor and as a cholera sufferer by a biomedical doctor, but this does not mean that these two concepts are equal to each other. By definition, *kakuran* focuses on a pattern of symptoms (watery diarrhoea), whereas cholera always refers to a specific bacterial cause (*Vibrio cholera*) in a biomedical context. Generally speaking, a biomedical diagnosis remains stable during the course of a disease (unless it was the wrong diagnosis initially), whereas a *kanpō* pattern may change over time into a different pattern of symptoms.

2 Stability of ema designs and purposes over time

The literature on religious healing in Japan emphasises that health-related benefits were sometimes adapted to changing medical or social needs (e.g., asthma instead of flu and cancer instead of boils) [EO-149; RT-57]. *Hōsōgami* (the Japanese deity of smallpox) would spread epidemics of smallpox (*hōsō*) but could also be invoked to prevent or mitigate such epidemics. Although smallpox ceased to be endemic in Japan in 1951 [7], he is still worshipped at *Honkōji* (Ichikawa City, Chiba Prefecture) to pray for *kodomo no seichō* (growth of children). Such adaptations may even bring the usefulness of a figure of worship or *ema* design completely outside the health-related realms of *byōki no kaifuku* (recovery from illness) and *hito no isshō* (human life issues). An *ema* example is the representation of *hina* (dolls) that served in the past for the healing of *fujinbyō* (women's illnesses), but are now used for *enmusubi* = joining two people together in love/marriage (see the entry on *hina* dolls on p.193).

However, such changes have apparently not been the rule. Many health-related *ema* designs and purposes were already well-established in the first half of the 20th century and remained largely stable in its second half. As a result, they may be associated with old epidemiological patterns

Japanese term	Meaning
Te	Hand, hands, arm or arms (depending on context)
Ashi	Foot, feet, leg or legs (depending on context)
Hara	Refers to the area of the stomach and abdomen
Shaku and *senki*	Refer to disorders causing stomach, intestinal, or back pain. *Shaku* seems to have been used for more acute problems and *senki* for more chronic conditions.
Katakori	Can be roughly translated as neck/shoulder discomfort or neck/shoulder pain, but there is no English term which has precisely the same meaning.
Yonaki	Sleep-related night-time crying of infants and young children. It occurs most often after midnight, when infants have been asleep for some time, whereas colics tend to peak in the late afternoon and early evening.
Kannomushi	Stands for short-temperedness, nervousness and convulsions in children. In the past, it was attributed to a *mushi* (bug, worm) thought to cause or increase *kan* (temper, nerves).

Table 10 Japanese health-related terms for which it is difficult to offer an equivalent biomedical label [6]

Sanctuary	Benefit offered
Nariaiji 成相寺 (Miyazu, Kyoto Prefecture)	Sells a *yubiwa mamori* (finger ring charm) which inter alia lowers blood pressure [GG2-2013/11]
Fushigi Fudōin 不思議不動院 (Kita Ward, Kyoto)	Can be visited for *hone no byōki chiyu* (healing of bone disease)
Meguro Ōtori Jinja 目黒の大鳥神社 (Meguro Ward, Tokyo)	Offers benefits concerning *tōnyōbyō* (diabetes mellitus) and *seikatsushūkan-byō* (lifestyle diseases) [GK]
Rakuyaji 櫟野寺 (Koka, Shiga Prefecture)	Its statue of *Jūichimen Kannon* (Eleven Faces *Kannon*) is imputed with the power to prevent and cure diabetes

Table 11 Shrines and temples offering benefits for modern chronic conditions

rather than with current ones. In this respect, it is noteworthy that two of the modern chronic conditions for which *ema* are available (stroke and dementia in Table 9) were already important causes of death before World War II [US; PH05]. This does not mean, however, that every major disease in pre-war Japan had its own *ema* design(s). For instance, no small *ema* have been unearthed for infectious diarrhoeal diseases (such as enteritis, cholera and dysentery). There is a French source that alludes to the existence of small *ema* for dysentery, but it does not offer any concrete example [8].

3 The benefits of health-related ema are regularly connected to a legend or word play

The purpose of various health-related *ema* can be traced to an *engi* (foundation legend) or some other legendary story (e.g., about a miraculous cure) or to some kind of pun (e.g., between the name of an illness and the name of a food from which the worshipper promises to abstain). A predilection for such cultural triggers may have hampered epidemiological motives.

4 Modern health-related ema can have a very broad scope

Modern health-related *ema* can have such a broad purpose (e.g., *byōki heiyu* = recovery from illness) that they cannot be accommodated into a specific complaint-related category [9].

The use of such general *ema* for a specific modern disease will remain unnoticed (unless it is possible to take the writings on the reverse into consideration as well). A good example may be the *ema* design of two *Niō* statues from a temple that offers a ritual act to prevent stroke (*nōsocchū*). Yet this *ema* is not specifically associated with cerebrovascular disease, as one of its inscriptions refers to the much broader concept of bodily health (*shintai kenzen*) (see p.143).

5 New health-related benefits may be invented without creating a corresponding ema

Some sanctuaries offer *goriyaku* (divine favours) for modern chronic conditions (Table 11). However, they may do so without selling a specific accompanying *ema*. For instance, *Iwamasan Shōhōji* (Otsu, Shiga Prefecture) sells an *ema* that portrays *Kannon* as a protector from thunder, while the main benefit it offers today is *boke fūji* (prevention of senility) (see p.49).

Table 12 Non-biomedical healthcare approaches in present-day Japan [13]

Traditional Japanese medicine (TJM) TJM undeniably belongs to the professionalised sector. It developed by a unique adaptation of traditional Chinese medicine (TCM) to Japanese cultural conditions while retaining much of the original Chinese flavour. The term *kanpō* (commonly spelled as kampo in English sources) can refer to TJM as a whole but is often used more specifically for herbal TJM. Other forms of TJM treatment are: acupuncture, moxibustion and manipulative therapies. Acupuncture (*hari*) is based on the concept that vital energy (*ki* in TJM after *qi* in TCM) flows through the body along specific interconnected channels commonly designated as meridians (*keiraku*). Moxibustion (*okyū*) involves the treatment of acupuncture points (or certain other areas of the body surface) with burning *mogusa* herb (moxa or mugwort in English).	**Medicine based on *shinshūkyō* (new religions)** The so-called new religions developed in the 19th and 20th centuries. Healing is a prominent feature in their teachings, and testimonials of members who have recovered from illness after the performance of prescribed practices are a recurrent theme.
Medicine based on Shinto and Buddhism Besides many opportunities for self-care (such as praying to an enshrined deity or procuring a health-promoting amulet), these institutions offer special ceremonies carried out by priests. Some shrines and temples exhibit famous statues or stones that are believed to provide relief when rubbed, while others offer special festivals or foodstuffs to ward off illness.	**Foreign alternative medicine** In recent years, alternative therapies from other parts of the world (such as chiropractic, osteopathy, homoeopathy, reflexology, and yoga) have gained popularity in Japan. Some of these treatments belong to the professionalised sector, while others belong to the folk sector or lay sector.
	Folk medicine Folk healers such as shamans, mediums, *kitōshi*, herbal drug peddlers, and other itinerant care providers once played a prominent role but have now become much less important. *Kitōshi* were faith healers who used prayers and incantations to drive out evil spirits and to cure illnesses. They are sometimes portrayed as priests or monks specialised in healing, but they could also be laymen with the ability to heal through praying.

In the 1980s, a pilgrimage centring on the worship of *Boke Fūji Kannon* (*Kannon* for prevention of senility) was constructed in western Japan. Thirty-three temples established a pilgrimage association together and commissioned the production of scrolls and pilgrims' books that could be stamped at each temple, as well as guidebooks and amulets that could be commercially sold to pilgrims [10]. The question may be raised, however, how many of these temples actually started to offer *ema* for *boke fūji* as well [11].

Another example is that the Fukushima Daiichi nuclear disaster did not result in the production of any *ema* to protect against radiation effects. The only practice that was retrieved from the internet is the presentation of *ema* with livestock on them at *Sōma Kodaka Jinja* (Minamisoma, Fukushima Prefecture) to offer condolences to the livestock that had to be killed because of contamination with radioactivity.

Place of health-related *ema* in Japanese healthcare

Early Western accounts of non-Western medical systems tended to focus on healers, their varied beliefs and skills, and their often exotic practices. They paid no or relatively little attention to the views and actions of the patients themselves. This changed in the 1970s, when anthropologists started to look together with patients at the healthcare decisions patients make. This perspective yielded two important insights. The first one was that patients often have a choice between different healers and different types of healing, which gives them (together with the persons close to them) control over their own therapeutic process. The second insight concerned the high prevalence and relative importance of self-treatment.

As a result of these findings, anthropologists nowadays categorise healthcare systems into three major sectors [12]:

a) The *professionalised sector*, which comprises the well-organised healing systems, such as Western biomedicine and the great Asian medical traditions (Ayurveda, Unani, traditional Chinese medicine, traditional Japanese medicine).
b) The *folk sector*, which encompasses all types of folk healing that are not derived from a scholarly medical tradition and therefore cannot be classified in the professionalised sector (e.g., unlicensed herbalism, bone-setting, midwifery, shamanism, and so on).
c) The *lay sector*, which accommodates popular health beliefs and activities at non-professional levels (individual, family, social network or community). This sector comprises a wide range of self-prescribed therapies, such as diets, licensed over-the-counter drugs, unlicensed herbal and vitamin supplements, exercises, non-professional massage, etc.

The literature about *ema* occasionally mentions that *ema* could be prescribed by a folk healer. In the Tsugaru region (now in Aomori Prefecture) there was a strong belief in *itako*

Type of practice used in preceding year	Percentage of respondents reporting use
Pain relief patches	32.8%
Massage (by self or family)	32.0%
Praying for own health	18.3%
Attending traditional healing ceremony (temples, shrines, etc.)	16.8%
Massage device	16.4%
Dietary therapy	11.2%
Wearing talisman for health or recovery	10.8%
Electrotherapy device (not massage)	9.2%
Hot-spring therapy	7.9%
Yoga	5.4%
Aromatherapy	4.8%
Tai Chi/Qigong	1.0%
Moxibustion	0.8%
Zen/meditation	0.8%
Cupping	0.6%
Other	1.3%

Table 13 Non-biomedical self-help practices, as reported by 519 visitors to rural Japanese family medicine clinics in 2013.

After: Shumer G. et al. Complementary and alternative medicine use by visitors to rural Japanese family medicine clinics: results from the international complementary and alternative medicine survey. BMC Complement Altern Med 14 (2014): 360

(blind female shamanic mediums) and *gomiso* (ascetic females with the power to prophesy, exorcise and heal). When they were consulted by someone with an illness, they would first communicate with the gods and then tell that person what kind of *ema* to offer. They would sell several *ema* to him that had been made either by themselves or on their instructions. Their popularity could be gauged by the number of votive pictures in their houses [OT].

However, it must have been much more common to purchase the *ema* of one's choice directly, e.g., after advice from a relative, friend or *ema* seller. Today, it is also possible to consult a guidebook or website to find the right sanctuary for the *goriyaku* (divine favour) one is looking for. This places the offering of health-related *ema* firmly in the lay sector.

How does the religious offering of *ema* compare to other treatment modalities in Japanese healthcare? Today, the leading healthcare system is unquestionably Western biomedicine. It was introduced by the Dutch in the 18th century and has become dominant since the government imposed German medical care and education in the Meiji period. It is universally covered by social health insurance. However, when Japanese fall ill or want to prevent illness, they can choose from a variety of non-biomedical healthcare modalities to complement or substitute the biomedical approach (see Table 12).

In two large surveys undertaken just after the turn of the 21st century, the overall use of non-biomedical treatments in Japan was substantial: 76.0% in 1000 adults in general and 49.6% in almost 500 patients visiting a general urban hospital. The respondents appeared to be more interested in material treatments than in spiritual therapies (such as meditation or relaxation techniques). Most prominent was the use of nutritional drinks/dietary supplements/vitamins, which outranked forms of Japanese traditional medicine as well as certain foreign therapies (chiropractic/osteopathy, aromatherapy, homoeopathy). However, neither of these two surveys was informative about religion-based healing, because they did not specifically inquire into this type of healing [14].

Religion-based healing

Questions about religion-based practices were included in a recent survey carried out among 649 patients visiting rural primary care clinics. Out of 519 respondents, 95 (18.3%) had prayed for their own health in the preceding year; 87 (16.8%) had attended a traditional healing ceremony (e.g., at a shrine or temple) for health recovery/promotion; and 56 (10.8%) had worn a charm for health recovery/promotion (Table 13). When prayers and religious ceremonies were excluded, the number of respondents reporting at least one non-biomedical practice decreased only slightly from 415 to 403 (from 80.0% to 77.6%). In other words, most respondents who had turned to religious healing had combined it with one or more other non-biomedical practices. Unfortunately, the study questionnaire did not separate the offering of *ema* from other forms of Japanese religious behaviour and did not make a clear distinction between Shinto/Buddhist healing and healing through *shin shūkyō* (new religions). It would also be important to repeat the study in an urban

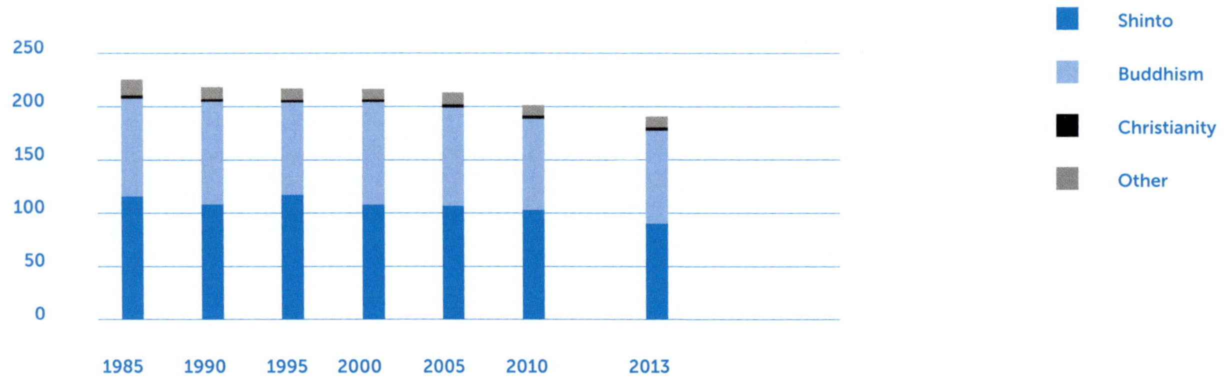

Figure 3 Affiliations with religions in Japan (1985-2013) expressed in millions

Based on Chapter 23 Religion of the Japan Statistical Yearbook 2015 and Chapter 26 of the Japan Statistical Yearbook 2016 (Statistics Bureau, Ministry of Internal Affairs and Communications, Tokyo)
Available at: http://www.stat.go.jp/english/data/nenkan/back64/1431-23.htm and http://www.stat.go.jp/english/data/nenkan/1431-26.htm [accessed 27 May 2016]

setting. Since more than 90% of Japanese now live in urban areas, rural studies are not representative for the whole of Japan.

Estrangement from religion (*shūkyōbanare*)

Official Japanese statistics counted 190 million affiliations to religions in 2013, while the total population in the same year was only 127 million (Figure 3). The major reason for this excess is that many Japanese feel affiliated with Shinto as well as with Buddhism. For instance, they visit Shinto shrines for childbirths and the growing up of their children while turning to Buddhist temples for funerals. However, these traditions seem to have more the character of a social practice than of a religious act. When surveys about religion in Japan phrase their questions differently (e.g., by asking whether one believes in religion or whether one considers religion to be important), only a quarter to a third of respondents answer positively. These lower levels of actual belief correspond to higher levels of education and urbanisation and are particularly seen in younger people (in their twenties). Interest in traditional religious practices, such as buying charms, keeping household altars and making pilgrimages may very well be declining in parallel. Present-day materials promoting pilgrimages tend to emphasise their profane benefits (such as beautiful scenery, photogenic sights and local delicacies), while avoiding more religious topics (such as miracles, salvation and healing) [15].

Living tradition or relics of the past

There are no reliable figures about the extent to which health-related *ema* are still in use today. More likely than not, the custom of offering such *ema* has not escaped the general trend of secularisation. When we visited *Hibiya Jinja* (Minato Ward, Tokyo) a few years ago to collect its *saba* (mackerel) *ema* for tooth problems, we found that it was no longer for sale, because it was no longer in demand. Recently, we sent a letter to *Karube Jinja* (Soja City, Okayama Prefecture) to ask for its *chichi* (breasts) *ema* for a safe child birth, abundant lactation and the healing of breast cancer (see p.191). An attentive villager living near the shrine responded that she was writing back to us because there was no longer a Shinto priest at the shrine and that she and her fellow villagers were now keeping the shrine clean. According to the Japan Statistical Yearbook 2016, the number of Shinto clergymen in Japan was 22% lower in 2013 than it had been in 1990 [SY16].

It may also be telling that many of the contemporary *ema* in this catalogue are late 20th century copies of earlier designs for the sake of *ema* collectors and for the Naito Museum of Pharmaceutical Sciences and Industry. Some of these earlier designs are still being sold by shrines and temples today (often in a modernised format). However, the question seems justified how many of these early designs have become relics of the past.

It is true that the presentation of *ema* is still common for certain purposes, e.g. when one faces an important exam or job interview, when one is looking for a suitable life companion, or when one celebrates a special occasion, such as *shōgatsu* (New Year). However, most Japanese do not seem to consider these practices as expressions of a deeply rooted faith. Remarkably, the shift from religious objects to cultural relics may already have started in pre-war times. There is a comment in a Japanese source from 1930 that *ema* were no longer about belief but were merely interesting objects [HS-51].

More than 75 years later, health-related *ema* still deserve to be put in the limelight by an exhibition and an accompanying catalogue. It is worthwhile not only to study the private messages on the reverses of contemporary *ema* but also to consider the pictures and pre-printed inscriptions on the fronts. The latter can be done without any concern about privacy, and an additional advantage is that many designs have not substantially changed over time. As a result, they not only offer a rich view at the present, but also testify about days gone by, when the majority of believers could not yet rely on their own writing skills and had to put their trust in pictorial images and professional help to appreciate the intended purposes of *ema*.

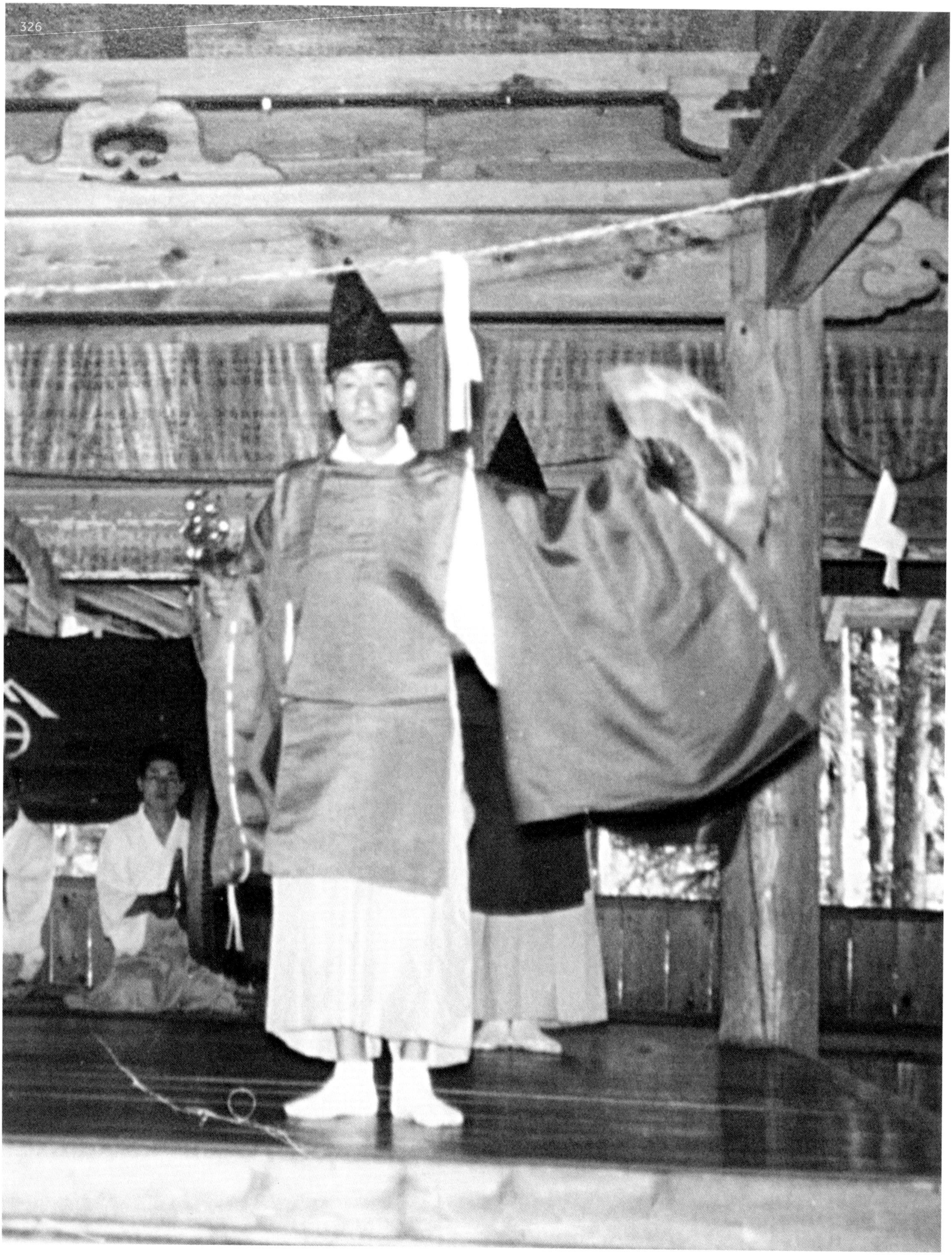

6 解説

326
日本の神社仏閣は我が身の安全を願うところというだけではなく、専門的な癒しを無料で与えるところでもある。この写真は、裏面の記載によると長崎県のどこかで行われたもので、古代神道の賽の神に病気平癒を祈願した奉納の舞を撮影したものであるという。

ご利益を得るため神仏に祈り、あるいはそれが成就したときにお礼を申し述べるために絵馬を神社仏閣に奉納する行為は、日本の伝統として今日まで至っている。祈願で最も多いのは、人の一生のうちで健康に関するもの、病気の平癒、病気の予防である。これらのご利益は人間に限らず家畜にも及んでいる。家畜に対しては殺してしまったことに対する謝罪や、ぼけ封じ、延命、ぽっくり（突然死）にまで及ぶことがある。

人の一生	
絵馬に託す健康に関する願い事	関連すると思われる生物医学的な病因および死因
子宝	性感染症による不妊症
安産	出産時の出血または感染による母の死
子育て	乳幼児死亡の高リスク

病気平癒	
絵馬に託す健康に関する願い事	関連すると思われる生物医学的な病因および死因
眼病	感染病による失明（トラコーマ、淋病、天然痘）
逆まつげ	トラコーマ
足の病	脚気 梅毒
頭痛 腹の病 肩こり	抑うつ症（プライマリケアを受ける日本の抑うつ病の患者は米国の抑うつ病患者より頭痛、腹痛、首や肩の痛みを訴えている（159ページ参照））
けいれん	脳卒中
呼吸器疾患	伝染性肺疾患（結核、インフルエンザ、肺炎、百日咳）
皮膚病	症状は天然痘、梅毒、結核などの全身感染症の場合もある。
皮膚色素の部分損失（白斑）	二期梅毒

表8　絵馬に託す健康に関する願い事と医学的な病因との関連可能性[1]

絵馬の詞書にあるようにこれは奉納されたもので、このようなものを奉納額という。奉納は、祈り、その祈りに答えてくれた神への感謝をささげる聖域訪問（礼参り）、聖なるものの加護を求めてする何らかの断食（断ちもの）、祈りの前の冷水による祓い清め（水垢離）などの慣行とともに、往古より行われている。

　この最終討論では健康を願う絵馬を主に検討することとする。そのような絵馬を見るときには、その絵柄に込められた直接的な意味（絵馬の表に書かれている願主や願い）と究極の願い（絵馬がどのようなご利益なり感謝の気持ちで聖域に奉納されたのか）を区別する必要がある。これは同じ絵馬の絵柄が時間の経過とともに変化し、場所が違えば（しかも同じ場所でさえも）ご利益も違ってくることがあるので重要な点である。たとえば蛸の描かれた絵馬がときと場所によっては子供の疱瘡よけ、婦人病、小児病、眼病、脱腸、腫れ物、いぼ、丘疹や発疹、咳、大漁（皮膚病および消化器系疾患の項を参照）などに使われている。[1]　また参拝者が、表の絵柄の意味するものとは異なる願文を裏面に書くこともある。

継続と変化

前節では現代日本の絵馬が、健康に関する事項を相当広範囲にカバーすることを明らかにした。このような絵柄と使用目的は既に20世紀前半に確立し、それ以降ほとんど変わっていないか不動といえる。このような連続性とともに、20世紀においてはAIDS保護、水子供養、ぽっくり願望、ペットの健康などの新たな医療および社会的な関心事が明らかになり、新たに健康に関する絵馬が出現したことも特徴的である。さらに神社仏閣の中には、病のパターンの変化に合わせ医療問題での重点をこれまでの問題から新しい問題へと移行しているところがある。たとえば京都で毎年行われる「やすらい祭」は、その昔に疫神を退散させるために始められたものであるが、今日では一般的に健康を願う場となっている。

生物医学的見解

健康に関する絵馬で目立つ特徴は、医学的な診断ではなく、症状（たとえば麻痺、頭痛、咳）やもう少し広範な症状（たとえば胃病、眼病、婦人病）を対象にしていることである。しかしそのような症状を日本の戦前の死因と比較すると、両者には関連性が認められそうである（表8）。

疫学的パターンの差

健康に関する絵馬について医学的に見て最も特徴的なのは、絵柄に描かれているものではなく、そこにあまり描かれていないもの、あるいはまったく描かれていないものである。日本における死亡原因は20世紀に伝染性のものから非伝染性のものへと大きく変化した（例として図2を参照）。このような変化は現在入手できる絵馬の絵柄にその一部が見て取れるだけである。がんは病気としては多いものの描かれている絵柄数は、特に多いわけではない。インターネットを検索しても特に心疾患、高血圧性疾患、脳血管疾患を予防するための絵馬デザインは出てこない。とりわけ中風の予防にはかぼちゃを描いた絵馬が用いられるが、これは間接的に脳血管疾患と関連している（167ページ参照）。これとは別に仁王像の絵馬は寺院に由来するもので、参詣者は仁王像の股の間を這いくぐり、脳卒中、くも膜下出血、麻痺のな

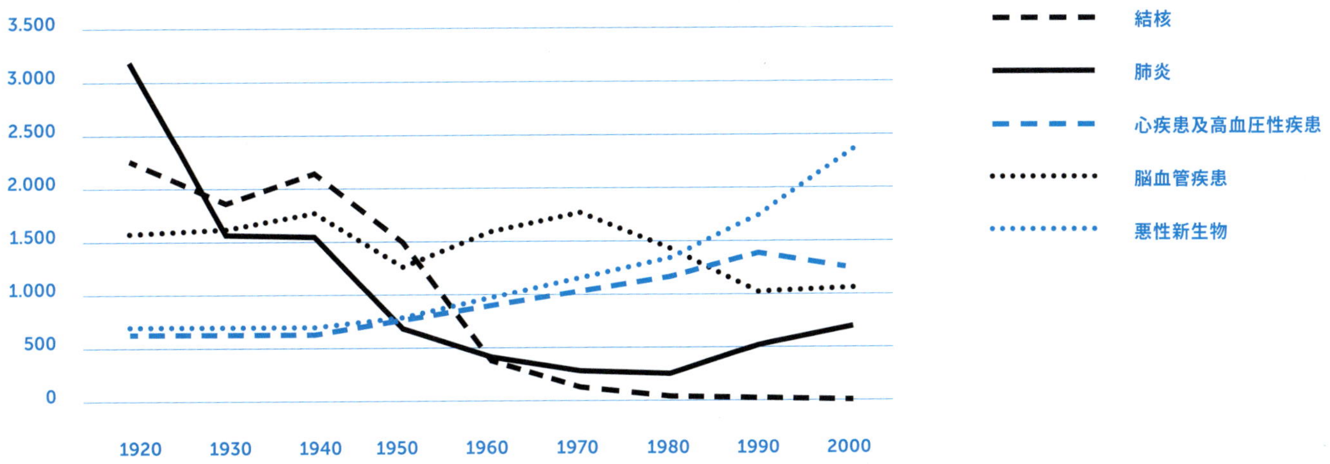

図2　日本における1920年から2000年までの主要死因別年間死亡率（100万人当たり）の推移[2]「日本の保健医療の経験 ー 途上国の保健医療改善を考える」による。東京、日本、国際協力機構、2005年：第1章および別紙

出所： https://www.jica.go.jp/jica-ri/IFIC_and_JBICI-Studies/english/publications/reports/study/topical/health/index.html [2016年5月27日アクセス]

いことを願う。しかしこの絵馬が特に脳卒中のないことを祈願するだけに用いられたとすることはできない。絵馬に記載されている言葉は広く健康（身体健全）を願うものであるからである（143ページ参照）。

表9　高齢化社会で健康で丈夫であるために避けたい15の慢性疾患に対応する絵馬の有無[4]

慢性病	対応する絵馬の有無
聴力損失	耳の病気に対する絵馬
心不全	なし
高血圧	なし
冠動脈疾患	なし
心房細動	なし
変形性関節症	そのような絵馬はないが筋骨格系疾患用のものがある
骨粗しょう症	なし
脳卒中	そのような絵馬はないが中風のためのものがある
認知症	絵馬には呆け用のものがある
抑うつ症	なし（ただし日本の抑うつ症患者が訴えている腹痛、頭痛、首や肩の痛みなどの身体の不調についての絵馬が存在する）[5]
慢性閉塞性肺疾患	そのような絵馬はない（咳や喘息に対する絵馬はあるが、咳を伴う慢性閉塞性肺疾患に関する呼吸困難についてのものではない）
床擦れ	なし
床擦れ	なし（ただし糖尿病末期にみられる眼合併症に対しては眼病除けの絵馬が使われることがある）
尿失禁	下の世話にならない絵馬あり
慢性腎不全	なし

日本で障害調整生命年（DALY）を短くする原因を見ても同様のことがいえる。[2] 第1の原因（腰痛）は絵馬の願い（腰痛）に直接対応しており、第2の原因（脳血管疾患）の対応は間接的で（上記参照）、第3のもの（虚血性心疾患）はまったく対応していない。[3] また健康に関する絵馬の願い事を高齢化社会での大きな関心事である糖尿病のような慢性病と並置しても、医学的パターンとの関連性はあまりない（表9）。

相違の理由

絵馬の健康に関するご利益が現在の疫学的パターンと一対一で対応しないのはなぜか。この現象にはさまざまな理由が考えられる。

1　健康に関するご利益は医学的な概念ではない

上述のように健康に関するご利益は庶民の言葉で表現された症状に関するものであって、医学的な診断用語ではない。このような庶民の表現はしばしば不正確で、対応する医学用語を見つけるのが困難なことがある（表10）。また医学的な診断用語は日本の伝統医学である漢方における疾患に用いられる用語にも当てはまる。水様性下痢症の患者は漢方医では霍乱と診断され西洋医学ではコレラと診断されるかもしれないが、この2つの概念が同一であるわけではない。定義上は霍乱が症状（水様性の下痢）に注目するのに対し、西洋医学のコレラは常に原因となる特定のバクテリア（コレラ菌）を指す。一般に西洋医学での診断は（当初の診断に誤りがない限り）病気の経過中に変わることはないが、漢方のパターンは時間とともに別の症状パターンに変わることがある。

2　時を超えても変わらない絵馬の絵柄とご利益

宗教による癒しに関する日本の文献では、健康に関するご利益が医療や社会的ニーズに適応する場合があることを強調している（たとえばインフルエンザのかわりに喘息、腫れ物のかわりにがん、というように）。

疱瘡神（天然痘に関する日本の神）は天然痘の災厄をもたらすが、そのような疫病を防いだり和らげるためにも呼び出される。日本では1951年に天然痘は流行性ではないとされたが、[7] 千葉県市川市の本光寺では疱瘡神が子供の成長のために依然として信仰の対象となっている。そのような適応によって、信仰される神仏や絵馬の絵柄は病気の回復や人の一生といった健康に関係する分野とはまったく異なる分野にも使われることになる。絵馬では、かつて婦人病を癒すために描かれたお雛様が、今日では縁結びを象徴しているという例がある（お雛様に関する記述p.193を参照）。

しかしそのような変化が一般的というわけではない。健康に関する絵馬の絵柄やご利益は20世紀前半には既に定まり、そのまま20世紀後半に続いているのである。その結果そのような絵柄やご利益は現在の医学のパターンではなく従来の疫学的パターンに関連付けられる。この点で、慢性病のうち絵馬がある2つ（脳卒中と認知症 表9）は既に第二次世界大戦前において主な死亡原因になっていたことに注意しておく必要がある。ただしこのことは、戦前の日本で主な病気に対するそれぞれの絵馬の絵柄があったことを意味するものではない。たとえば伝染性の下痢（腸炎、コレラ、赤痢など）除けの小型の絵馬は見つかっていない。赤痢除けの小型絵馬の存在を示唆するフランスの情報源があるが、そこに実例は示されていない。[8]

3　健康に関する絵馬のご利益は普通、言い伝えや語呂合わせに結びついている

健康に関する絵馬の願い事は、縁起（創設の言い伝え）、その他の伝説（たとえば奇跡的な治癒）、または何らかの語呂合わせ（たとえば病気の名

日本の用語	意味
手	手、両手、腕、両腕（状況による）
足	足、両足、脚、両脚（状況による）
腹	胃および腹部を指す
癪および疝気	胃腸または背中の痛みによる不調を指す癪は急性の症状に、疝気は慢性の症状に使われる傾向があるようである。
肩こり	大まかには首から肩にかけての不快感または痛みであるが、英語でまったく同じ意味の言葉はない。
夜泣き	乳幼児が睡眠に関連し夜に泣くこと。大抵幼児がしばらく寝てから夜中を過ぎて始まる。これに対してコリックといわれる大泣きは一般に午後遅くと夜の早い時間に起こる。
疳の虫	子供のかんしゃく、神経質、ひきつけを指す。かつては疳（気性、神経）の原因となる、またはそれを増大させる虫がいるとされた。

表10　医学用語と対応しにくい日本の健康関連用語

神社仏閣	ご利益
成相寺 （京都府宮津市）	とりわけ血圧を下げるといわれる指輪お守りを販売する
不思議不動院 （京都市北区）	骨の病気を治癒するといわれる
目黒の大鳥神社 （東京都目黒区）	糖尿病と生活習慣病に対するご利益があるとされる
櫟野寺 （滋賀県甲賀市）	十一面観音には糖尿病の予防と治癒の力があるとみなされている

表11　現代の慢性病に対するご利益をうたう社寺[6]

前と食べ物の名前で願い主が摂らないことにするもの）に由来していることがある。そのような文化的な機縁を好む傾向が疫学的動機を消極的にしてきた可能性がある。

4　現代の健康に関する絵馬はきわめて広範囲に及ぶ

現代の健康に関する絵馬にはさまざまな目的があり（たとえば病気平癒）、特定の症状と結びつけて区分することはできない。[9]

そのような一般的な絵馬が特定の現代の病気に利用されていることはまだ注目されていない（絵馬の裏面にある記載も考慮されない限り）。好例は脳卒中を防ぐ儀礼的なしぐさをして並び立つ2つの仁王像を描いた寺院の絵馬であろう。しかしこの絵馬が特に脳血管疾患に関連しているわけではない。祈願の文字を見ればもっと広く身体の健康（身体健全）を願っているからである（143ページ参照）。

5　健康に関する新たなご利益は対応する絵馬を作らなくとも生み出せる

寺社の中には現代の慢性病に対するご利益を掲げているところもある（表11）。しかし対応する絵馬を売らずにそうすることも可能である。たとえば滋賀県大津市の岩間山正法寺は、雷除けとしての観音を描いた絵馬を売っているが、同寺が今日掲げる主たるご利益はボケ封じである（信仰の対象としての仏像の項にある観音の説明を参照）。

日本の伝統医学(TJM)
TJMが専門療法に属することは疑いを容れない。これは伝統中国医学 (TCM) をその考えを残しつつ日本の文化状況に合わせ独自に発展させたものである。漢方(kanpō、英語では一般にkampoと表記)は概してTJMを指すが、特に漢方薬を指すことも多い。TJM治療にはその他に鍼、灸、手技療法がある。鍼は、生命エネルギー(TJMでもTCMにならい気という)が経絡とよばれる相互につながる道を伝い身体の中を流れるという考えを基盤にしている。お灸はもぐさを経穴(またはその他の身体表面部位)の上に置いて燃やす治療である。

神道および仏教に基づく医療
祀られている神仏に祈ったり健康増進のお守りを買い求めるようなさまざまな自己療法に加え、神社仏閣では神官僧侶が特別な儀式を行っている。神社仏閣によっては撫でると救済されると信じられている有名な彫像や石を開陳しているところがあり、病気を追放する特別な祭礼を催したり食物を供するところもある。

新宗教による治療
いわゆる新宗教は19、20世紀に創始された。新宗教の教えでは治癒というのは大きな特徴で、教えに従ったところ病気が治ったという信者の証言がしばしば出てくる。

海外の代替医療
近年、カイロプラクティック、整骨療法、ホメオパシー、リフレクソロジー、ヨガなど、世界各地の代替療法が日本でも盛んに行われている。これらの治療の中には専門療法になるものもあれば民間療法や素人療法になるものもある。

民間医療
シャーマン、霊能者、祈祷師、ハーブ薬の行商人など旅をしながら治療を行う民間のヒーラーは、かつて大きな役割を果たしたが、現在ではその重要性を減じている。祈祷師は邪悪な霊を追い出し病気を治すために祈祷やまじないを行う、信仰治療師であった。このような祈祷師は癒しを専門とする僧侶や御師の姿をとることもあるが、祈りによって治癒させる能力を備えた俗人であることもある。

表12 現代日本における医学以外のヘルスケアアプローチ[13]

1980年代に主として呆け封じ観音を参拝する巡礼が西日本で組織された。33箇寺が霊場巡りを組織し、参拝者に売る掛け軸、集印帳、ガイドブック、お守りを作成した。[10] しかしどれだけの寺が呆け封じの絵馬も売り始めたのかという疑問が出てくるかもしれない。[11]
別の例としては福島第一原子力発電所事故で放射能汚染除けの絵馬が作られなかったことが挙げられる。インターネットで発見できた唯一の事例は、放射能汚染で屠殺された家畜の冥福を祈る相島小高神社(福島県南相馬市)の牛を描いた絵馬である。

日本のヘルスケアにおける健康に関する絵馬の占める位置

西洋が西洋以外の医療制度を見るとき、以前はヒーラー、そのさまざまな信仰、技術、そしてしばしば見られる奇妙な慣行に注目しがちであった。西洋の研究者は患者自身の考え方や行動にはほとんど注意を払っていなかった。これが変わったのは1970年代で、人類学者は医療上の判断をする患者も観察するようになった。このような見方により大きな発見が2つあった。第1は患者が治療者および治療のタイプを選べることで、それにより患者(およびその近親者)は治療経過を自分で管理できるのである。第2は自分で治療することが広く行われ、それがかなり重要であるという発見である。

このような発見の結果、人類学者は現在ではヘルスケアシステムを3つの部門に分けている。[12]
a) 専門療法:西洋医学やアジアの伝統医療(アーユルヴェーダ、ユナニ医学、中国の伝統医療、日本の伝統医療)のように体系立てられた治療制度。
b) 民間療法:学問的な医療の伝統に基づくものでなく、専門的なものとは分類されない、民間で行われているさまざまなタイプの療法(たとえば認可されていないハーブ治療、接骨、助産術、シャーマニズムなど)を含む。
c) 素人療法:専門レベルではない健康に関し普及している考えや実践(個人、家族、ソーシャルネットワーク、コミュニティー)。この部門には、ダイエット、認可されている市販の薬、未認可のハーブやビタミンのサプリメント、エクササイズ、専門家以外の者によるマッサージ等さまざまな自己療法がある。

絵馬に関しては民間のヒーラーが絵馬を指定することがあると触れている文献が散見される。

青森県の津軽地方ではイタコ(口寄せをする盲目の女性)とゴミソ(予言、お祓い、治癒の力を持つ巫女)が広く信じられている。病気に苦しむ人から相談を受けるとイタコやゴミソは神と交信してその人にどのような絵馬を捧げるべきかを伝えるのである。イタコたちは自分で作ったまたはその指示で作らせておいた絵馬をその人に売るのである。彼女らの評判は自分の家にある奉納額の数で測られる。

しかし親族や友人、絵馬を売る者などの助言を得たうえで自分で選んだ絵馬を買うことの方が一般的であろう。今日ではガイドブックやウェブサイトで自身が求めるご利益が適切に得られる霊場を探すこともできる。これによって健康に関する絵馬の奉納が庶民の間に定着するのである。

絵馬の奉納を日本の医療で行われている他の治療法と比較するとどうなるであろうか。今日の日本における主要なヘルスケアシステムが西洋医学であることは疑いない。西洋医学は18世紀にオランダ人によって伝えられ、明治時代に政府がドイツの医学と教育を採用して以来主流となっている。これは健康保険制度であまねくカバーされている。しかし日本人が病気になり、あるいは

前年に行った行為	していると回答した者の比率
消炎鎮痛の貼り薬	32.8%
自分または家族によるマッサージ	32.0%
自分の健康祈願	18.3%
寺社等の伝統的な癒しの儀式に出席	16.8%
マッサージ器具	16.4%
食事療法	11.2%
健康維持またはその回復のためにお守りを身に着ける	10.8%
電子治療器具(マッサージ器以外	9.2%
温泉療法	7.9%
ヨガ	5.4%
アロマセラピー	4.8%
太極拳／気功	1.0%
灸	0.8%
禅／瞑想	0.8%
吸角法	0.6%
その他	1.3%

表12 医学によらない自助の慣行：日本の地方における家庭診療所への通院者519人に関する2013年調査報告

病気を予防したいときには、医学的アプローチを補完しまたは代替する、医学によらないさまざまな手段を選ぶことができる(表12参照)。

21世紀となった直後に行われた2つの大規模調査によると、日本では医学によらない治療がかなり行われ、全体では成人1000人のうち76.0%が、都市部の総合病院に通院する患者ほぼ500人のうちの49.6%が利用していた。回答者は瞑想やリラクセーション法などの精神的療法よりも実質的療法により関心を持っている。最も顕著であったのは栄養ドリンク／栄養補助食品／ビタミンの利用で、伝統的な各種日本医療や海外の療法(カイロプラクティック／整骨療法、アロマセラピー、ホメオパシー)などを上回っていた。しかし2つの調査のいずれも、宗教に基づく癒しについては特に質問をしていなかったため、このようなヒーリングに関する情報は得られていない。[14]

宗教に基づく癒し

宗教に基づく癒しに関する質問は、地方のプライマリーケア診療所に通う649人の患者を対象に2013年に実施した調査の中に含まれていた。519人の回答者のうち、95人(18.3%)はその前年に自らの健康を祈願し、87人(16.8%)は神社仏閣にて健康回復／増進を願う伝統的な癒しの儀式に参加し、56人(10.8%)は健康回復／増進のお守りを身に着けていた(表 12)。祈祷と宗教儀式を除外しても、医学によらないものを少なくとも1つは実践している回答者の数は、415人から403人(80.0%から77.6%)へとわずかに減少しただけである。これは宗教的ヒーリングを行っている回答者の多くが、その他にも医学によらない療法を実践していることになる。残念ながらこの調査の質問では絵馬の提供を日本の他の宗教的な行動と区別しておらず、神道／仏教のヒーリングと新宗教のヒーリングについても明確に区別していない。またこの研究を都市部でも繰り返すことが必要であろう。現在は日本人の90%超が都市部に住んでいるので、地方での調査では日本の全体を表すことにならないからである。

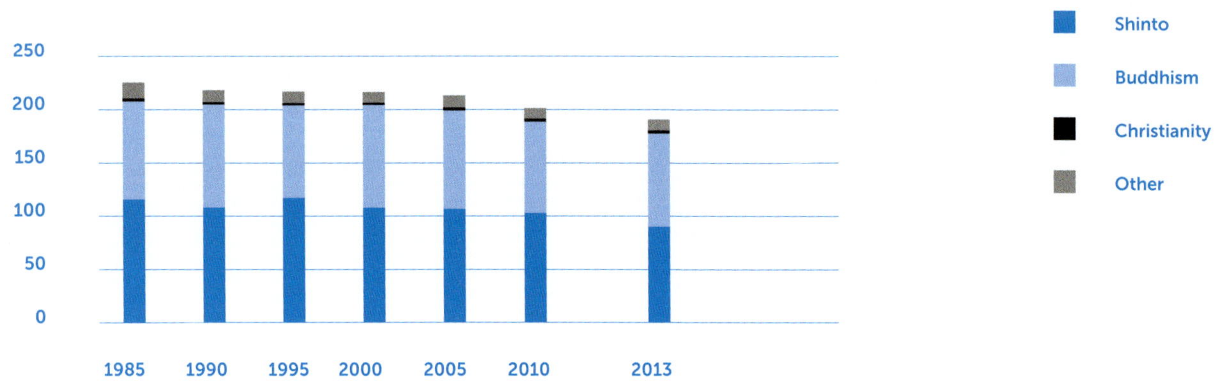

図3　日本の宗教人口（1985-2013、単位：100万人）

2015年日本統計年鑑第23章宗教および2016年日本統計年鑑第26章（総務省統計局、東京）による
出所：http://www.stat.go.jp/english/data/nenkan/back64/1431-23.htm および http://www.stat.go.jp/english/data/nenkan/1431-26.htm [2016年5月27日アクセス]

宗教離れ

日本の公式統計では2013年の宗教信者数は1億9000万人であるが、同年の総人口は1億2700万人である（図3）。このような超過が生ずる主な理由は、日本人の多くが神道にも仏教にも結びついているからである。たとえば日本人は出産や子供の成長については神社に参詣し、葬式については寺院に連絡を取る。しかしながらこのような伝統は宗教的行動というより社会慣行としての特徴を持っていると見られる。

日本での宗教に関する調査では質問の仕方が異なる（たとえば宗教を信ずるかと質問したり、宗教を大切なものと考えるかと質問したりしている）ものの、積極的に回答した者は1/4から1/3しかいない。実際に信じていないという回答は、教育程度が高まるにつれ、また都市部になるほど多くなり、特に若年層（20代）に多く見られる。これと並行してお守りを買う、神棚を置く、霊場巡りをするなどといった伝統的な宗教的慣習に対する関心も下がっている。昨今の霊場巡りを呼びかける資料では、世俗的な魅力（美しい風景、絵になる場所、地元のおいしい料理）を強調し、宗教的なもの（奇跡、救済、癒しなど）には触れないようにしている。[15]

伝統や過去の遺産とともに生きる

健康に関する絵馬が今日どの程度使われているかについて信頼できる数字はない。どちらかといえばそのような絵馬を供える習慣も世俗化という一般の流れを免れてはいない。数年前我々が日比谷神社（東京都港区）を訪ね、歯の問題についての鯖絵馬を収集しようとしたところ、そのような絵馬は需要がないのでもはや販売していないことが明らかになった。最近軽部神社（岡山県総社市）に安産と乳の出を願い乳がんの治癒を祈願する乳の絵馬を求める手紙を送った（000ページ参照）。同神社の傍の住人から返事があり、神社にもはや神主がいなくなり彼女や村の人々が神社を守っているとのことであった。2016年の日本統計年鑑によると日本の神主の数は1990年と比較すると2013年には22％減少している。

また絵馬の収集家や内藤記念くすり博物館が収集しこのカタログに収めた現代の絵馬は昔の絵柄をもとに20世紀後半に製作された可能性がある。このような昔の絵柄の絵馬（現代に合わせていることがよくあるが）は今でも神社仏閣で販売されている。しかしこのような昔の絵柄のうちのどれだけが過去の遺物になったのかと問うても不思議ではない。

絵馬の奉納は、大切な受験や就職面接のとき、相応しい人生の伴侶を探しているとき、正月のような特別な行事を祝うときなど、目的によっていまだ広く行われていることは事実である。しかしこのような習慣が信仰に深く根差した表現であると多くの日本人は考えていないように見受けられる。信仰の対象から文化財への変化は驚くべきことに戦前に始まっていたと考えられる。1930年の日本のある資料には、絵馬は信仰に関するものではなく単に興味ある対象物となったという記述がある。

75年後の今日でも健康に関する絵馬は展覧会やカタログによって注目に値するものとなっている。現代の絵馬の裏面にある個人の願いを研究するだけでなく、表の絵柄や予め印刷された文字を検討することも価値あることである。絵馬の表を検討する際にはプライバシーを心配する必要がなく、さらに多くの絵柄が時の経過にもかかわらず大きく変わっていないというメリットもある。その結果これらの品々は、単に現在見ごたえのあるものになっているだけでなく、信仰にすがる者の多くが自ら書く力を持たず絵馬本来のご利益を得るため絵柄を信頼し専門家の助力を求めねばならなかった往時を語るものにもなっているのである。

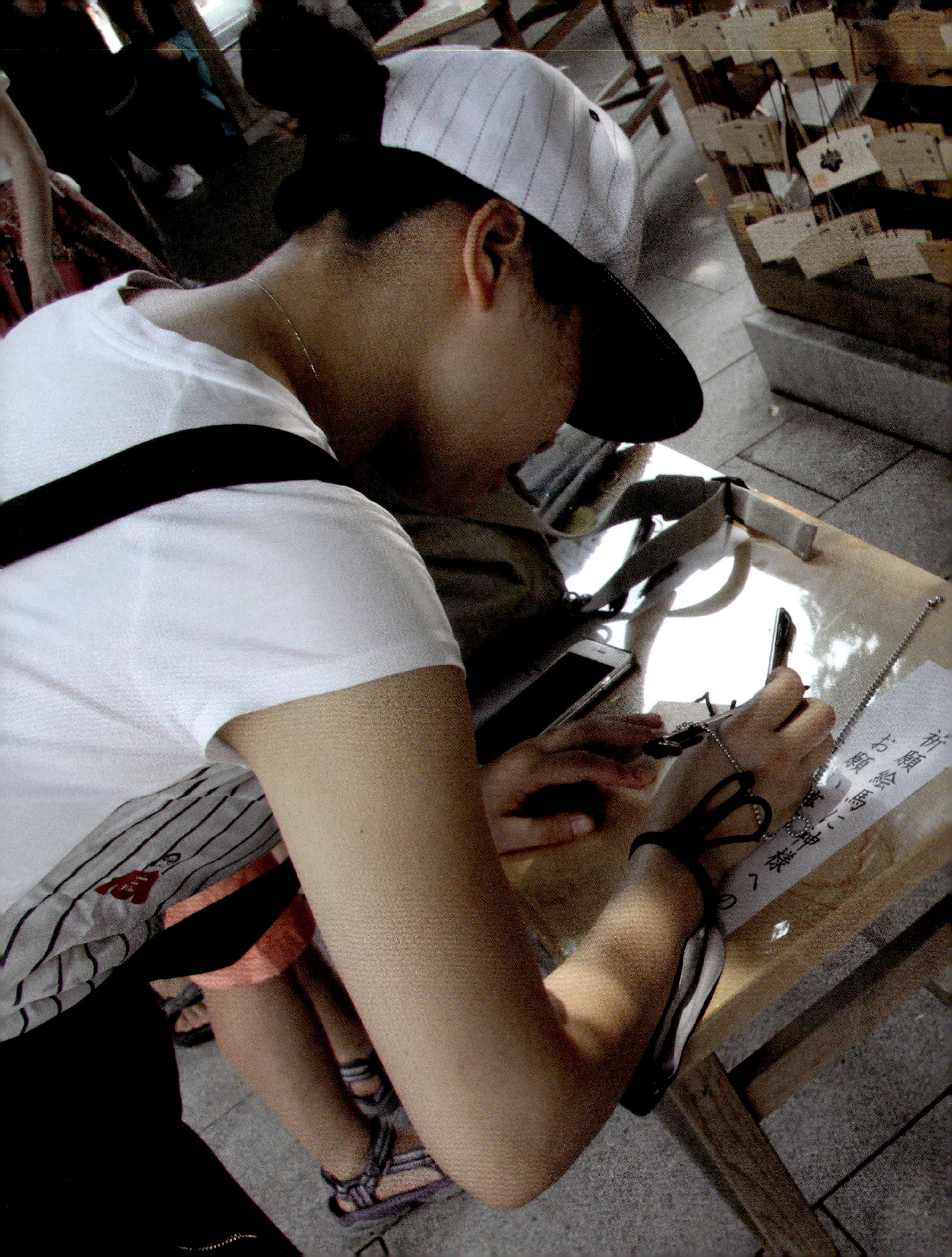
祈願絵馬

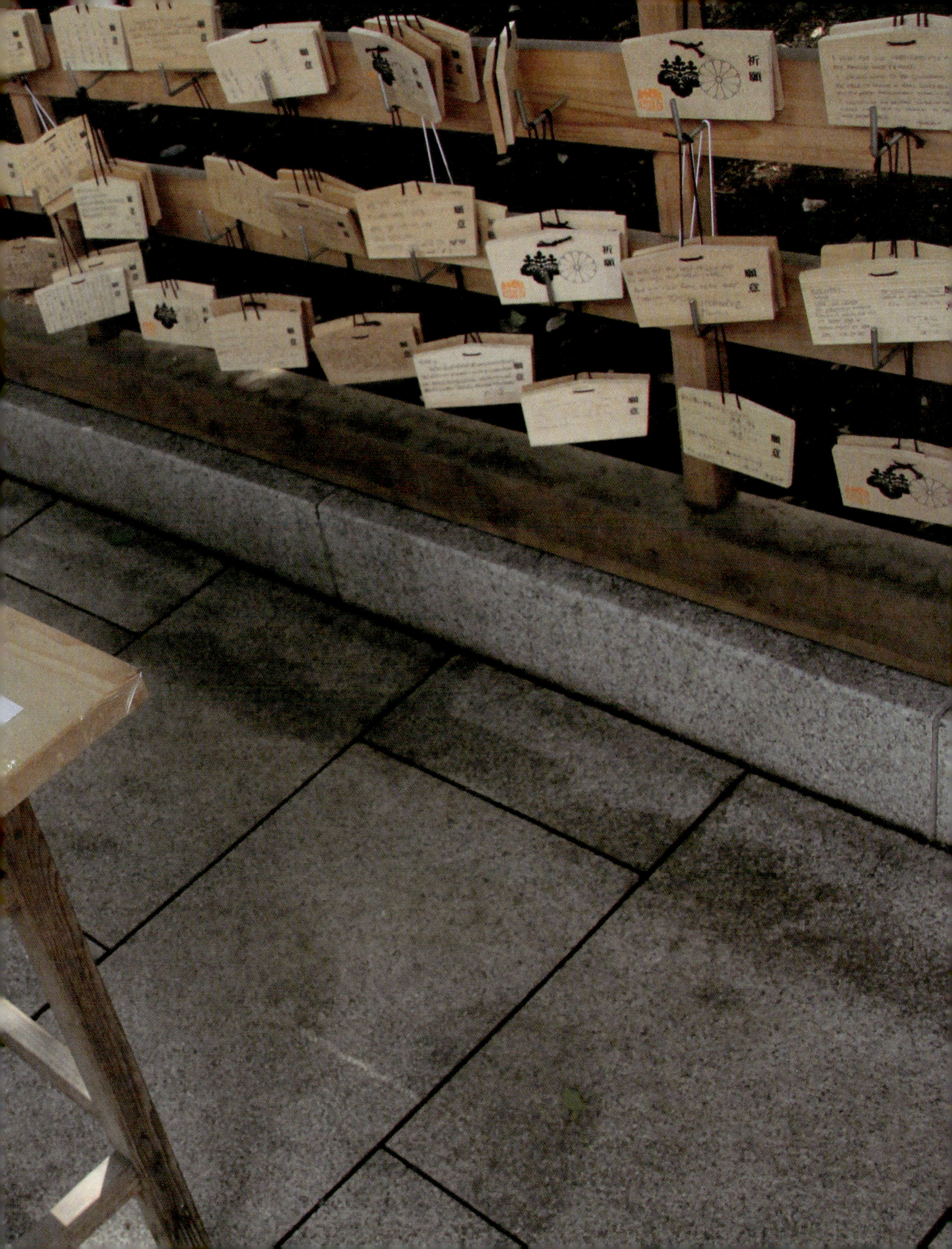
祈願

Acknowledgements

The authors would like to thank the following individuals and organisations for their faith in an exhibition with accompanying book about health-related votive tablets from Japan and/or for their valuable contributions to the realization of this project:

– Kris Schiermeier (director), Teatske Kramer, Dick Raatgever, Kuniko Forrer, Marjolijn Goos, Elizabeth van der Wind and Sandra Bouhuis (Japanmuseum SieboldHuis, Leiden)
– Anniek Meinders (publisher) and Romy Uijen (Leiden University Press, Leiden)
– Eva Trimp for her translations of *ema* inscriptions
– Manon van Rookhuijzen for the professional quality of her photography
– Haico Beukers and Marga Scholma for their creative design
– Prof. Kiichiro Tsutani for his crucial support
– The Association for Health Economics Research and Social Insurance and Welfare, Tokyo, for financial support.

They also would like to thank the museums, institutions and companies listed in the credit sections of the colophon for their permission to reproduce *ema*, images or data.

Unless stated otherwise, the *ema* in this catalogue come from the collections of the authors. Peter De Smet would like to acknowledge Lida Teng, Koji Akai, Ryuto Masuda, Ryosuke Kizaki, Steve and Makiko Kotake, and above all Manabu Fukuzawa, for their indispensable help in building his *ema* collection. He also would like to thank the various shrines and temples that responded to a written request to send him their *ema*. Ian Reader would like to acknowledge the generosity of the family of the late Jan van Bremen, anthropologist of Japan and *ema* collector, in passing on to him Jan's *ema* collection.

Last but not least, Peter De Smet would like to acknowledge the usefulness of Google Images and Google Translate in the finding and reading of relevant websites in Japanese.

Notes

1 Introduction 紹介 (*Shōkai*)

1 Based on https://en.wikipedia.org/wiki/History_of_Japan and http://afe.easia.columbia.edu/timelines/japan_timeline.htm [both accessed 28 Dec 2015]

2 Shinzo O, Takao O. Votive pictures depicting horses – "ema". Daruma Magazine 1994;38-40 • Ohnuki-Tierney E. The monkey as mirror: symbolic transformations in Japanese history and ritual. Princeton: Princeton University Press, 1987:48-49 • Piggott JR. Mokkan: wooden documents from the Nara period. Monumenta Nipponica 1990; 45:449-470 • Groemer G. Female shamans in Eastern Japan during the Edo period. Asian Folklore Studies 2007;66:27-53 • Anonymous. Japan's oldest votive tablets showing monkey leading a horse, and a cow are unearthed. Okayama University e-Bulletin 2013;4

3 Anderson W. Descriptive and historical catalogue of a collection of Japanese and Chinese paintings in the British Museum. London: Longmans & Co., 1886:401-402 • Clark T. Ukiyo-e paintings in the British Museum. London: British Museum Press, 1992:131

4 Yakuwa T. Report on surveys of literacy rates in Meiji Japan. In Rubinger R, (ed): New materials for the study of literacy in history: report of the Indiana Conference on literacy in Japanese history. Bloomington: Indiana University, 2008:63-73. Available at: http://www.indiana.edu/~easc/publications/doc/CRJEHVolume3.pdf [accessed Dec 31 2015]

5 Zeng K. Prayer, luck, and spiritual strength: the desecularization of entrance examination systems in East Asia. Comparative Education Review 1996;40:264-279

6 Mizutani M, Dorsey J, Moor JH. The internet and Japanese conception of privacy. Ethics and Information Technology 2004;6:121-128 • Orito Y, Murata K. Privacy protection in Japan: cultural influence on the universal value. Electronic Proceedings of Ethicomp 2005;5 Available at: http://www.kisc.meiji.ac.jp/~ethicj/Privacy%20protection%20in%20Japan.pdf [accessed Dec 31 2015]

7 The changing face of ema votive tablets. Available at: http://newsonjapan.com/html/newsdesk/article/111876.php [accessed 29 Jan 2016]

8 Embree JF. Notes on the Indian God Gavagrīva (Godzu Tennō) in contemporary Japan. Journal of the American Oriental Society 1939;59:67-70

9 Smyers KA. "My own Inari": personalization of the deity in Inari worship. Japanese Journal of Religious Studies 1996;23:85-116

10 This catalogue follows the anthropological convention of labelling disorders as illnesses when they are cultural concepts and as diseases when they are biomedical concepts.

11 http://www.kith.no/upload/2705/ICPC-2-English.pdf [see http://www.kith.no/upload/2705/ICPC-2-Japanese.pdf for the translation into Japanese]

2 Health-related images 健康関連画像 (*Kenkō kanren gazō*)

Figures of worship 礼拝の姿 (*Reihai no sugata*)

1 The label 'Buddhist deities' is frequently used in the consulted literature but some scholars do not like this term, because in theory not all of them are deities. It has therefore been replaced here by the label 'Buddhist figures of worship' (abbreviated as 'Buddhist figures').

2 Willemen C. Bhaisajyaguru, the Medicine Buddha. In Van Alphen J, Aris A, (eds): Oriental medicine: an illustrated guide to the Asian arts of healing. Boston: Shambhala, 1997:261-265

3 Suzuki Y. Medicine master Buddha: the iconic worship of Yakushi in Heian Japan. Leiden: Brill, 2012

4 Derived from: EO-150 • MS • GK • Bays JC. Jizo Bodhisattva: guardian of children, travelers, and other voyagers. Shambhala, 2003:33-34 • Clark JRK. Guardian of the sea: Jizo in Hawai'i. Honolulu: University of Hawai'i Press, 2007:23-24

5 Clement EW. Japanese medical folk-lore. Transactions of The Asiatic Society of Japan 1907;35:15-32 • Weinstein S. Aristocratic Buddhism. In Whitney Hall JW, (ed): The Cambridge history of Japan. Volume 2: Heian Japan. Cambridge: Cambridge University Press, 1999:449-516

6 Schwarz KM. Netsuke subjects: a study on the netsuke themes with reference to their interpretation and symbolism. Wien: Böhlau Verlag, 1992:32 • Kobayashi T. An enduring vision: 17th-20th-century Japanese painting from the Gitter-Yelen collection. New Orleans: New Orleans Museum of Art, 2002:289

Festivals 祭 (*matsuri*)

1 Plutschow HE, O'Neill PG. Matsuri: the festivals of Japan. Japan Library, 1996

2 Plutschow HE. Introducing Kyoto. Tokyo: Kodansha International, 1979:37

3 Bauer H, Carlquist SJ. Japanese festivals. Garden City: Doubleday, 1965: 137 • McMullin N. On placating the gods and pacifying the populace: the case of the Gion *goryō* cult. History of Religions 1988;27:270-293 • Ikegami E. Bonds of civility: aesthetic networks and political origins of Japanese culture. Cambridge: Cambridge University Press, 2005:88

Charms 守り (*mamori*)

1 Born W. Fetish, amulet and talisman. Ciba Symp 1945;7:102-132 • Paine S. Amulets: a world of secret powers, charms and magic. London: Thames & Hudson, 2004

2 Kyburz JA. *Omocha*: things to play (or not to play) with. Asian Folklore Studies 1994;53:1-28

3 Human life 人の一生 (*Hito no isshō*)

The treasure that is children 子宝 (*kodakara*)

1 Richie D, Ito K. The erotic gods: phallicism in Japan. Tokyo: Zufushinsha, 1967 • Clark TT, Gerstle CA, Ishigami A, Yano A. Shunga: sex and pleasure in Japanese art. London: British Museum Press, 2013 • Turnbull S. Japan's sexual gods: shrines, roles and rituals of procreation and protection. Leiden: Brill, 2015

2 Cornell LL. Infanticide in early modern Japan? Demography, culture, and population growth. Journal of Asian Studies 1996;55:22-50

3 Shinagawa SN. A short history of reproductive medical problems in Japan. Eubios Journal of Asian and International Bioethics 1996;6:158-159 • Kubo H. Epidemiology of infertility and recurrent pregnancy loss in society with fewer children. Jap Med Assoc J 2009; 52:23-28

4 Cornell 1996 (see note 2) • Kurosu S. Studies on historical demography and family in early modern Japan. Early Modern Japan 2002;10:3-21 • Johnston WD. Sexually transmitted diseases and demographic change in early modern Japan. East Asian Science, Technology, and Medicine 2009;30:74-92

5 Numazawa K. The fertility festival at Tagata Shinto Shrine, Aichi Prefecture, Japan. Acta Tropica 1959;16:193-217

Abortion 流産 (*ryūzan*)

1 Muramatsu M. Effect of induced abortion on the reduction of births in Japan. Milbank Memorial Fund Quarterly 1960;38:153-166 • Goto A, Fujiyama-Koriyama C, Fukao A, Reich MR. Abortion trends in Japan, 1975-95. Studies in Family Planning 2000;31:301-308 • Sato R, Iwasawa M. Contraceptive use and induced abortion in Japan: how is it so unique among the developed countries. Japanese Journal of Population 2006;4:33-54 • Sedgh G, Henshaw SK, Singh S, Bankole A, Drescher J. Legal abortion worldwide: incidence and recent trends. Perspectives on Sexual and Reproductive Health 2007;39:216-225

2 Brooks AP. "*Mizuko kuyō*" and Japanese Buddhism. Japanese Journal of Religious Studies 1981;8:119-147 • LaFleur WR. Liquid life: abortion and Buddhism in Japan. Princeton: Princeton University Press, 1994 • Tanabe Jr. G. Liquid life: abortion and Buddhism in Japan by William R. LaFleur. Japanese Journal of Religious Studies 1994;21: 437-440 • Hardacre H. Marketing the menacing fetus in Japan. Berkeley: University of California Press, 1997 • Reader I. Review of: Helen Hardacre, Marketing the menacing fetus in Japan. Asian Folklore Studies 1998;57:152-155

3 Drixler F. Mabiki: infanticide and population growth in Eastern Japan, 1660-1950. Berkeley: University of California Press, 2013:153-156 • Brooks 1981, Tanabe Jr. 1994, and Hardacre 1997 (see note 2).

Easy childbirth 安産 (*anzan*)

1 Nagaya K, Fetters MD, Ishikawa M, Kubo T, Koyanagi T, Saito Y, Sameshima H, et al. Causes of maternal mortality in Japan. JAMA 2000;283:2661-2667 • Göhlert C. *Anzan kigan*: rituelle Geburtspraktiken Japans im Wandel der Zeit. Asiatische Studien 2014;68: 189-232 • Maeda K. Highly improved perinatal states in Japan. J Obstet Gynaecol Res 2014;40:1968-1977

2 Shrine and temple guide. Available at: http://www.kaiun-goriyaku.com/spots [accessed 25 Mar 2016]

3 Swanger ER. A preliminary examination of the *omamori* phenomenon. Asian Folklore Studies 1981;40:237-252 • Reader I. Religion in contemporary Japan. Honolulu: University of Hawai'i Press, 1991:150

Breastfeeding 授乳 (*junyū*)

1 Takeuchi M. Breastfeeding in Japan: historical perspectives and current attitudes and practices. Jpn Hosp 1992; 11:79-92 • Segawa M. Buddhism and breastfeeding. Breastfeeding Medicine

2008;3:124-128 • Haku M. Breastfeeding: factors associated with the continuation of breastfeeding, the current situation in Japan, and recommendations for further research. Journal of Medical Investigation 2007;54:224-234 • Inoue M, Binns CW, Otsuka K, Jimba M, Matsubara M. Infant feeding practices and breastfeeding duration in Japan: a review. Int Breastfeed J 2012;7:15
2 See note 1
3 Fig.1 in Segawa 2008 (see note 1)

Child rearing 子育て (*kosodate*)

1 Handa M. *Ginkgo biloba* in Japan. Arnoldia 2000;60:26-34

4 Illnesses 病気 (*Byōki*)

Recovery from illness 病気平癒 (*byōki heiyu*)

1 *Ema* [in Japanese]. Available at: http://www.kitanet.ne.jp/~murai/ema.htm [accessed 27 May 2016]
2 Ashkenazi M. Handbook of Japanese mythology. Santa Barbara: ABC-CLIO, 2003:204

Epidemics 疫癘 (*ekirei*)

1 Kyōko I. Disease prevention prints. Daruma 2003;No.40 (Autumn):13-27 • Salter R. Japanese popular prints: from votive slips to playing cards. Honolulu: University of Hawaii Press, 2006:120-124

Neoplasms 新生物 (*shinseibutsu*)

1 Parkin DM, Bray F, Ferlay J, Pisani P. Global cancer statistics, 2002. CA Cancer J Clin 2005;55:74-108 • Torre LA, Bray F, Siegel RL, Ferlay J, Lortet-Tieulent J, Jemal A. Global cancer statistics, 2012. CA Cancer J Clin 2015;65:87-108

Tooth and mouth symptoms/complaints 歯と口の症状／愁訴 (*ha to kuchi no shōjō/ shūso*)

1 Nakahara S. Manners and customs of dentistry in ukiyoe (Ukiyoe ni miru shika fu zoku shi). Tokyo: Ishiyaku Publishers, 1980:133-134 • Sugisaki M. The dawn of modern dentistry in Japan. Japanese Dental Science Review 2013;49:57 • https://www.jda.or.jp/park/histry/index11.html [accessed 29 Jan 2016]
2 Suddick RP, Harris NO. Historical perspectives of oral biology: a series. Critical Reviews in Oral Biology and Medicine 1990;1:135-151 • Miyazaki H, Morimoto M. Changes in caries prevalence in Japan. European Journal of Oral Sciences 1996;104:452-458 • Fujita H. Dental caries in Japanese human skeletal remains. J Oral Biosci 2009;51:105-114
3 Breen J, Teeuwen MJ. A new history of Shinto. Chichester: Wiley-Blackwell, 2010:58 • Smyers KA. "My own Inari": personalization of the deity in Inari worship. Japanese Journal of Religious Studies 1996;23:85-116
4 Harada T. A brief history of dental education in Japan (2). Journal of Nihon University School of Dentistry 1962;4:193-199
5 https://www.jda.or.jp/park/knowledge/index12_8.html [accessed 29 Jan 2016] • http://www.dent-kng.or.jp/chishiki/museum/hakubutukan/edohaita/minkan2.htm [accessed 29 Jan 2016]

Digestive symptoms/complaints 消化器症状／愁訴 (*shōkaki shōjō/shūso*)

1 Tokuda Y, Takahashi O, Ohde S, Shakudo M, Yanai H, Shimbo T, Fukuhara S, et al. Gastrointestinal symptoms in a Japanese population: a health diary study. World J Gastroenterol 2007;13:572-578
2 Matsuda A, Matsuda T, Shibata A, Katanoda K, Sobue T, Nishimoto H. Cancer incidence and incidence rates in Japan in 2008: a study of 25 population-based cancer registries for the Monitoring of Cancer Incidence in Japan (MCIJ) project. Jpn J Clin Oncol 2014;44: 388-396 (fig.1) • Nagini S. Carcinoma of the stomach: A review of epidemiology, pathogenesis, molecular genetics and chemoprevention. World J Gastrointest Oncol 2012;4:156-169
3 Meyer Rochow VB, Okui K, Henshall K, Brooks DL. The mental concept of "worm/bug" in Japanese and English idioms. Suomen Antropologi 2000;25:25-49
4 Katsuyama O. Veterinary folk remedies in Japan. Rev Sci Tech 1994;13:453-463
5 *Muryō de kon'nani tanoshī nante!* Naito Museum of Pharmaceutical Science and Industry 2 [in Japanese]. Available at: http://blog.livedoor.jp/glucklichfamilie/archives/17666836.html [accessed 29 Jan 2016]

Eye symptoms/complaints 眼 症状／愁訴 (*me shōjō/shūso*)

1 Miyashita S. Das Trachom in Japan und den Grenzgebieten Chinas. Leiden: Boek- en Steendrukkerij Eduard IJdo, 1929 • Kamiya S. Mass treatment of trachoma: in Nara Prefecture, Japan, 1951-1954. Am J Ophthalmol 1956;42:269-283
2 Iwase A, Araie M, Tomidokoro A, Yamamoto T, Shimizu H, Kitazawa Y. Prevalence and causes of low vision and blindness in a Japanese adult population: the Tajimi Study. Ophthalmology 2006;113:1354-1362 • Yamada M, Hiratsuka Y, Roberts CB, Pezzullo ML, Yates K, Takano S, Miyake K, Taylor HR. Prevalence of visual impairment in the adult Japanese population by cause and severity and future projections. Ophthalmic Epidemiol 2010;17:50-57
3 Triplett K. Healing rituals in contemporary Japanese Esoteric Buddhism as acts of individual and cultural purification. In Martin GM, Triplett K, (eds): Purification: religious transformations of body and mind. London: Bloomsbury T&T Clark, 2013:107-118
4 Bays JC. Jizo Bodhisattva: guardian of children, travelers, and other voyagers. Shambhala, 2003:20 • De Visser MW. The Bodhisattva Ti-Tsang (*Jizō*) in China and Japan. Berlin: Oesterheld, 1914:175

Ear symptoms/complaints 耳症状／愁訴 (*mimi shōjō/shūso*)

1 Fujii K, Nagata C, Nakamura K, Kawachi T, Takatsuka N, Oba S, Shimizu H. Prevalence of tinnitus in community-dwelling Japanese adults. J Epidemiol 2011;21:299-304

Circulatory symptoms/complaints 循環器症状／愁訴 (*junkanki shōjō/shūso*)

1 Heine S. Dōgen, Zen master, Zen disciple: transmitter or transgressor? In Heine S, Wright DS, (eds): Zen masters. Oxford: Oxford University Press, 2010:117-146
2 Anonymous. Ji no kami. Japanese Journal of Proctology 1940;1:226
3 Ashcraft B. In Japan, there is a shrine for ... hemorrhoids. Available at http://kotaku.com/in-japan-there-is-a-shrine-for-hemorrhoids-1601066809 [accessed 05 Feb 2016]
4 Cf. the *ema* design from *Awashima Jinja* (Uto, Kumamoto Prefecture) on pp.192-193, which shows the actual crawling under a *mini torii* to ward off evil and illnesses and to grant *anzan* (easy childbirth).

Musculoskeletal symptoms/complaints 筋骨格 症状／愁訴 (*kinkokkaku shōjō/shūso*)

1 Carpenter KJ. Beriberi, white rice, and vitamin B: a disease, a cause, and a cure. Berkeley: University of California Press, 2000:xi • Moore Jr. MB. The epidemiology of syphilis. JAMA 1963;186:831-834
2 Suka M, Yoshida K. The national burden of musculoskeletal pain in Japan: projections to the year 2055. Clin J Pain 2009;25:313-319 • Takasawa E, Yamamoto A, Kobayashi T, Tajika T, Shitara H, Ichinose T, Mieda T, et al. Characteristics of neck and shoulder pain in the Japanese general population. J Orthop Sci 2015;20:403-409 • Yoshimura N, Muraki S, Oka H, Mabuchi A, En-Yo Y, Yoshida M, Saika A, et al. Prevalence of knee osteoarthritis, lumbar spondylosis, and osteoporosis in Japanese men and women: the research on osteoarthritis/osteoporosis against disability study. J Bone Miner Metab 2009;27:620-628

Nerve symptoms/complaints 神経症状／愁訴 (*shinkei shōjō/shūso*)

1 Tsuboi T. Epidemiology of febrile and afebrile convulsions in children in Japan. Neurology 1984;34:175-181 • Daidoji K. Water cures in Japan: the case of a health manual in the early nineteenth century. Asian Medicine 2009;5:80-107
2 Clay device used for helmet moxibustion, Japan, 1980-1995. Available at: http://www.sciencemuseum.org.uk/online_science/explore_our_collections/objects/index/smxg-8015546 [accessed 05 Feb 2016]

Mental/behavioural symptoms/complaints 精神的／行動的 症状／愁訴 (*seishinteki/kōdōteki shōjō/shūso*)

1 Ozawa C. Japanese indigenous psychologies concepts of mental illness in light of different cultural epistemologies. Anthropology & Medicine 1996;3:11-21 • Kitanishi K, Nakamura K, Miyake Y, Hashimoto K, Kubota M. Diagnostic consideration of Morita shinkeishitsu and DSM-III-R. Psychiatry Clin Neurosci 2002;56:603-608
2 Kawakami N, Takeshima T, Ono Y, Uda H, Hata Y, Nakane Y, Nakane H, et al. Twelve-month prevalence, severity, and treatment of common mental disorders in communities in Japan: preliminary finding from the World Mental Health Japan Survey 2002-2003. Psychiatry Clin Neurosci 2005;59:441-452
3 Ozawa 1996 (see note 1) • Waza K, Graham AV, Zyzanski SJ, Inoue K. Comparison of symptoms in Japanese and American depressed primary care patients. Fam Pract 1999;16:528-533 • Nakane Y, Jorm AF, Yoshioka K, Christensen H, Nakane H, Griffiths KM. Public beliefs about causes and risk factors for mental disorders:

a comparison of Japan and Australia. BMC Psychiatry 2005;5:33
4 Akira H. Psychiatry and religion in modern Japan: traditional temple and shrine therapies. In Harding C, Fumiaki I, Shin'ichi Y, (eds): Religion and psychotherapy in modern Japan. Oxon: Routledge, 2014:51-75
5 Eguchi S. Between folk concepts of illness and psychiatric diagnosis: *kitsune-tsuki* (fox possession) in a mountain village of western Japan. Cult Med Psychiatry 1991;15:421-451 • Akira 2014 (see note 4)
6 Fukumizu M, Kaga M, Kohyama J, Hayes MJ. Sleep-related nighttime crying (*yonaki*) in Japan: a community-based study. Pediatrics 2005;115:217-224
7 Osaki Y, Matsushita S, Shirasaka T, Hiro H, Higuchi S. Nationwide survey of alcohol drinking and alcoholism among Japanese adults [English abstract]. Nihon Arukoru Yakubutsu Igakkai Zasshi 2005;40:455-470
8 Higuchi S, Matsushita S, Maesato H, Osaki Y. Japan: alcohol today. Addiction 2007;102:1849-1862
9 Ueshima H, Choudhury SR, Okayama A, Hayakawa T, Kita Y, Kadowaki T, Okamura T, et al. Cigarette smoking as a risk factor for stroke death in Japan: NIPPON DATA80. Stroke 2004; 35:1836-1841
10 Suwaki H, Fukui S, Konuma K. Methamphetamin abuse in Japan: its 45 year history and the current situation. In Klee H, (ed): Amphetamine misuse: international perspectives on current trends. Amsterdam: Overseas Publishers Association, 1997:199-214
11 Vaughn MS, Huang FF, Ramirez CR. Drug abuse and anti-drug policy in Japan past history and future directions. British Journal of Criminology 1995;35: 491-524
12 Traphagan JW. Senility as disintegrated person in Japan. J Cross Cult Gerontol 2002;17:253-267 • Miyamoto M, George DR, Whitehouse PJ. Government, professional and public efforts in Japan to change the designation of dementia (*chihō*). Dementia 2011;10:475-486
13 Reader I. Pilgrimage in the marketplace. New York: Routledge, 2014:67-69

Respiratory symptoms/complaints 呼吸器 症状／愁訴 (*kokyūki shōjō/shūso*)

1 Suzuki T, Inoue T. Earliest evidence of spinal tuberculosis from the Aneolithic Yayoi period in Japan. Int J Osteoarchaeol 2007;17:392-402
2 Johnston W. The modern epidemic: a history of tuberculosis in Japan. Cambridge: Council on East Asian Studies, Harvard University, 1995 • Fukuda M. A cultural history of tuberculosis [Japanese]. Kekkaku 2004;79:655-658
3 http://blog.livedoor.jp/glucklichfamilie/archives/17666836.html [accessed 29 Jan 2016]

Skin illnesses 皮膚病 (*hifubyō*)

1 Fiumara NJ, Cahn T. Leukoderma of secondary syphilis: two case reports. Sex Transm Dis 1982;9:140-142
2 Namazu-e: earthquake catfish prints. Available at: http://pinktentacle.com/2011/04/namazu-e-earthquake-catfish-prints/ [accessed 16 Jan 2016]
3 瘡山 神社 (*Kasayama Jinja*). Available at: http://www.norichan.jp/jinja/kenkou2/kasayama.htm [accessed 16 Jan 2016]
4 Leroi-Gourhan A. Ema. Techniques & Culture 2011;57
5 The legend of Octopus Buddha. Available at: http://www.japannavigator.com/2013/07/the-legend-of-octopus-buddha-tako.html [accessed 16 Jan 2016]

Nutritional and metabolic symptoms/complaints 栄養と代謝の症状／愁 (*eiyō to taisha no shōjō/shūso*)

1 Inouye K, Katsura E. Etiology and pathology of beriberi. In Shimazono N, Katsura E, (eds): Review of Japanese literature on beriberi and thiamine. Kyoto: Vitamin B Research Committee of Japan, 1965:1-28 • Igata A. Clinical studies on rising and re-rising neurological diseases in Japan. A personal contribution. Proc Jpn Acad Ser B 2010; 86:366-376
2 Aoki K. Short history of epidemiology for noninfectious diseases in Japan. Part 1: Selected diseases and related episodes from 1880 through 1944. Journal of Epidemiology 2007;17:1-18 • Berkley JA. Nutrition. In Davidson R, Brent A, Seale A, (eds): Oxford handbook of tropical medicine. 4th ed. Oxford: Oxford University Press, 2014: 683-728
3 Inouye and Katsura 1965 (see note 1) • Aoki 2007 (see note 2)
4 Carpenter KJ. Beriberi, white rice, and vitamin B: a disease, a cause, and a cure. Berkeley: University of California Press, 2000:2
5 Neville SE, Boye KS, Montgomery WS, Iwamoto K, Okamura M, Hayes RP. Diabetes in Japan: a review of disease burden and approaches to treatment. Diabetes Metab Res Rev 2009;25: 705-716

Women's illnesses 婦人病 (*fujinbyō*)

1 Frühstück S. Then science took over: sex, leisure, and medicine at the beginning of the twentieth century. In Linhart S, Frühstück S, (eds): The culture of Japan as seen through its leisure. Albany: State University of New York Press, 1998:59-82 • Anesaki M. History of public health in modern Japan: the road to becoming the healthiest nation in the world. In Lewis MJ, MacPherson KL, (eds): Public health in Asia and the Pacific: historical and comparative perspectives. Oxon: Routledge, 2008: 55-72 • Johnston WD. Sexually transmitted diseases and demographic change in early modern Japan. East Asian Science, Technology, and Medicine 2009;30:74-92
2 Tanami Y, Yamamoto J. The venereal disease problem in Japan. Bull World Health Organ 1958;19:519-529 • Fukuda MH. Public health in modern Japan: from regimen to hygiene. In Porter D, (ed): The history of public health and the modern state. Clio medica. Rodopi, 1994: 385-402
3 Groemer G. A short history of the *gannin*: popular religious performers in Tokugawa Japan. Japanese Journal of Religious Studies 2000;27:41-72

Incontinence 失禁 (*shikkin*)

1 Danely JA. Departure and return: abandonment, memorial and aging in Japan. Dissertation. San Diego: University of California, 2008:59-60. Available at: http://escholarship.org/uc/item/1dv4s2nb [accessed 06 Feb 2016] • Takahashi,Y. Pokkuri-dera: the meaning of longevity among Japanese elderly. Available at: http://homepages.wmich.edu/~weinreic/GRN670/Japan/PokurriDera1.html [accessed 06 Feb 2016]
2 Young R, Ikeuchi F. Religion in 'the hateful age': reflections on pokkuri and other geriatric rituals in Japan's aging society. Japanese Religions 1995;20:167-200 • Takahashi (see note 1)

5 Animal health 動物の健康 (*Dōbutsu no kenkō*)

1 Katsuyama O. Veterinary folk remedies in Japan. Rev Sci Tech 1994;13:453-463
2 Katsuyama 1994 (see note 1)
3 Katsuyama 1994 (see note 1) • Smith RJ. Kurusu: the price of progress in a Japanese village, 1951-1975. Stanford: Stanford University Press, 1978:219 • Ryan LR. Horse trappings. Daruma 2005;48:28-39
4 Ohnuki-Tierney E. The monkey as mirror: symbolic transformations in Japanese history and ritual. Princeton: Princeton University Press, 1987:48-49
5 Anonymous. Japan's oldest votive tablets showing monkey leading a horse, and a cow are unearthed. Okayama University e-Bulletin 2013;4
6 Katsuyama 1994 (see note 1)
7 Pastoret P-P, Yamanouchi K, Mueller-Doblies U, Rweyemamu MM, Horzinek N, Barrett T. Rinderpest – an old and worldwide story: history to c.1902. In Barrett T, Pastoret P-P, Taylor WP, (eds): Rinderpest and peste des petits ruminants: virus plagues of large and small ruminants. London: Academic Press, 2006:86-104 • Spinage CA. Cattle plague: a history. New York: Kluwer Academic/Plenum Publishers, 2003:489
8 Fujiwara H. Votive tablets for short horned cattle in Hashino-Road, Iwate [in Japanese]. Japanese Journal of Veterinary History 1997;No.34:1-8
9 Kenney E. Pet funerals and animal graves in Japan. Mortality 2004;9:42-60 • Veldkamp E. The emergence of pets as family and the socio-historical development of pet funerals in Japan. Anthrozoos 2009;22:333 • Ambros B. Bones of contention: animals and religion in contemporary Japan. Honolulu: University of Hawaii Press, 2012
10 Kenney 2004 (see note 9).

6 Commentary 解説 (*Kaisetsu*)

1 *Kodakara* and eye illnesses: Johnston WD. Sexually transmitted diseases and demographic change in early modern Japan. East Asian Science, Technology, and Medicine 2009;30:74-92
Feet/leg illnesses: Moore Jr. MB. The epidemiology of syphilis. JAMA 1963;186:831-834 • Carpenter KJ. Beriberi, white rice, and vitamin B: a disease, a cause, and a cure. Berkeley: University of California Press, 2000:2
Somatic symptoms of depression: Waza K, Graham AV, Zyzanski SJ, Inoue K. Comparison of symptoms in Japanese and American depressed primary care patients. Fam Pract 1999; 16:528-533
Ingrown eyelashes: Bog H, Yorston D, Foster A. Results of community-based eyelid surgery for trichiasis due to trachoma. Br J Ophthalmol 1993;77: 81-83
Leukoderma: Fiumara NJ, Cahn T. Leukoderma of secondary syphilis: two case reports. Sex Transm Dis 1982; 9:140-142

2 The DALY or disability-adjusted life year is an international standardised unit in which the burden of disease is expressed as the sum of life years lost due to premature mortality and disability.

3 Gilmour S, Liao Y, Bilano V, Shibuya K. Burden of disease in Japan: using national and subnational data to inform local health policy. J Prev Med Public Health 2014;47:136-143

4 Min LC, Wenger NS, Fung C, Chang JT, Ganz DA, Higashi T, Kamberg CJ, MacLean CH, Roth CP, Solomon DH, Young RT, Reuben DB. Multimorbidity is associated with better quality of care among vulnerable elders. Med Care 2007;45:480-488

5 Waza et al. 1999 (see note 1)

6 *Hara*: EO-58,150
Shaku / senki: AJ
Katakori: Waza et al. 1999 (see note 1) • Fujii T, Matsudaira K, Yoshimura N, Hirai M, Tanaka S. Associations between neck and shoulder discomfort (*katakori*) and job demand, job control, and worksite support. Mod Rheumatol 2013;23:1198-1204
Yonaki: Fukumizu M, Kaga M, Kohyama J, Hayes MJ. Sleep-related nighttime crying (*yonaki*) in Japan: a community-based study. Pediatrics 2005;115:217-224
Kannomushi: ML-95

7 Fenner F, Henderson DA, Arita I, Jezek Z, Ladnyi ID. Smallpox and its eradication. Geneva: World Health Organization, 1988:343-344

8 US-67 • PH05 • Leroi-Gourhan A. *Ema*. Techniques & Culture 2011;57

9 More than one-third of the illness-related benefits in Table 2 (p.37) fall into the "general" category.

10 Reader I. Pilgrimage in the marketplace. New York: Routledge, 2014:67-69

11 The pilgrimage has more recently been disbanded, because the temples were too widely dispersed to make it practical for people to visit them. A more localised pilgrimage around the Kyoto area that incorporates ten temples with *Boke Fūji Kannon* (and includes temples initially on the larger route) has been developed. The most prominent temple of these (*Imakumano Kannonji*, Higashiyama Ward, Kyoto) sells special pillowcases for *boke fūji* (prevention of senility) and *zutsū fūji* (prevention of headache) but without offering a specific *ema* for the same purposes (see p.155).

12 De Smet PAGM. Different truths: ethnomedicine in early postcards. Amsterdam: KIT Publishers, 2010: 125-126

13 *General*: ML-14 • EO-123 • SH • Matsunaga L. Spirit first, mind follows, body belongs: notions of health, illness and disease in Sukyo Mahikari UK. In Clarke PB, (ed): Japanese new religions: in global perspective. Richmond: Curzon Press, 2000:198-239 • Saint Arnault D. Japanese. In Ember CR, Ember M, (eds): Encyclopedia of Medical Anthropology. Health and Illness in the World's Cultures. Volume 2 (Cultures). New York: Springer-Verlag, 2004:765-776
Medicine based on Shinto and Buddhism: RT • GK *Medicine based on shinkō shūkyō (new religions)*: Astley T. New religions. In Swanson PL, Chilson C, (eds): Nanzan guide to Japanese religions. Honolulu: University of Hawaii Press, 2006:91-114 • Shimazono S. Contemporary Japanese religions. In Swanson PL, Chilson C, (eds): Nanzan guide to Japanese religions. Honolulu: University of Hawaii Press, 2006:220-231
Foreign alternative medicine: Yamashita H, Tsukayama H, Sugishita C. Popularity of complementary and alternative medicine in Japan: a telephone survey. Complement Ther Med 2002;10:84-93 • Togo T, Urata S, Sawazaki K, Sakuraba H, Ishida T, Yokoyama K. Demand for CAM practice at hospitals in Japan: a population survey in Mie Prefecture. Evid Based Complement Alternat Med 2011;2011:591868
Folk medicine: Embree JF. Sanitation and health in a Japanese village. Journal of the Washington Academy of Sciences 1944;34:97-108 • Casal UA. The goblin fox and badger and other witch animals of Japan. Folklore Studies 1959;18:1-93 • Kalland A. Facing the spirits: illness and healing in a Japanese community. NIAS Report 1991;No.2

14 Yamashita et al. 2002 (see note 13) • Hori S, Mihaylov I, Vasconcelos JC, McCoubrie M. Patterns of complementary and alternative medicine use amongst outpatients in Tokyo, Japan. BMC Complement Altern Med 2008;8:14

15 Reader I. Secularisation, R.I.P.? Nonsense! The 'rush hour away from the Gods' and the decline of religion in contemporary Japan. Journal of Religion in Japan 2012;1:7-36 • Roemer MK. Japanese survey data on religious attitudes, beliefs, and practices in the twenty-first century. In Prohl I, Nelson JK, (eds): Handbook of contemporary Japanese religions. Leiden: Brill, 2012:23-58 • Tanaka K. Limitations for measuring religion in a different cultural context – the case of Japan. Soc Sci J 2010;47:845-852

6 エピローグ 見通

233頁にある英語版の記述を参照。

About the authors

Prof.dr. Peter A.G.M. De Smet
Scientific advisor of the Royal Dutch Pharmaceutical Association in The Hague and professor in Quality of Pharmaceutical Care at the Academic Medical Centre of the Radboud University Nijmegen, The Netherlands. (Co)author of 11 previous books and more than 350 scientific and professional articles and book chapters on drug therapy, pharmaceutical care, phytotherapy and ethnomedicine.

Prof.dr. Ian R. Reader
Professor emeritus and former head of Japanese Studies at the School of Arts, Languages and Cultures of the University of Manchester, United Kingdom. (Co)author of 9 previous books, co-editor of 7 volumes and author of over 100 scientific articles and book chapters on the historical and contemporary aspects of Japanese religion and pilgrimage.

Glossary 用語集 (*yōgoshū*)

Numbers are page numbers.

Akabeko: folk toy in the form of a red cow/ox 63
Aka-e: woodblock print against smallpox 117
Anmin: quiet sleep 161
Anzan: easy delivery 85
Ashi: foot; leg 147
Awabi: abalone shell which can be written on and presented as a votive object 153
Awase ema: two joint together votive tablets that can be closed and tightly bound after the message has been written down 21, 35

Bodhisattva: see *Bosatsu*
Boke: senility 167
Bosatsu (Bodhisattva in Sanskrit): has almost reached enlightenment but has temporarily renounced this transition to help living beings on earth to achieve salvation 45
Buddha: see *Nyorai*
Byōki heiyu: recovery from illness 113

Chichishibori: breasts spurting milk 95
Chōju: longevity 101
Chōmei: long life 101

Dacchō: abdominal hernia 131
Dembo: tumour 121
Dō: hall of sanctuary

Ekirei: epidemic 117
Ema: votive tablet
Emadō: special hall for hanging up large *ema* 17
Enmusubi: joining people together in love or marriage 35

Fuda: talisman 61

Gion Matsuri: *Gion* Festival 53
Gōkaku: realization of entry to school or university 33
Goriyaku: divine favour; benefit 33
Goryō Matsuri: *Goryō* Festival 53

Hachiman: god of warriors
Haiku: very short Japanese poem 31
Hara: area of stomach and abdomen 129
Haremono: swelling, tumour 175
Hari: acupuncture 214
Hashika-e: woodblock print against measles 117
Hina: dolls 193
Hina Matsuri (Dolls Festival) 193
Hito no isshō: human life 67
Hōju: wish granting jewel 19, 27
Hyakudo mairi: practice of walking around two marker stones a hundred times 121

Ibo: wart 173
Inari: god of rice
Inuhariko: folk toy in the form of a papier-mâché dog 63

Ji: Buddhist temple
Ji: haemorrhoid 143
Jingū: high-status Shinto shrine with connection to imperial family
Jinja: Shinto shrine
Jinmashin: urticaria 181
Jizō: *Bosatsu* patron of children, expectant mothers, firemen, travellers and pilgrims 47
Jō to uba: old man and old woman (symbol of longevity) 25
Jūnishi no dōbutsu: twelve animals of the zodiac system 29
Junyū: breastfeeding 93

Kahanshin: lower half of the body of a female worshipper 189
Kakke: beriberi 185
Kame: tortoise/turtle (symbol of longevity) 103
Kami: Shinto deity 41
Kannomushi: short-temperedness 161
Kannon: *Bosatsu* of mercy and compassion 49
Kanpō: traditional Japanese medicine (commonly spelled as kampo in English) 214
Kasa: boil; syphilis 175
Kata: model; Japanese type of wooden votive 145
Katakori: neck/shoulder pain 145
Katashiro: representation of a sacred object; Japanese type of wooden votive 145
Kenkō: health 105
Kishibojin: Buddhist goddess for fertility and childbirth 93
Kitōshi: faith healer 214
Kitsune: fox 27
Kodakara: the treasure that is children 69
Kosazuke: to be blessed with a child 69
Kosodate: child rearing 97
Kōtsū anzen: traffic safety 35
Koyasu: safe childbirth 85
Kusa: eczema 175

Mabiki: infanticide 81
Mame: blister, corn 99
Mamori: protective amulet usually worn on the person 61
Matsuri: festival 53
Me: *hiragana* character meaning eye or eyesight 137
Mikoshi: portable shrine in which *kami* is carried in procession during festivals 29
Miya: shrine
Mizuko: aborted, stillborn or miscarried foetus 81
Mukai me: two facing *me* characters, the left one is usually shown in reverse 137

Nadeushi: cow/ox statue to be rubbed 113
Nanakusa no sekku: Festival of Seven Herbs 53
Niō: guardian *Deva* kings 111
Nyonin shugo: guardian of women 51
Nyorai (Buddha in Sanskrit): Buddhist figure of worship who has attained enlightenment 45

Odeki: boil 173
Ōkuninushi: Shinto god of healing and marriage 41
Okyū: moxibustion (treatment of certain points or of the body surface with burning mugwort) 214
Omamori: see *mamori*
Oni: demon 157

Pokkuri: sudden painless death 199
Pokkuridera: temple where one can pray for *pokkuri* 197

Sakamatsuge: ingrown eyelashes 139
Sanada matsuri: *Sanada* Festival 171
Sanzaru: three monkeys that speak, hear and see no evil 51
Sarukomahiki: monkey leading a horse 203
Seibyō: venereal disease 187
Seikatsu no hanei: prosperity in life 33
Sekidome: cough-stopping 169
Sesshu: moderation in drinking 163
Setsubun: celebration associated with Lunar New Year 57
Setsuen: moderation in smoking 163
Sha: shrine (usually Shinto)
Shamoji: wooden rice scoop 23
Shichifukujin: Seven Gods of Good Fortune 51
Shichigosan: annual festival in November when girls aged seven and three, and boys aged five are taken to the shrine or temple for ritual purification and to pray for their healthy growth 59
Shinshūkyō: new religions 214
Shugendō: path of ascetic training practiced by *yamabushi* (mountain priests) 25
Shinnō: Japanese name of Chinese god of agriculture and medicine 51
Shironamazu: leukoderma (localized loss of skin pigmentation) 179
Shitsū: toothache 125
Shōki: a Demon Queller protecting against evil spirits and illness 117
Shōmen-Kongō: health-related deity in Japanese Taoism 51
Shūkyōbanare: estrangement from religion 216
Somin Shōrai: charm based on legend that *Somin Shōrai* lodged the deity *Susanoo-no-mikoto* 65
Sukunahikona: dwarf deity of healing and sake brewing 43

Taisha: grand shrine
Te: hand; arm 145
Tera: Buddhist temple
Tomoe: abstract emblem consisting of comma-like shape(s) 123
Torahariko: papier-mâché tiger 63
Torii: Shinto gateway through which one enters the shrine 27
Tōsu: toilet in Zen monastery 199
Tsūkōtegata: travel pass 25
Tsuru: crane (symbol of longevity) 101

Yakushi Nyorai: Medicine Buddha 45
Yakuyoke: protection from danger 35
Yamabushi: mountain priests practicing *Shugendō* 25
Yashiro: shrine (usually Shinto)
Yasurai Matsuri: *Yasurai* Festival 55
Yonaki: night-time crying of infants and young children 161

Zutsū: headache 157

Index of designs
デザインのインデックス (*dezain no indekkusu*)

This index covers the health-related *ema* designs discussed in Parts 2 to 5. The numbers are page numbers.

Index of sanctuaries
聖域のインデックス
(*seiiki no indekkusu*)

This index covers the sanctuaries offering the health-related *ema* designs discussed in Parts 2 to 5. They are arranged from north to south in regions and prefectures. The numbers are page numbers.

Colophon

Japanese translation Akebono Translation Service
Design Beukers Scholma
Printed by Graphius, Gent (Belgium)

Photography
Manon van Rookhuijzen

Unnumbered images
p.6: see image 006 (p.16)
p.8: *Fushimi Inari Taisha* 伏見稲荷大社, Fushimi Ward, Kyoto
p.10-11: *Kōfukuji* 興福寺, Nara
p.228-229: *Meiji Jingū* 明治神宮 Shibuya Ward, Tokyo
The latter three images provided by Beukers Scholma

Numbered image credits
British Museum, London: 008
Cultural Properties Division, Ota City Hall, Ota, Gunma Prefecture: 124
Fg2: 176 [photograph in public domain; downloaded from Wikimedia Commons: https://upload.wikimedia.org/wikipedia/commons/f/f6/Shakuzoji_Kuginuki_Jizo-3588.jpg]
Ian Reader: 019, 189, 251, 252, 255, 257, 316
Kris Schiermeier: 015
Nagasaki University Library, Nagasaki (Akihiko Kanamaru): 196
Naito Museum of Pharmaceutical Sciences and Industry, Kakamigahara, Gifu Prefecture (Hiroshi Morita and Kyoko Ito): 027, 186, 205, 206, 215, 223, 224, 264, 284, 285, 293, 294, 299
Nakano Ward Museum of History and Folklore, Tokyo: 206
Nigensha Publishing Company, Tokyo for reproductions from Hiromi Iwai. Ema ni negai 2007: 185, 201, 216, 305
Nippon Boehringer Ingelheim, Tokyo (Robert Reinsma and Emi Futakuchi): 275
Peter De Smet: 013, 014, 020, 021, 022, 032, 035, 077, 090, 106, 121, 139, 146, 163, 174, 178, 184, 198, 230, 277, 278, 297
Tenri University Sankokan Museum, Tenri, Nara Prefecture: 188, 250, 258, 260, 288, 292
Wellcome Library, London: 282 [photograph in public domain; downloaded from: http://wellcomeimages.org/indexplus/image/%20L0074708.html]

Table and Figure credits
BMC Complementary and Alternative Medicine: Table 13 (p.215)
Cambridge University Press, Cambridge: Table 3 (p.41)
Japan International Cooperation Agency, Tokyo: Figure 2 (p.211)
Tokyo: Statistics Bureau, Ministry of Internal Affairs and Communications, Tokyo: Figure 1 (p.121) and Figure 3 (p.216)

isbn 978 90 8728 252 3
nur 644

This book is distributed in North America by the University of Chicago Press (www.press.uchicago.edu).

JAPANMUSEUM SieboldHuis